Human Papillomavirus Infections

Clinical Practice of Gynecology

Michael S. Baggish, MD, *Series Editor*

Forthcoming Issues

Pediatric and Adolescent Gynecology

Donald P. Goldstein, Editor

DES Update

Kenneth L. Noller, Editor

Premalignant Lesions of the Lower Genital Tract

Albert Singer, Editor

Laser Endoscopy

Michael S. Baggish, Editor

Clinical Practice of

Gynecology

Series Editor: Michael S. Baggish, MD

Human Papillomavirus Infections

Editors:

Barbara Winkler, MD and
Ralph M. Richart, MD

Volume 1, Number 2, 1989

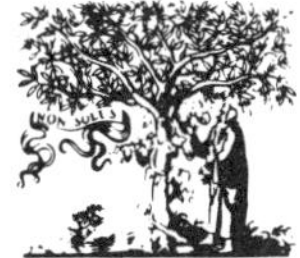

Elsevier

New York • Amsterdam • London

Clinical Practice of Gynecology is abstracted in *Excerpta Medica.*

Clinical Practice of Gynecology is published three times a year by Elsevier Science Publishing Co., Inc., 655 Avenue of the Americas, New York, NY 10010. Subscription price: institution $65.00, individual $55.00. Please add $19.00 for surface delivery outside the U.S., Canada, and Mexico. Claims for missing issues can be honored only up to three months for domestic addresses or six months for foreign addresses. Duplicate copies will not be mailed to replace ones lost through failure to notify Elsevier of change of address. Single copy and back volume information available on request.

Postmster: please send address changes to *Clinical Practice of Gynecology*, Elsevier Science Publishing Co., Inc., 655 Avenue of the Americas, New York, NY 10010.

Please direct orders for this series, change of address, and claims for missing issues to: Journals Fulfillment Department, Elsevier Science Publishing Co., Inc., 655 Avenue of the Americas, New York, NY 10010.

Human Papillomavirus Infections

CONTENTS

Human Papillomavirus Infections

CONTRIBUTORS

Michael S. Baggish, MD, FACOG, FACS Professor and Chairman, Department of Obstetrics and Gynecology, SUNY Health Science Center, 736 Irving Avenue, Syracuse, New York 13210

Renzo Barrasso, MD, Unité papillomavirus, Institut Pasteur and Colposcopy Clinic, Hospital Pasteur, 24 Rue du Docteur Roux, 75015 Paris, France

Christine Bergeron, MD, PhD, Institut de Pathologie et Cytologie Appliquées, 53 Rue des Belles Feuilles, Paris, France

Matthias Dürst, PhD, Institut für Virsuforschung, Deutsches Krebsforschungzcntrum im Neuenheimer Feld 280, 6900 Heidelberg, West Germany

Alex Ferenczy, MD, Professor of Pathology and Obstetrics and Gynecology, The Sir Mortimer B. Davis-Jewish General Hospital, 3755 Chemin de la Cote St. Catherine, Montreal, Quebec, Canada H3T 1E2

Yao-Shi Fu, MD, Professor of Pathology, Department of Pathology, UCLA School of Medicine, Center for the Health Sciences, Los Angeles, California 90024

Lee H. Hilborne, MD, MPH, Robert Wood Johnson Clinical Scholar and Instructor, Department of Pathology, UCLA School of Medicine, Los Angeles, California 90024

Larry S. Hirschfield, MD, Department of Pathology, Long Island Jewish Medical Center, New Hyde Park, New York 11042

Stephania Jablonska, MD, Department of Dermatology, University of Warsaw School of Medicine, U1. Koszykowa 82A, PL–02008, Warsaw, Poland

Alexander Meisels, MD, FRCPC, FIAC, Professor of Pathology, Department of Anatomic Pathology and Cytology, Hopital du Saint-Sacrament, 1050 Chemin Ste-Foy, Quebec, Canada G1S 4L8

GERARD J. NUOVO, MD, Department of Pathology P&S 16–404, Columbia-Presbyterian Medical Center, New York, New York 10032

JOEL PALEFSKY, MD, Assistant Professor of Laboratory Medicine and Stomatology, University of California at San Francisco, San Francisco, California 94143-0100

RALPH M. RICHART, MD, Professor of Pathology, Columbia University College of Physicians & Surgeons, Director, Division of Ob/Gyn Pathology, The Sloane Hospital for Women, New York, New York 10032

MICHEL ROY, MD, FRCS, Gynecologic Oncology, Hotel-Dieu De Quebec, 11 Cote du Palais, Quebec, Canada G1R 2J6

BETTIE M. STEINBERG, MD, PhD, Head, Section Otolaryngology Research, Long Island Jewish Medical Center, New Hyde Park, New York 11042

JEFFREY L. STERN, MD, University of Wisconsin Medical School Milwaukee, Clinical Campus, Sinai Samaritan Medical Center, Mount Sinai Campus, 950 North 12th Street, Milwaukee, Wisconsin 53233

DUANE E. TOWNSEND, MD, FACOG, Professor and Vice Chairman, Department of Obstetrics and Gynecology, University of California, Davis, School of Medicine, 1621 Alhambra Blvd., Suite 2500, Sacramento, California 95816

STEPHEN K. TYRING, MD, PhD, Assistant Professor, Departments of Microbiology and Dermatology, University of Texas Medical Branch at Galveston, Galveston, Texas 77550-2782

LINDA VAN LE, MD, Assistant Professor, Department of Obstetrics and Gynecology, University of North Carolina, Chapel Hill, School of Medicine, Chapel Hill, North Carolina 27599

BARBARA WINKLER, MD, Kyto Diagnostics, 216 Congers Road, New City, New York 10956

Human Papillomavirus Infections

CHAPTER 1

Human Papillomavirus Infections: Introduction

Barbara Winkler, MD and Ralph M. Richart, MD

The epidemic of genital human papillomavirus (HPV) infection is obvious to anyone working in gynecology. The U.S. estimates for infected individuals exceeded 2 million in 1982,[1] and screening studies using molecular techniques suggest a latency pool of some 10–30% of young women.[2] The clinical impact of this widespread infection is only now being appreciated in the rising incidence of cervical intraepithelial neoplasia (CIN), vulvovaginal carcinoma, and endocervical adenocarcinoma in young women. Despite the epidemic of genital wart infection and its attendant morbidity, the public knows little about these diseases, and the role of HPV as one of the most common sexually transmitted diseases is still greatly underappreciated.

The evolution of our current understanding of genital HPV infection began only in the past decade when the involvement of HPV in genital neoplasia was recognized. The association between HPV and cervical dysplasia/neoplasia was first reported in cytomorphologic studies by Meisels and Fortin,[3] and Purola and Savia in 1977.[4] These now classic studies in cytology set the stage for all subsequent research in this area. The authors first recognized that flat, colposcopically identifiable, aceto-white CIN lesions of the cervix were HPV-related. Furthermore, they pointed out that the cytopathic effect of HPV infection—koilocytosis—could be identified in cervicovaginal smears and could be used to diagnose HPV infection and squamous intraepithelial neoplasia. Soon thereafter, histologic and immunohistochemical studies documented that koilocytosis—the presence of superficial and intermediate cells with distinct perinuclear clear spaces and irregular cytoskeletons—could be identified in almost all CIN and that these flat, plaquelike lesions were uniformly HPV-associated. Furthermore, clinicopathologic studies related HPV-associated architectural and cytologic changes as the common denominator between a variety of genital squamous abnormalities, including condyloma acuminatum, verrucous carcinoma, in-

Clinical Practice of Gynecology: **2**, 1–3, 1989
© 1989 Elsevier Science Publishing Co., Inc.
655 Avenue of the Americas, New York, NY 10010
ISSN 1043-3198/89/$3.50

traepithelial neoplasia (IN), Bowen's disease, bowenoid papulosis, and squamous cell carcinoma.

Koilocytotic atypia had previously been described by Koss and Durfee in 1956,[5] but its recognition as a virus-caused cytopathy associated with squamous precancers and cancers eluded researchers for over 20 years. Similarly, other harbingers of the importance of HPV in genital squamous pathology—the report by Dunn and Oglivie of the electron microscopic identification of intranuclear viral particles in genital warts in 1968[6] and the report by Oriel on the high rate of contagion and venereal transmission of genital wart infection in 1971[7]—went unappreciated.

Once the association of HPV with lesions other than the typical vulvar condyloma was recognized, the widening of the clinical spectrum of HPV-induced lesions became apparent, as did the true extent of the genital HPV epidemic. Colposcopic evaluation of the female genitalia led to the description of a number of previously unrecognized manifestations of HPV infection, including flat condyloma, spiked condyloma, and condylomatous vaginitis and vulvitis. The multifocal and multicentric nature of HPV infection became clear as more women were carefully examined and followed. In 1984, the application of colposcopic examination to the male partner was reported, documenting an unsuspected pool of penile HPV infection in the form of subtle, flat, papular lesions and intraurethral condylomata.[8] Subsequent clinical studies in men further emphasized the multicentric nature of genital HPV infection and its high rate of sexual transmission. Infection of the perianal region and anorectal "transformation zone" was also recognized.

Along with the explosion of clinical studies relevant to genital HPV infection, there was a revolution in molecular technology, which, for the first time, allowed investigators to study the microbiology of the papillomaviruses. Studies of animal papillomaviruses in the 1930s and 1940s formed the basis of tumor virology, first elucidating models of viral cocarcinogenesis as developed by Rous and coworkers.[9] Studies of human papillomaviruses, however, were long hampered by the inability to grow the virus in in vitro culture systems and by the lack of any diagnostic techniques for the virus other than cervical and histologic examination. Advances in recombinant DNA technology in the 1970s and 1980s, however, have now permitted the beginning of the detailed study of HPVs, including their genomic organization and mechanisms of action. DNA diagnostics are becoming available and can be used for the identification of HPV DNA in clinical specimens.

With the advent of molecular biologic study, it became apparent that the HPVs were a unique and diverse group of viruses. They are epitheliotropic, specifically infecting squamous epithelia and mucus membranes and producing lesions typified by papillomatosis and epithelial hyperplasia, exemplified by the usual exophytic condyloma and common hand wart.

Viral replication is tied, in an unknown manner, to squamous epithelial maturation, requiring terminal squamous differentiation for whole virus production. Particular HPV types, as defined by DNA hybridization, produce a variety of squamous lesions distinguished by body site, clinical presentation, and oncogenic potential. Human papillomavirus 1, eg, is specific for the cornified epithelium of the soles of the feet, producing plantar warts with a distinctly benign, albeit aggravating, clinical course. Other HPV types are specific for the genital skin and mucosa. In the genitalia, the HPV segregate into two groups. Some types, such as HPV 6 and 11, have a predilection for the mature epithelium and are associated with benign condylomata, whereas others—particularly types 16, 18, and 31—are principally associated with IN and carcinoma. It has become apparent that HPVs play a pivotal role in the pathogenesis of lower anogenital tract carcinoma in women and in men and that they represent the sexually transmissible agent long thought to be responsible for cervical neoplasia.

Studies are now underway to define the structural and functional properties of the HPVs, particularly with respect to the mechanisms of viral oncogenesis.

The topics covered by the articles collected were chosen to provide a comprehensive exposition of what is known about the classification of HPVs and their molecular biology, histology, and cytology, as well as the application of this basic knowledge to clinical diagnosis and management. This is a complex, emerging area of investigation, and the clinician must be aware of the molecular aspects of the diseases caused by HPV in order to evaluate and use the newer diagnostic tests in clinical management. Reading and understanding the material collected in this book will provide a foundation on which further knowledge can be built.

REFERENCES

1. Centers for Disease Control: MMWR 1983;32:306.
2. Schneider A, Kraus H, Schumann R, Gissman L: Papilloma virus infection of the lower genital tract. Detection of viral DNA in gynecologic swabs. Int J Cancer 1985;35:443.
3. Meisels A, Fortin R: Condylomatous lesions of the cervix and vagina. Cytologic patterns. Acta Cytol 1976;20:505.
4. Purola E, Savia E: Cytology of gynecologic condyloma acuminatum. Acta Cytol 1977;21:26.
5. Koss LG, Durfee GR: Unusual patterns of squamous epithelium of the uterine cervix: Cytologic and pathologic study of koilocytotic atypia. Ann NY Acad Sci 1956;63:1235.
6. Dunn AEG, Ogilvie MMJ. Intranuclear virus particles in human genital wart tissue: Observations on the ultrastructure of the epidermal layer. J. Ultrastuct Res 1968;22:282.
7. Oriel JD: Natural history of genital warts. BRJ Vener Dis 1971;47:1.
8. Levine RM, Crum CP, Herman E, et al.: Cervical papillomavirus infection and intraepithelial neoplasia: A study of male sexual partners. Obstet gynecol 1984;64:16.
9. Rous P, Kidd JG, Smith WE: Experiments on the cause of rabbit carcinomas derived from virus-induced papillomas. J Exp. Med 1953;96:159.

CHAPTER 2

The Papillomaviruses: Structure and Function

Joel Palefsky, MD

Diseases caused by papillomaviruses have long been recognized as distinct clinical entities. The first written records of diseases associated with human papillomaviruses (HPVs) date back to the Roman Empire. Diseases caused by animal papillomaviruses, such as equine papillomaviruses, were described in the ninth century AD by a stablemaster of the Caliph of Baghdad.[1] Perhaps the most eloquent historical description of the clinical manifestations of papillomaviruses came from John Astruc[2] in 1737:

> There remains a fourth species of venereal disease to be added to those which we have already described, viz., warty excresences of the genitals, which sometimes succeed impure coition, but for the most part follow other pocky disorders that have been ill managed. Sometimes they wither of themselves and fall off, leaving a root behind them, from whence they spring up afresh; sometimes they are permanent, but are flaccid, soft, and almost void of sense; sometimes hard, dry, rigid, horny, destitute of sense, and perfectly callous; but sometimes they are painfull, having an ichorous discharge from their heads, and seem to be of a cancerous nature.[2]

This elegant discourse of the disease manifestations of HPV highlights two important features that have led to a resurgence of interest in HPV, and papillomaviruses in general: 1) its nature as a sexually transmitted agent, and 2) its association with the development of epithelial cancer.

Long before these features of HPV were fully appreciated, animal papillomaviruses were the focus of interest for tumor virologists. Beginning at the turn of the century, most of these studies, were conducted on Shope papillomavirus, also known as cottontail rabbit papillomavirus (CRPV), and bovine papillomavirus (BPV), as well as the tumors generated by these viruses. With the recent appreciation of the pathogenic potential of HPV, it is clear that the information generated by these early studies can offer valuable insight into the mechanisms of human disease.

Clinical Practice of Gynecology: **2,** 4–28, 1989
© 1989 Elsevier Science Publishing Co., Inc.
655 Avenue of the Americas, New York, NY 10010
ISSN 1043-3198/89/$3.50

Animal papillomaviruses occupy an important place in the history of tumor virology. Cottontail rabbit papillomavirus was the first oncogenic deoxyribonucleic acid (DNA) virus to be isolated and characterized.[3] One of the first experimental models of viral carcinogenesis was described when Rous and Beard observed the progression of benign CRPV-induced papillomas to invasive cancer.[4] The utility of this model was further expanded when Kidd and Rous showed that the tumors could be transplanted from one rabbit to another.[5] The concept of viral cocarcinogenesis was largely developed using models of CRPV-induced tumors, when Rous et al showed that irradiation and chemical mutagens could both act as cofactors in the progression to malignancy.[6,7] Cofactors that were investigated in this manner included methylcholanthrene or tar,[7] hydrocarbons,[8] and x-ray irradiation.[9] It was subsequently shown[10] that the malignant conversion of benign rabbit papillomas did not occur until approximately 12 months after infection, suggesting that the process requires multiple steps and that viral infection alone may not be sufficient for tumor induction.

Animal papillomaviruses have become valuable agents in the study of pathogenesis of human disease for several reasons: First, the genomic organization of animal papillomaviruses is very similar to those of HPVs. Second, diseases produced by animal papillomaviruses, such as bovine fibropapillomas, bear some similarity to human diseases. Third, papillomaviruses, including HPV, cannot be passaged in tissue culture, precluding in vitro studies of the viral life cycle and its interactions with host cells. Therefore, the purification of large quantities of virus for study has been difficult. However, serial passage of CRPV-induced carcinomas in cottontail rabbits has proven to be very useful in this regard, providing a steady source of experimental material,[5,11] and purification of CRPV DNA from these tumors has allowed the genome to be studied and characterized.[12,13] Similarly, reproducible sources of experimental material derived from BPV-induced fibropapillomas have allowed physicochemical characterization of bovine papillomaviruses. Fourth, animal papillomaviruses permitted the first studies of the role of infection in the development of cancer. Evidence for the role of papillomaviruses in tumor development in vivo was first provided by the demonstration that CRPV was transcriptionally active in skin tumors of the cottontail rabbit.[14–16] In vitro models of eukaryotic cell transformation were first developed using CRPV[17] and BPV.[18,19] With the advent of the tools of molecular biology in the 1970s and 1980s, these in vitro model systems provided the first opportunities to define precisely the roles of different papillomavirus proteins in the regulation of viral DNA replication, RNA transcription, and malignant transformation.

At the current level of knowledge, an understanding of the role of papillomaviruses in the pathogenesis of benign and malignant disease requires familiarity with terminology frequently used by molecular biologists.

The following section is designed to describe some of the concepts essential to this understanding.

CONCEPTS IN MOLECULAR BIOLOGY

Deoxyribonucleic acid contains the information that specifies the sequence of proteins. It is composed of four different deoxyribonucleotides, deoxyadenosine (A), deoxyguanosine (G), deoxycytidine (C), and thymidine (T), arranged in a double-stranded molecule, in which the A molecules of one strand are bound to the T molecules of the other, and the G molecules are bound to the C molecules. Thus, knowledge of the sequences of one strand of DNA permits the prediction of the sequence of the complementary strand. For example, if the sequence of part of one of the strands is AATGCTTA, the complementary strand will include the sequence TTACGAAT. Ribonucleic acid (RNA) is similar to DNA, with the exception that it is composed of ribonucleotides instead of deoxyribonucleotides, and thymidine is replaced by uridine (U). In both DNA and RNA, nucleotides are linked to each other through a 3′,5′ phosphodiester bond. Both DNA and RNA have an orientation in which the 5′ end is the first nucleotide in the sequence, and the last nucleotide of the sequence is at the 3′ end of the molecule. A sequence that is closer to the 5′ end of the piece of DNA than another sequence is therefore considered to be "upstream" of the latter. In contrast, the sequence that is closer to the 3′ end is "downstream" of the former.

Deoxyribonucleic acid is copied in the cell nucleus into messenger RNA (mRNA) by enzymes known as RNA polymerases in a process known as transcription. During this process, the DNA strands are separated, and the mRNA is copied off one of the strands, in a 5′ to 3′ direction. Therefore, the mRNA sequence will be identical to that of the complementary strand, which is known as the sense strand. In contrast, the strand that is used as the template for the mRNA is known as the antisense strand. Messenger RNA is transported to the cell cytoplasm, where it becomes physically associated with ribosomes and transfer RNA (tRNA). In the process known as translation, the binding of transfer RNA bearing specific amino acids to the messenger RNA permits the building of amino acid sequences that constitute the polypeptide or protein.

The genetic code that specifies the precise amino acid sequence is organized into sets of three deoxynucleotides, known as codons. A combination of any of the four nucleotides at the three positions, when copied into mRNA, will result in the binding of tRNA, through three nucleotides complementary to the mRNA codon, known as the anticodon. The tRNA molecule with this specific anticodon sequence always carries the same amino acid. Thus, a given series of codons, copied off one of the DNA strands into mRNA will determine the same specific amino acid sequence (Figure 2–1). In the following example, amino acids are designated by their three

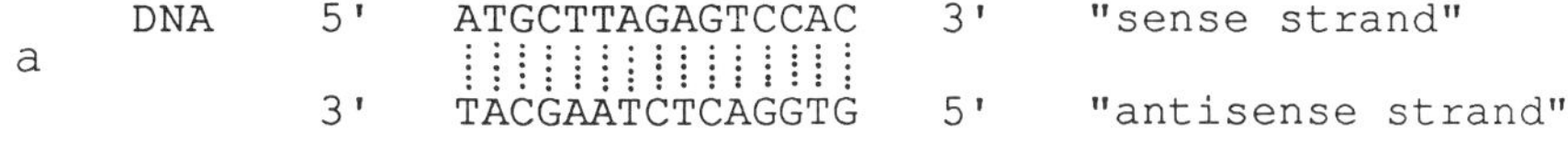

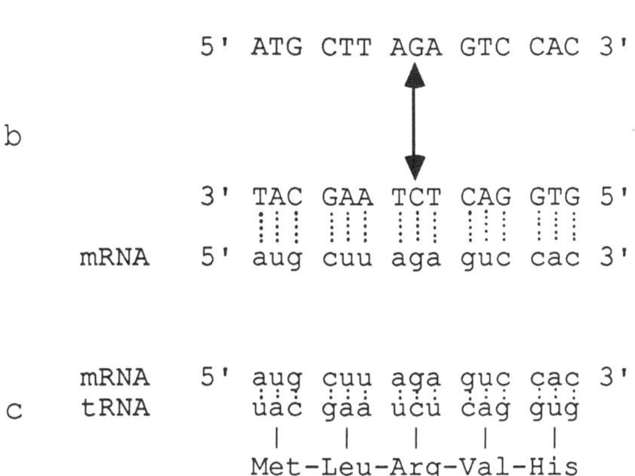

FIGURE 2–1 Transcription and translation of DNA. a) Double-stranded DNA sequence (upper-case letters). b) Transcription of DNA: strands come apart, and serve as template for mRNA strand (lower-case letters). c) Translation of DNA: anticodons of tRNA bearing a specific amino acid bind to complementry mRNA sequences. Amino acids join together through peptide bonds to form a polypeptide. (Amino acids are referred to by their three letter code).

letter codes, DNA nucleotides are in upper cases, and RNA nucleotides are in lower case.

Each amino acid is specified by a specific DNA codon. In some cases, an amino acid may be specified by more than one codon. For example, the amino acid cysteine may be encoded by the codons ugu or ugc; this is known as redundancy. The beginning of the protein sequence is known as the amino-terminus, and the end of the protein is known as the carboxy-terminus.

By definition, any sequence of DNA capable of encoding a polypeptide is known as an open reading frame (ORF). Most proteins begin with the amino acid methionine, specified by the codon aug, and, therefore, most open reading frames will begin with this sequence. Polypeptide chain termination is also specified by the specific codons uaa, uag, or uga, and many ORFs will contain this signal to terminate the sequence. Typically, the transcripts are cleaved by a specific enzyme known as an endonuclease, which recognizes the sequence AATAAA; therefore, these sequences specify $3'$ cleavage and polyadenylation of viral transcripts. In BPV, several of these sites may be found within the genome. Following cleavage, an enzyme known as polyA polymerase adds a number of A residues, resulting in the addition of a poly A tail, the function of which is not yet known.

As can be seen, each piece of DNA theoretically can be translated into three different polypeptides, depending on the site at which transcription begins. For example, the sequence TAC GAA TCT CAG GTG, shown above, could also be read as T ACG AAT CTC AGG TG, or TA CGA ATC TCA GGT G, and would result in Thr-Asn-Leu-Arg or Arg-Ile-Ser-Gly, respectively. Each of these sets of codon sequences is known as reading frames, and use of one or more of these frames is one of the means by which a given piece of DNA may be used to generate different pieces of information.

In addition to what is described above, eukaryotes and many viruses utilize another system to generate different amino acid sequences from the same DNA sequence, known as RNA splicing (Figure 2–2). When this occurs, mRNA is transcribed off the DNA strand as above but is processed prior to protein translation such that pieces of the sequence are deleted, and the remaining pieces of RNA are spliced together to form a new strand of mRNA. The result is a mRNA sequence that is different from the original DNA sequences, and, consequently, a different polypeptide will be encoded.

Viewed schematically, in Figure 2–2c, that part of the mRNA sequence complementary to part B of the DNA sequence, has been deleted through splicing, and only parts A and C will be translated. When this occurs, part B is known as an intron. Parts A and C are known as exons, as these are the parts being translated. In addition to permitting the translation of new amino acid sequences from the same piece of DNA, the downstream piece of RNA may be spliced onto the upstream segment in any of the three reading frames, resulting in the possibility of translating three new proteins. Another method used in nature to generate diverse proteins from the same DNA sequence is called posttranslational modification. In this case, proteins are modified after they have been translated from the mRNA sequence; parts of the protein may be cleaved, and some of the amino acids, such as tyrosine or serine may be phosphorylated, or other groups such as carbohydrates may be added.

Some RNA and DNA sequences serve specific functions, and because the same, or very similar, sequences are used for the same purpose in many different species, these sequences are termed consensus sequences. For example, the sites at which RNA is deleted, the splice sites, are not determined at random. Rather, it appears that a specific sequence is needed at the $3'$ end of the upstream segment, the consensus donor sequence, and a specific sequence is needed at the $5'$ end of the segment to which the upstream sequence is spliced, the consensus acceptor sequence. Thus, examination of a given DNA sequence will reveal those sites at which splicing

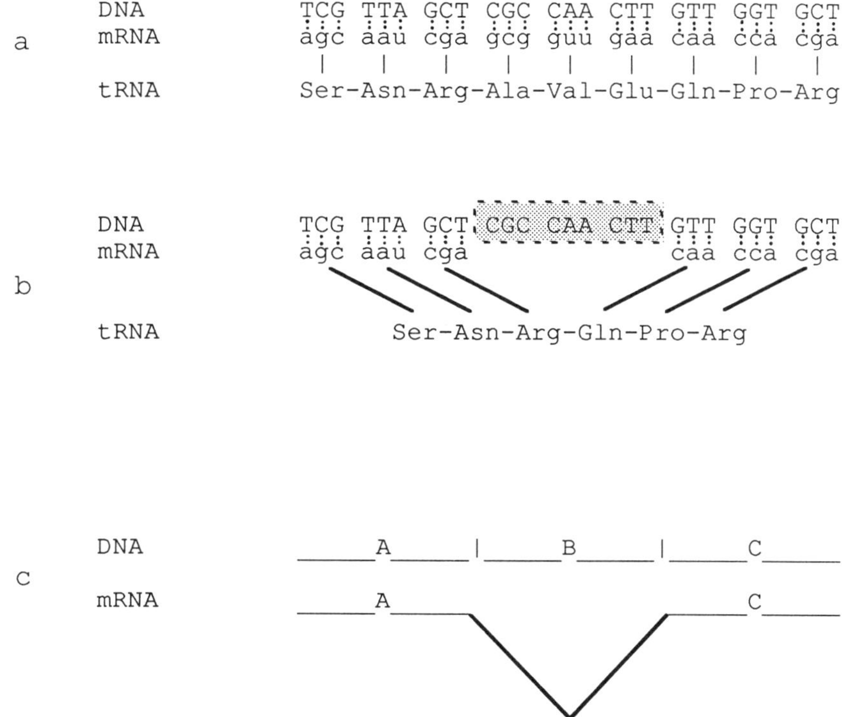

FIGURE 2-2 Splicing of mRNA. a) Messenger RNA transcription and translation proceed as in Figure 2-1. b) The middle three codons in this hypothetical example of splicing are deleted from the mRNA transcript, resulting in the translation of a different polypeptide from Figure 2-1c. c) Schematic depiction of Figures 2-2a and 2-2b.

could theoretically, but not necessarily, occur. For example, splicing has been shown to occur at the sequence 5′ . . . CAG/GTA, in which the last nucleotides of the donor sequence is CAG. Acceptor sequences vary between papillomavirus species, occurring at the site AG/CA . . . 3′ in HPV 6 and 11, in which the first two nucleotides of the 5′ end of the acceptor sequence is CA.[20]

Consensus sequences also exist for the site at which RNA polymerases bind DNA in order to begin transcription of mRNA. Such sequences are known as promoters, and these occur typically in papillomaviruses with the sequence TATAAA, also known as a TATA box; they are upstream of the start point for RNA transcription. Many promoters also exhibit another sequence about 75 nucleotides upstream of the transcription start-site, containing the sequence CAAT. In order to recognize the promoter site and initiate mRNA transcription off the DNA strand, RNA polymerases generally require the presence of other specific proteins, known as transcription factors; several examples of these DNA-binding proteins have been demonstrated in papillomaviruses, as described below. In human papillomaviruses, the location of these promoters is different. For example, the 5′ end of the transcripts of papillomaviruses derived from genital condyloma is located in the E7 region.[20]

Another kind of consensus sequence is known as an enhancer. These sequences, which may be thousands of nucleotides away from the gene that is being transcribed, are capable of greatly stimulating the promoter of that gene. These sequences have no promoter activity of their own and may be upstream, downstream, or even in the midst of a transcribed gene, and they may be found on either the coding DNA strand or the noncoding DNA strand. Enhancers tend to be effective only in certain kinds of cells, and the restricted host range of papillomaviruses may in part be a consequence of the existence of species-specific and host cell-specific enhancers, eg, keratinocyte-specific enhancers. In the case of bovine papillomavirus, the enhancer sequence contains the motif ACC__N6__CGGT, in which the identities of the middle nucleotides designated N are not critical to the enhancer function. Papillomavirus enhancer sequences will be described in greater detail below. It is hypothesized that enhancers serve as the docking site for the assembly of initiation complexes containing RNA polymerase. Presumably, these sites, which are thousands of nucleotides apart, are brought into proximity through the binding of transcription factors and other regulatory proteins that may induce DNA bending. Thus, transcription factors interact cooperatively with a variety of regulatory sequences in giving RNA polymerase access to specific genes.

The influence of one gene over the expression of another may occur in one of two ways. In cis-activation, a gene that is influencing the expression of another gene is upstream of the latter, usually in close proximity. Presumably, the gene product of the former is acting directly on the gene that is being influenced, and the relative orientation of these genes is critical to their function. Another means of gene activation is called trans-activation. When trans-activation occurs, the position of the activating gene relative to the gene sequence that is being influenced is not important. This is due presumably to the fact that the gene product of the activating gene is a soluble factor that can migrate to its site of action. Thus, the activating gene and its target do not even have to be on the same molecule. As described below, much of the regulatory activity of papillomaviruses occurs through trans-activation.

In general, papillomaviruses exist as closed circular, double-stranded DNA molecules. As such, they may be considered to be plasmids, much as a bacterium contains plasmids that exist separately from the host chromosome. When papillomaviruses exist in the plasmid state, they are considered to be episomal, meaning that they are not integrated into the host cell chromosome. While in this state, papillomavirus DNA replicates itself separately from the host DNA, although host and viral regulatory factors result in a complex interaction between the two.

Viruses such as papillomaviruses are classified as tumor viruses on the basis of their ability to induce tumors in laboratory animals or to transform cell in tissue culture. In general, experimental induction of tumors requires injection of large amounts of virus into hosts that have varying degrees of immunodeficiency, such as newborn mice; frequently, the ability of a virus to cause tumors under these circumstances does not correlate with the ability of the virus to cause a tumor under natural conditions. Likewise, in vitro cell transformation is a very inefficient process.

In the study of in vitro transformation, it is assumed that many of the properties of a virus that confer the ability to transform are relevant to the pathogenesis of naturally occurring cancer. This model is supported by the observation that transformed cells share many of the properties of cancer cells. Among the properties that distinguish transformed cells from non-transformed cells are 1) altered cell density and morphology of the former when they are growing on a plastic or glass surface; 2) the ability of trans-formed cells to grow in low concentrations of fetal calf serum that would not support the growth of nontransformed cells; 3) formation of dense colonies of cells (foci); and 4) the ability to form large cell colonies in a semisolid medium, without anchorage to a solid support. Of these charac-teristics, the latter correlates best with tumorigenicity of the transformed cells.

In addition to alterations in growth characteristics, transformed cells exhibit alterations of the cell surface, such as alterations in surface glycoproteins, increased trans-membrane rate of nutrient transport, and alterations in agglutinability by plant lectins. Other characteristics in-clude increased secretion of proteases and modification of the cell cytoskeleton.

Much of our understanding of the functions of papillomavirus pro-teins and their role in the pathogenesis of malignancy has been derived from various kinds of transformation assays. In these assays, papillomavi-rus DNA, such as whole genomic BPV, or one or more different papillo-mavirus ORFs, is introduced in plasmid form into mammalian cells in tissue culture, by the use of a process known as DNA transfection. The BPV genome replicates itself and produces proteins that contribute to development of the transformation phenotype. Further evidence to sup-port the role of these proteins is provided by mutation studies, in which the ORF in question is altered, and the effect of the modified protein is observed.

STRUCTURE AND FUNCTION OF PAPILLOMAVIRUSES

Papillomaviruses are closed circular, double-stranded DNA viruses that are classified as members of the papovavirus group, standing for *pa*pilloma, *po*lyoma, simian *va*cuolating virus.[21] Members of the papovavirus group include mouse polyomavirus, simian vacuolating virus (SV40), the human BK virus, and the human JC virus.[22] Recent studies at the biochemical and genetic levels have indicated that this taxonomic classification is incorrect; both the papillomavirus capsid and DNA genome are approximately 50% larger than those of the SV40-polyomavirus group, and the genetic organization of the two groups bears little similarity. Furthermore, the clinical manifestations of viral infection of these two groups are different; members of the SV40-polyoma group may infect a wide variety of tissues, including visceral and neural tissues, and they are not tumorigenic during natural infection in vivo. In contrast, papillomaviruses grow primarily in epithelial tissues at specific anatomic locations and may be associated with malignant transformation in vivo.

Papillomaviruses have been isolated from a wide variety of vertebrates. These include humans, cattle, sheep, goats, deer, elk, horses, rabbits, mice, dogs, monkeys, pigs, opossums, elephants, and chaffinches.[23-26] Multiple types and subtypes of papillomaviruses have been isolated from some species, such as five types of BPV,[27] and, to date, over 58 types of HPV have been described.[28]

Virion Structure

Papillomavirus particles from diverse animal origins have been shown to have remarkable structural similarity (Figure 2–3). Electron microscopic examination has revealed that the virus capsid consists of 72 capsomeres or subunits, arranged in an icosahedral structure. Unlike some of the larger DNA viruses, such as the herpesviruses, papillomaviruses have no lipid envelope surrounding the capsid.

Viral protein represents 88% of the mass of the viral particle.[29,30] The proteins that constitute the capsid are the major protein with a molecular weight of 50,000–60,000 daltons, as well as a number of minor proteins with molecular weights of 43,000–53,000 daltons. In addition, purified virions have been shown to contain four histones, possibly of cellular origin, in association with the viral DNA.[31,32] Studies have shown that the tail of L1 itself may bind to DNA in a manner similar to that of a histone.[33] Immune sera against whole virus particles show no cross-reactivity between heterologous viruses, and, thus, the surface antigenic determinants, which are derived from the L1 protein, are papillomavirus species-specific. However, antibodies to disrupted viral capsids are capable of broad cross-reactivity among species; these genus-specific determinants, located internally in the capsid, are also thought to be on the major capsid protein.[34,35]

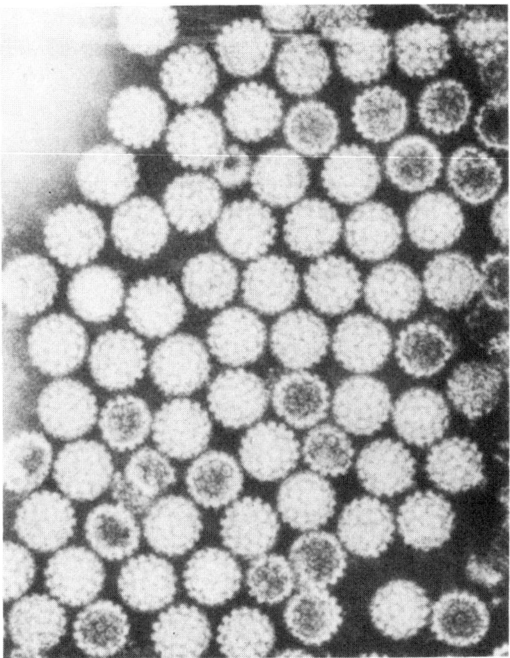

FIGURE 2–3 Electron micrograph of human papillomavirus particles. Dark particles probably lack DNA. Reprinted with permission from *Virology*, Fraenkel-Conrat H, and Kimball P, Englewood, NJ: Prentice-Hall, Inc.

Genetic Organization of the Papillomavirus Genome and Function of Papillomavirus Proteins

Papillomavirus DNA recovered from virions consists of covalently closed circular, double-stranded DNA of about 7,900 base pairs, with a guanosine:cytosine percent ranging from 41% for HPV to 50% for *Mastomys natalensis* (multimammate mouse papillomavirus).[36,37] Full particles, containing the DNA genome, have a buoyant density in cesium chloride of 1.34 g/mL, and empty particles, without the genome, have a buoyant density of 1.29 g/mL.[36]

The complete DNA sequences of a number of the human papillomavirus genomes, BPV-1, and CRPV, have now been determined.[38–46] Alignment of these sequences has revealed similarity in the organization of the ORFs (Figure 2–4). To date, mRNA transcription has been detected from only one of the DNA strands, the other encoding only very small ORFs. Because of the similarity of organization, information derived from the study of one species of papillomavirus, such as BPV, may often be generalized to the

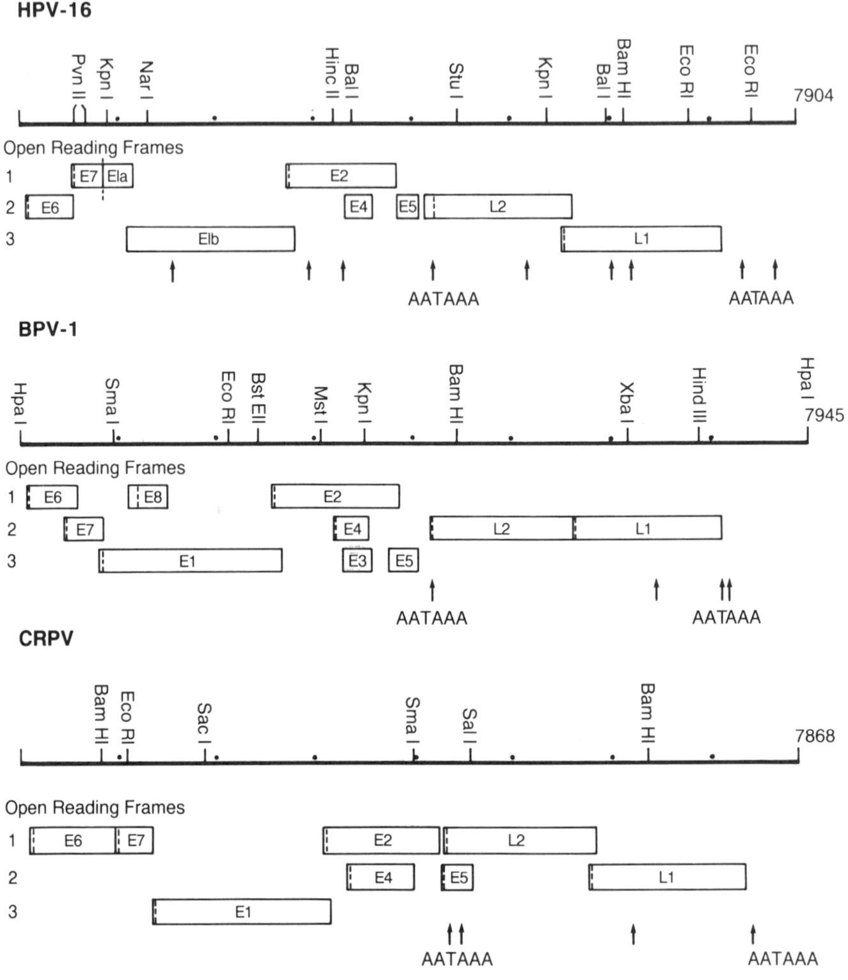

FIGURE 2–4 Genome organization of HPV 16, BPV 1, and CRPV.

other species. However, while similarities in function between analogous ORFs in different species of papillomaviruses do exist, it is also clear that in some cases, analogous ORFs in different species do not encode the same functions.

Analysis of the genomic organization of papillomaviruses has allowed the genome to be divided into two regions, operationally defined by the time after infection that these portions of the genome are thought to be expressed. Thus, in the process of transforming mouse cells, only the ORFs contained in a subgenomic fragment comprising 69% of the BPV genome are expressed,[47,48] and they are believed to be expressed soon after infection; this fragment is called the early region (E region). In contrast, two long ORFs in the remainder of the BPV genome are not expressed in transformed mouse cells,[49,50] but they are considered to be part of the late region (L region) because they encode the viral capsid proteins found only in productive bovine fibropapillomas. Thus, the numbers assigned to the ORFs have the prefix E or L, and the number following the prefix denotes the length of that ORF relative to the others in that region.

The study of the function of the proteins encoded by these ORFs has been hampered by the absence of a tissue culture system capable of supporting the virus through its complete replicative cycle. However, introduction of BPV DNA (transfection) into some cell lines, such as mouse fibroblast C127 and rat fibroblast NIH 3T3 cells, has resulted in the stable maintenance of the viral genome and, under certain circumstances, cell transformation. With the use of the techniques of genetic engineering, portions of the BPV 69% subgenomic fragment (the E region) have been modified to study the contributions of each ORF to this process. Further modifications, such as site-directed mutagenesis, deletions, or terminal mutations, have allowed researchers to further define those portions of the ORF that contribute to this process. In addition to being useful for the study of the role of individual papillomavirus proteins in transformation, these in vitro systems have been used to study the regulation of papillomavirus DNA copy number and the regulation of expression of other papillomavirus proteins. Increasingly, studies are also being performed that will analyze the interaction between papillomaviruses, host cell factors, and the host genome.

THE UPSTREAM REGULATORY REGION

The upstream regulatory region (URR), also known as the long control region (LCR) or noncoding region (NCR), is that part of the papillomavirus genome that lies between the end of the L1 ORF and the beginning of the E6 ORF. The LCR does not contain any ORFs, but it is thought to be important in the regulation of viral replication and transcription. This region contains one of two viral sequences known as plasmid maintenance sequences, known respectively as PMS-1 and PMS-2; PMS-1 is found within the URR, and PMS-2 is found within the E1 ORF replication of viral DNA is initiated at these sites.[51,52]

In addition to plasmid maintenance sequences, the URR contains promoters for initiation of mRNA synthesis, and it also contains the 5′ exons for some of these species of mRNA.[49] Thus, transcription of many of the early region ORFs begins in this region. In addition, the URR contains several AATAAA signals for the cleavage of mRNA transcripts.

The URR also contains several enhancer elements, which are present in one or more copies. These elements appear to be the target for the E2 protein. Of some interest was the observation that the E2 product of a given papillomavirus was able to transactivate enhancer sequences of other, distantly related papillomaviruses, suggesting conservation of the enhancer elements. The search for such an element revealed a motif ACCN6GGT or ACC-A/G N6C/T-GGT that was found repeated several times in the URR of all the papillomaviruses for which the URR sequence is known; DNA protection studies have confirmed that this is the motif to which the E2 protein binds.[54–58] The binding of the E2 protein to the enhancer is thought to result in the stimulation of transcription of early region messages, and, as described below, enhancement is mediated by the binding of the carboxy-terminal part of the E2 protein to the enhancer sequence.[58] Of note, duplication of the enhancer sequence in tandem was shown to result in increased ability to stimulate transcription. In conjunction with the observation that the enhancer sequence in some HPVs isolated from invasive cancers was present in tandem duplications, this suggests that the tumorigenic potential of these viruses may be correlated with the potentially augmented transcriptional activity.[58]

The mechanism by which the binding of E2 stimulates transcription appears to vary among papillomavirus species. Whereas E2 binding to the enhancer element is sufficient to stimulate transcription in BPV, it appears that binding to this sequence is not sufficient in HPV 6b and 11. In the latter, about 150 base pairs of the URR are necessary in addition to the 12-base-pair motif for full-enhancer activity, and the multiple components may be recognized by factors other than E2. Like the cell specificity of the enhancer element, these cellular factors may also be responsible for the cell tropism and specificity of papillomavirus infection. In summary, the URR, which is the region of the viral genome likeliest to be divergent among papillomaviruses, may be responsible for both cell specificity and for differences in virulence and malignant potential among species.[59,60]

THE E6 ORF

The E6 ORF clearly is involved in the process of cell transformation. Mutations within the BPV E6 ORF yield attenuated transformation in mouse C127 cells,[61,62] whereas introduction of expression vectors containing the E6 ORF into cell culture results in their transformation.[63,64] The E6 protein was found to be associated with cell nuclei and membranes in transformed cells;[56] this protein is highly basic and has repeating cys-x-x-cys motif, which is found in many DNA-binding proteins.[65,66] However, in some systems, such as mouse C127 cells, the expression of the E6 protein alone was not sufficient to efficiently induce transformation but instead required the presence of E7 ORF expression as well.[53]

In addition to its role in transformation, the E6 protein may play a role alone or in conjunction with the E7 ORF in the maintenance of a high episomal DNA copy number.[67,68]

Analysis of the E6 ORF sequences of several genital HPVs has revealed that splice donor and acceptor sites exist that allow for the transcription and translation of a truncated version of the E6 protein, known as E6*.[69] Of interest was the observation that this splice donor/acceptor site was found only in the papillomaviruses that are associated with a high risk of cervical cancer. Although the E6* protein has now been isolated,[70] its role in the process of malignant transformation, if any, is not yet clear.

THE E7 ORF

The E7 ORF is thought to play a role in conjunction with the E6 ORF in the regulation of the episomal DNA copy number, possibly by influencing the rate of replication initiation.[68,71] Accordingly, mutations in the E6^E7 region of the genome have been shown to result in substantial reduction in the number of episomal plasmids per cell.[67,68] In some transformation assays performed with HPV 16, the E7 ORF was shown to be capable of inducing transformation independent of E6.[72] Consistent with an important role in oncogenesis, the E7 ORF, like the E6 ORF, is consistently maintained and expressed in human cervical carcinomas and cervical carcinoma-derived cell lines.[73] In the latter, the E7 ORF is expressed as a 20,000-dalton phosphorylated protein.[74]

THE E1 ORF

The E1 ORF is the largest of the papillomavirus ORFs and has been shown to play an important role in the extrachromosomal regulation of DNA replication.[61,67] The 3′ end of the E1 ORF is thought to be important in maintenance of the episomal state. The protein encoded by this portion of the ORF is known as the E1-R, or replication, protein. Homology at the amino acid level has been shown between the 3′ end of the ORF and the ATP-binding domains of SV40 and polyoma large-T antigens.[75] Consistent with its role in the maintenance of the episomal state, mutations at the 3′ end of this ORF have been shown to result in integration of the viral genome into the host chromosome. The mechanism by which the E1-R protein maintains the episomal state is not yet known but appears to be a trans-acting function. Proof for this comes from experiments in which the addition of wild-type E1 ORF to the mutant E1 ORF permits normal episomal replication, even though its gene product is being encoded by a separate molecule.

As described previously, the E1 ORF has been shown to contain one of the two plasmid maintenance sequences, PMS-2, which is found in the middle of the ORF. PMS-2 can act independently of the URR PMS-1 as an origin of DNA replication.[51]

In contrast to the 3′ end of the E1 ORF, the 5′ end of the ORF appears to encode a negative regulator of plasmid replication,[76] which is known as the E1-M, or modulator, protein. This is a 23-kilodalton phosphoprotein[77] that is encoded by a spliced RNA transcript distinct from that encoding the E1-R protein.

Recent studies have shown that the E1 ORF may also play a role in regulation of E2 ORF activity, distinct from the functions described above. Mutations in both the 3′ and 5′ ends of the E1 ORF were shown to result in increased rates of viral transcription initiation, as well as increased levels of E2 transactivation activity.[78] These mutants demonstrated improved efficiency of transformation, confirming earlier studies that suggested that efficiency of transformation may be a consequence of increased viral gene expression.

THE E2 ORF

Like the gene products of the E1 ORF, the E2 protein is thought to encode a group of trans-acting proteins. The targets for the full-length E2 protein are thought to be enhancer sequences, such as those described previously in the URR. Deletion analysis studies have shown that E2 transactivation requires binding of the E2 protein to at least two of these binding sites at least 100 base pairs apart;[79] DNA looping may therefore be necessary for enhancer activity.[80] Support for this notion comes from studies that have shown that the binding of the E2 protein to the enhancer induces significant changes in the enhancer's conformation,[81] similar to the bending induced by other regulatory proteins, eg, SV40 large T antigen upon binding the Drosophila heat shock transcription factor.[82,83] Further genetic dissection of the E2 protein has also shown that the carboxy-terminus end of the full length protein contains the DNA-binding domain.[81,84,85]

The E2 protein is important in the process of cell transformation; in the absence of either the enhancer, or the E2 product that stimulates it, the efficiency of cell transformation is greatly reduced. Presumably, the result of E2 enhancer stimulation is increased transcription from the promoter initiation site for the E6 and E7 ORFs, and it is the gene products of the latter that are involved most directly in cell transformation. In addition to its effect on E6 and E7 transcription, BPV E2 transactivation has also been shown to enhance transcriptional activity of the promoter from which the E2 protein is itself transcribed, thus rendering the protein autoregulatory.[86]

Studies in the cottontail rabbit papillomavirus system have shown that the E2 protein expressed in COS-7 cells is phosphorylated and expressed primarily in the nucleus,[87] consistent with its function as a DNA-binding protein. The significance of the phosphorylation is not yet known, but it may play a role in the regulation of the trans-activating potential of the protein, similar to that seen in the large T antigen of SV40.[88]

Like the E1 ORF, a separate protein is encoded by the 3′ end of the ORF, as is known as the E2-C protein. In contrast to the full length E2 protein, the E2-C protein has a negative effect on transformation, possibly through a negative effect on the enhancer.[52] Thus, the E2 protein likely has three domains: the C-terminal domain, which contains the DNA binding activity and has an enhancer–repressor function; the N terminal domain, which may be required for interaction with other elements of the transcription complex; and the middle part, which is structurally flexible and may allow the other parts of the protein to interact with their respective elements.

THE E4 ORF

In contrast to the E6, E7, E1, and E2 proteins, no function has yet been assigned to the E4 protein; mutational analysis of this ORF has revealed that it is not required for cell transformation.[89,90] Despite this, more messenger RNA is transcribed from this ORF than any other, and in human plantar warts, the E4 protein was found to constitute 30% of the total protein mass.[91–93] Because of its abundance, it has been postulated that it may be a structural protein or that it may possibly play a scaffolding role in the viral capsid.

THE E5 ORF

Like the BPV E6 ORF, the BPV E5 ORF plays an important role in transformation of BPV-infected mouse cells.[94,95] Mutations of this protein have also been shown to result in deficient DNA replication.[96,97] Translation of the E5 ORF appears to initiate at a methionine in the middle of the ORF, resulting in a polypeptide with a molecular weight of 7000 daltons, and, as such, E5 is the smallest known transforming protein.[98] Thus, the transforming activity resides in the 3′ portion of the ORF. Structurally, the majority of the protein consists of a hydrophobic region embedded in the cell membrane in the form of homodimers and a hydrophilic tail that is found on the cell surface.[99] Dimerization has been shown to be essential for the transforming activity, because replacement of two cysteine residues thought to be important in dimerization resulted in diminished transforming efficiency.[100] Further analysis using microinjection techniques has demonstrated that induction of DNA synthesis may require only the last 13 amino acids of the carboxy terminus.[101] Recently, it has been shown that the expression of the E5 ORF is dependent on transactivation functions of the E2 ORF, thereby constituting one of the regulatory circuits in which the E2 ORF influences the efficiency of cell transformation.[102] Because of the small size of the E5 protein and its lack of homology with other known transforming proteins, it has been postulated that E5 may induce transformation through a novel, as yet uncharacterized mechanism.

Unlike the E5 protein of BPV, the E5 proteins of the HPVs investigated thus far have not been shown to be transforming, which demonstrates that caution in assigning similar functions to analogous ORFs in different papillomaviruses is in order. In some HPV types, the E5 ORF does not exist at all, and, in others, the putative E5 ORF varies considerably in structure. Moreover, the E5 ORF has been found to be deleted in some cervical carcinoma cell lines, and, therefore, the function of this ORF in HPV is not yet known.

OTHER EARLY REGION ORFs

Other ORFs can be found in the genomes of the papillomaviruses, and these vary from species to species. Notable examples are the E8 and E3 ORFs of the BPV genome, to which no function has yet been assigned.

THE L1 AND L2 ORFs

The L2 ORF encodes the minor capsid protein, with a molecular weight of approximately 76,000 daltons.[103] The L1 ORF encodes the major capsid protein with a molecular weight of approximately 54,000 daltons.[104] The L2 protein demonstrates considerable variability among papillomaviruses, but it is not highly antigenic, presumably because its antigenic epitopes are in the internal part of the viral capsid.[103,105] The migration of the L2 proteins detected in virion preparations on gels indicates a larger size than would be predicted by the ORF sequence, suggesting that some form of posttranslational modification may be occurring.[105]

In contrast to the L2 protein, the L1 protein is quite highly conserved among papillomaviruses, and antisera directed against disrupted BPV capsid antigen particles are used clinically as the group-specific antigens. These antigens are detected in the cell nuclei of differentiated epithelial cells infected with HPV or BPV, indicating productive viral infection and formation of complete virions, which are presumably infectious. Clinically used most often in immunohistochemical assays, the presence of capsid antigens in tissues indicates HPV infection but cannot distinguish between papillomavirus species or types.

In addition to the potential use for L1 antibodies as diagnostic reagents, L1 proteins have been used as immunogens for a vaccine against BPV.[106] With the use of L1 ORF DNA genetically engineered into *Escherichia coli* bacteria, large amounts of the purified L1 protein have been made and used as a vaccine to protect young calves from the development of warts;[107,108]

preliminary tests revealed good efficacy, and this vaccine was licensed in 1988 for use in cattle.

PATHOGENESIS OF LESIONS ASSOCIATED WITH HPV INFECTION

In order for papillomavirus to infect the epithelium, it is likely that some form of disruption of the integrity of the surface is needed, such as abrasions or wounds. Although it has not yet been proven, it is likely that papillomavirus infection is first established in the basal cell layer of the epithelium, which is the only dividing cell layer; thus, infection of these cells would constitute a reservoir for continuing infection of keratinocytes.

Upon infection, viral DNA is transported to the nucleus, where it replicates at a low level. As the keratinocyte matures, viral DNA replication is greatly augmented, and viral DNA becomes detectable using in situ hybridization techniques. In addition to enhanced replication, the more mature keratinocytes are also permissive for viral transcription and translation, such that the great majority of viral proteins are expressed only in the most mature cell layers of the epithelium. Therefore, capsid antigen is only expressed in this cell layer, and the number of cells demonstrating productive infection at one time is very small and highly focal. Of note is the observation that even in tumors with prominent fibroblastic proliferation, such as BPV-induced fibropapillomas, viral particles, and capsid antigen, are seen only in epithelial cells.

Papillomaviruses may infect either epithelial cells, fibroblasts, or both, depending on the species (Table 2–1). Whereas human papillomaviruses only infect skin and mucus membranes, and do not infect fibroblasts, BPV can infect both epithelial cells and fibroblasts, resulting in a fibropapilloma. Deer papillomaviruses, in contrast, predominantly infect fibroblasts and may produce fibromas without extensive epithelial abnormalities.[109]

A variety of changes occurs at the cellular level in association with papillomavirus infection. The spinous cell layer may enlarge (acanthosis), with an increased number of desmosomes, whereas other cells may show degenerative changes with nuclear atypia and cytoplasmic vacuolization. In the more mature cell layers, these changes become even more pronounced, with the development of nuclear degeneration. Koilocytosis or cytoplasmic vacuolization of cells may occur, in which the cells display a large perinuclear cavitation or halo, associated with an enlarged, irregular nucleus.

Infectivity studies of papillomaviruses have revealed that the skin's first reaction to infection is fibroblastic stimulation in the dermis, with an inflammatory response consisting of neutrophilia, congestion, and edema. Approximately 1 later, the inflammatory response begins to subside, but fibroblast proliferation and invasion of the papillary layer continue. The epithelium overlying this area begins to proliferate and demonstrate signs

TABLE 2–1. Animal Papillomaviruses

Virus	Host	Site	Histology	Reference
Bovine papillomavirus				
Type 1	Cattle	Cutaneous	Fibropapilloma	111
Type 2	Cattle	Cutaneous	Fibropapilloma	111
Type 3	Cattle	Cutaneous	Papilloma	112
Type 4	Cattle	Alimentary Tract	Papilloma	113
Type 5	Cattle	Teat	Papilloma	114
Cottontail rabbit (Shope) papillomavirus	Cottontail rabbit	Cutaneous	Papilloma	3
Equine papillomavirus	Horse	Cutaneous	Papilloma	115
Canine oral papillomavirus	Dog	Oral mucosa	Papilloma	116, 117
Sheep papillomavirus	Sheep	Cutaneous	Fibropapilloma	118
European elk papillomavirus	Elk	Cutaneous	Fibropapilloma	119
Deer fibromavirus	Deer	Cutaneous	Fibroma	109, 120
Mastomys natalensis papillomavirus	Multimammate mouse	Cutaneous	Papilloma	37
Chaffinch papillomavirus	Bird	Cutaneous	Papilloma	26, 121

Adapted with permission from *Animal Papillomaviruses*, Lancaster W. and Olsen C. Microbiol Rev 192;46:191–207, Table 1.

of acanthosis and hyperkeratosis. The epithelium contains localized hyperplasia, an intact basement membrane, an irregularly thickened prickle cell layer, and a granular layer containing koilocytes; the manner in which viral gene products stimulate cellular proliferation is not yet known. At this stage, the lesion may be clinically recognizable as a wart.

In general, papillomavirus infection results in benign, self-limiting tumors that regress after a period of time. However, in addition to stimulation of benign epithelial hyperplasia, papillomaviruses may induce dysplastic changes in infected cells, as well as invasive carcinomas. Evidence derived from BPV-related carcinoma suggests that factors in addition to viral infection may be necessary for malignant conversion. Such factors may be genetic or environmental, as in the case of alimentary tract papillomas in cattle caused by BPV-4; these have been shown to become cancerous in those regions of the world where the cattle ingest bracken fern as part of their diet.[25,110] Similarly, HPV can induce dysplasia and invasive carcinoma, probably in conjunction with one or more host or environmental factors. In many cases, the development of invasive cancer is accompanied by integration of the previously episomal viral genome into the host chromosome. The exact significance of this change is not yet clear, in part because integration has not been a consistent finding in all tumors. The site of viral integration in the host chromosome is variable, and the effect of viral integration on host gene expression is not yet understood. Likewise, viral integration results in the disruption of the papillomavirus genome, most often occurring in the E1 or E2 ORF, and frequently resulting the deletion of these ORFs. Although the idea is not yet proven, it is tempting to speculate that the disruption of these ORFs can result in aberrant regulation of viral gene transcription, which may in turn lead to augmented malignant potential.

SUMMARY

Papillomaviruses represent a group of DNA viruses from diverse sources in the animal kingdom. Despite this diversity, papillomaviruses retain remarkable similarity of structure and organization, with the early region gene products responsible for regulation of DNA replication and transformation, and late region products responsible for structural proteins. In addition, despite their diverse sources, papillomaviruses are associated with a stereotypic set of tissue responses upon infection, ranging from benign papillomas to invasive carcinomas. It is primarily in the context of the latter that papillomaviruses derive their considerable clinical importance. Recent work on the mechanisms of viral replication and transformation have contributed greatly to our understanding of the role of papillomaviruses in the pathogenesis of these diseases, and to host–virus interactions. It is expected that research on papillomaviruses at the molecular level will continue to contribute to our understanding of general biochemical principles, such as regulation of DNA replication, and mechanisms of cell transformation; in the future, such research will also contribute greatly to the development of diagnostic reagents for papillomavirus detection, as well as potential vaccine candidates.

REFERENCES

1. Erk N: A Study of Kitab al-Hail wal-Baitara by Muhammed Ibu ahi Hazam. Historica Medicinae Veterinariae 1976;1:101–104.
2. Astruc J: Of Porri, verucae, and condylomata of the pudenda. Treatis of venereal diseases in nine books. 1737.
3. Shope RE, Hurst EW: Infectious papillomatosis of rabbits; with a note on the histopathology. J Exp Med 1935;58:607–624.
4. Rous P, Beard JW: The progression to carcinoma of virus-induced rabbit papilloma (Shope). J Exp Med 1935;62:523–548.
5. Kidd JG, Rous P: A transplantable rabbit carcinoma originating in a virus-induced papilloma and containing the virus in a masked or altered state. J Exp Med 1940;71:813–838.
6. Rous P, Friedewald WF: The effect of chemical carcinogens on virus-induced carcinomas. J Exp Med 1944;79:511–537.
7. Rous P, Kidd JG: The carcinogenic effect of a virus upon tarred skin. Science 1936;83:468–469.
8. Rogers S, Rous P: Joint action of a chemical carcinogen and a neoplastic virus to induce

cancer in rabbits. Results of exposing epidermal cells to a carcinogenic hydrocarbon at time of infection with the Shope papilloma virus. J Exp Med 1951;93:459–488.

9. Syverton JT, Harvey RA, Berry GP, et al: The Roentgen radiation of papilloma virus (Shope) 1. The effect of X-rays upon papillomas on domestic rabbits. J Exp Med 1941;73:243.

10. Syverton JT: The pathogenesis of the rabbit papilloma-to-carcinoma sequence. Ann NY Acad Sci 1952;54:1126–1140.

11. Rogers S, Kidd JG, Rous P: Relationships of the Shope papillomavirus to the cancers it determines in domestic rabbits. Acta Union Int Contra Cancrum 1960;16:129–130.

12. Favre M, Jibard N, Orth G: Restriction mapping and physical characterization of the cottontail rabbit papillomavirus genome in transplantable VX2 and VX7 domestic rabbit carcinomas. Virology 1982;119:298–309.

13. Watson JD, Littlefield JW: Some properties of DNA from Shope papillomavirus. J Molec Biol 1960;2:161–165.

14. Georges E, Breitburd F, Jibard N, et al: Two Shope papillomavirus-associated VX-2 carcinoma cell lines with different levels of keratinocyte differentiation and transplantability. J Virol 1985;55:246–250.

15. McVay P, Fretz M, Wettstein, F, et al: Integrated Shope virus DNA is present and transcribed in the transplantable rabbit tumor VX-7. J Gen Virol 1982;60:271–278.

16. Nasseri M, Wettstein F: Differences exist between viral transcripts in cottontail papillomavirus-induced benign and malignant tumors as well as non-virus producing and virus-producing tumors. J Virol 1984;51:706–712.

17. Ito Y, Evans CA: Induction of tumors in domestic rabbits with nucleic acid preparations from partially purified Shope papilloma virus and from extracts of papillomas of domestic and cottontail rabbits. J Exp Med 1961;114:485–500.

18. Black PH, Hartley JW, Rowe WP, et al: Transformation of bovine tissue culture cells by bovine papillomavirus. Nature 1963;199:1016–1018.

19. Thomas M, Borion M, Tanzer J, et al: In-vitro transformation of mice cells by bovine papilloma virus. Nature 1964;202:709–710.

20. Chow L, Nasseri M, Wolinsky S, et al: Human papillomavirus types 6 and 11 mRNAS from genital condyloma acuminata. J Virol 1987;61:2581–2588.

21. Melnick JL: Papova virus group. Science 1962;135:1128–1130.

22. Melnick JL, Allison AC, Butel JS, et al: Papovaviridae intervirology 1974;3:106–120.

23. Rangan SRS, Gutter A, Baskin GB, et al: Virus associated papillomas in colobus monkeys (Colobus guereza). Lab Anim Sci 1980;30:885–889.

24. Sundberg JP, Russell WC, Lancaster W: Papillomatosis in Indian elephants. JAMA 1981;179:1247–1248.

25. Lancaster W, Olsen C: Animal papillomaviruses. Microbiol Rev 1982;46:191–207.

26. Osterhaus AMDE, Ellens DJ, Horzinek MC: Identification and characterization of a papillomavirus from birds (Frigillidae). Intervirology 1977;8:351–359.

27. Pfister H: Biology and biochemistry of papillomaviruses. Rev Physiol Biochem Pharmacol 1984;99:111–182.

28. deVilliers E-M: Human papillomaviruses reference chart. Burlington, NC, and Roche Diagnostic Systems, Montclair, NJ: Roche Biomedical Laboratories, 1989.

29. Crawford LV: Nucleic acids of tumor viruses. Adv Virus Res 1969;14:89–152.

30. Kass SJ, Knight CA: Purification and chemical analysis of Shope papilloma virus. Virology 1965;27:273–281.

31. Favre M, Breitburd F, Croissant O, et al: Structural polypeptides of rabbit, bovine and human papillomaviruses. J Virol 1975;15:1239–1247.

32. Howley PM: Molecular Biology of SV40 and the Human Polyomaviruses BK and JC. *In:* Klein G, ed. Viral oncology. New York: Raven Press, 1980:489–550.

33. Larsen PM, Storgaard L, Fey S: Proteins present in papillomavirus particles. J Virol 1987;61:3596–3601.

34. Jenson A, Rosenthal J, Olsen C, et al: Immunological relatedness of papillomaviruses from different species. J Nat Cancer Inst 1980;64:495–500.

35. Orth G, Breitburd F, Favre M: Evidence for antigenic determinants shared by the structural polypeptides of (Shope) rabbit papillomavirus and human papillomavirus type 1. Virology 1979;91:243–255.

36. Crawford LV, Crawford EM: A comparative study of polyoma and papilloma viruses. Virology 1963;21:258–263.

37. Muller H, Gissmann L: *Mastomys natalensis* papillomavirus (MnPV), the causative agent of epithelial proliferations: Characterization of the virus particle. J Gen Virol 1978;41:315–323.

38. Chen EY, Howley PM, Levinson AD, et al: The primary structure and genetic organization of the bovine papillomavirus type 1 genome. Nature 1982;299:529–534.

39. Giri I, Danos O, Yaniv M: Genomic structure of the cottontail rabbit (Shope) papillomavirus. PNAS 1985;82:1580–1584.

40. Cole ST, Streek RE: Genome organization and nucleotide sequence of human papillomavirus type 33, which is associated with cervical cancer. J Virol 1986;58:991–995.

41. Cole ST, Danos O: Nucleotide sequence and comparative analysis of the human papillomavirus type 18 genome: Phylogeny of papillomaviruses and repeated structure of the E6 and E7 gene products. J Mol Biol 1987;193:599–608.

42. Danos O, Engel LW, Chen EY, et al: A comparative analysis of the human type 1a and bovine papillomavirus type 1 papillomavirus genomes. J Virol 1983;46:557–566.

43. Dartmann K, Schwarz E, Gissmann L, et al: The nucleotide sequence and genome organization of human papillomavirus type 11. Virology 1986;151:124–130.

44. Fuchs PG, Iftner T, Weninger J, et al: Epidermodysplasia verruciformis-associated human papillomavirus 8: Genomic sequence and comparative analysis. J Virol 1986;58:626–634.

45. Schwarz E, Durst M, Demkowski C, et al: DNA sequence and genome organization of human papillomavirus type 6b. EMBO J 1983;2:2341–2348.

46. Seedorf K, Krammer G, Durst M, et al: Human papillomavirus type 16 DNA sequence. Virology 1985;145:181–185.

47. Heilman CA, Engel L, Lowy DR, et al: Virus-specific transcription in bovine papillomavirus-transformed mouse cells. Virology 1982;119:22–34.

48. Lowy DR, Dvoretzky I, Shober R, et al: In vitro tumorigenic transformation by a defined subgenomic fragment of bovine papilloma virus DNA. Nature 1980;287:72–74.

49. Baker CC, Howley PM: Differential promoter utilization by the bovine papillomavirus in transformed cells and productively infected wart tissues. EMBO J 1987;6:1027–1035.

50. Engel LW, Heilman CA, Howley PM: Transcriptional organization of the bovine papillomavirus type 1. J Virol 1983;47:516–528.

51. Lusky M, Botchan MR: Characterization of the bovine papillomavirus type 1 plasmid maintenance sequences. Cell 1984;36:391.

52. Lambert P, Spalholz BA, Howley PM: Evidence that bovine papillomavirus type 1 may encode a negative transcriptional regulatory factor. *In:* Steinberg BM, Brandsma JL, Taichman LB, eds. Cancer cells. Cold Spring Harbor, NY: Cold Spring Harbor Laboratory, 1987;5:15–22.

53. Neary K, DiMaio D: Open reading frames E6 and E7 of bovine papillomavirus type 1 are both required for full transformation of mouse C127 cells. J Virol 1989;63:259–266.

54. Spalholz BA, Yang YC, Howley PM: Transactivation of a bovine papillomavirus transcriptional regulatory element by the E2 gene product. Cell 1985;42:183–191.

55. Yang YC, Spalholz BA, Rabson MS, et al: Dissociation of transforming and transactivating functions for bovine papillomavirus type 1. Nature 1985;318:575–577.

56. Androphy EJ, Lowy DR, Schiller JT: Bovine papillomavirus E2 transactivating gene product binds to specific sites in papillomavirus DNA. Nature 1987;325:70–73.

57. Moskaluk C, Bastia D: The E2 "gene" of bovine papillomavirus encodes an enhancer binding protein. PNAS 1987;84:1215–1218.

58. Giri I, Yaniv M: Study of the E2 gene product of the cottontail rabbit papillomavirus reveals a common mechanism of transactivation among papillomaviruses. J Virol 1988;62:1573–1581.

59. Boshart M, zur Hausen H: Human papillomaviruses in Buschke-Lowenstein tumors: Physical state of the DNA and identification of tandem duplication in the noncoding region of human papillomavirus 6 subtype. J Virol 1986;58:963–966.

60. Rando RF, Lancaster WD, Han P, et al: The noncoding region of HPV 6VC contains two distinct transcriptional enhancing elements. Virology 1986;155:545–556.

61. Sarver N, Rabson MS, Yang YC, et al: Localization and analysis of bovine papillomavirus type 1 transforming functions. J Virol 1984;52:377–388.

62. Schiller JT, Vass WC, Lowy DR: Identification of a second transforming protein inbovine papillomavirus DNA. PNAS 1984;81:7880–7884.

63. Schiller JT, Androphy EJ, Vass WC, et al: The bovine papillomavirus E6 gene: Identification of its transforming function and protein product. In: Howley PM, Broker TR, eds. Papillomaviruses: Molecular and clinical aspects. UCLA Symposia on Molecular and Cellular Biology. New York; Alan R. Liss, 1985;32:457–472.

64. Yang YC, Okayama H, Howley PM: Bovine papillomavirus contains multiple transforming genes. PNAS 1985;82:1030–1034.

65. Friedman T, Doolittle RT, Walter G: Amino acid sequence homology between polyoma and SV40 tumor antigens deduced from nucleotide sequences. Nature 1978;274:291–293.

66. Wain-Hobson S, Sonigo P, Danos O, et al: Nucleotide sequence of the AIDS virus, LAV. Cell 1985;40:9–17.

67. Lusky M, Botchan MR: Genetic analysis of bovine papillomavirus type 1 *trans*-activating replication factors. J Virol 1985;53:955.

68. Berg LJ, Singh K, Botchan MR: Complementation of a bovine papillomavirus low-copy-number mutant: Evidence for a temporal requirement of the complementing gene. Mol Cell Biol 1986;6:859.

69. Schneider-Gadicke A, Schwarz E: Different human cervical carcinoma cell lines show similar transcription patterns of human papillomavirus type 18 early genes. EMBO J 1986;5:2285–2292.

70. Schneider-Gadicke A, Kaul S, Schwarz E, et al: Identification of the human papillomavirus type 18 E6* and E6 proteins in nuclear protein fractions from human cervical carcinoma cells grown in the nude mouse or in-vitro. Cancer Res 1988;48:2969–2974.

71. Lusky M, Botchan M: Transient replication of bovine papilloma virus type 1 plasmids: Cis and trans requirements. PNAS 1986;83:3609–3613.

72. Smotkin D, Wettstein F: Transcription of human papillomavirus type 16 early genes in a cervical cancer and a cancer-derived cell line and identification of the E7 protein. PNAS 1986;83:4680–4684.

73. Smotkin D, Wettstein FO: Transcription of human papillomavirus type 16 early genes in a cervical cancer and a cancer derived cell line and identification of the E7 protein. PNAS 1986;83:4680–4684.

74. Smotkin D, Wettstein FO: The major human papillomavirus protein in cervical cancers is a cytoplasmic phosphoprotein. J Virol 1987;61:1686–1689.

75. Clertant P, Seif I: A common function for polyoma virus large-T antigen and papillomavirus E1 proteins? Nature 1984;311:276–279.

76. Berg LJ, Lusky M, Stenlund A, et al: Repression of BPV replication is mediated by a virally encoded *trans*-acting factor. Cell 1986;46:753–762.

77. Thorner L, Bucay N, Choe J, et al: The product of the bovine papillomavirus type 1 modulator gene (M) is a phosphoprotein. J Virol 1988;62:2474–2482.

78. Lambert P, Howley PM: Bovine papillomavirus type 1 E1 replication-defective mutants are altered in their transcriptional regulation. J Virol 1988;62:4009–4015.

79. Spalholz BA, Lambert PF, Yee CL, et al: Bovine papillomavirus transcriptional regulation: localization of the E2-responsive elements of the long control region. J Virol 1987;61:2128–2137.

80. Schleif R: Why should DNA loop? Nature 1987;327:369–370.

81. Moskaluk C, Bastia D: DNA bending is induced in an enhancer by the DNA-binding domain of the bovine papillomavirus E2 protein. PNAS 1988;85:1826–1830.

82. Ryder K, Silver S, DeLucia AL, et al: An altered DNA conformation in Origin Region 1 is a determinant for the binding of SV40 large T antigen. Cell 1986;44:719–725.

83. Shuey DJ, Parker CS: Bending of promoter DNA on binding of heat shock transcription factor. Nature 1986;323:459–461.

84. Giri I, Yaniv M: Structural and mutational analysis of E2 trans-activating proteins of papillomaviruses reveals three distinct functional domains. EMBO J 1988;7:2823–2829.

85. McBride A, Schlegel R, Howley PM: The carboxy-terminal domain shared by the bovine papillomavirus E2 transactivator and repressor proteins contains a specific DNA binding activity EMBO J 1988;7:533–539.

86. Hermonat PL, Spalholz BA, Howley PM: The bovine papillomavirus P2443 promoter is E2 *trans*-responsive: evidence for E2 autoregulation. EMBO J 1988;7:2815–2822.

87. Barbosa M, Wettstein F: E2 of the cottontail rabbit papillomavirus is a nuclear phospho-protein translated from an mRNA encoding multiple open reading frames. J Virol 1988;62:3242–3249.

88. Simmons DT, Chow W, Rodgers K: Phosphorylation downregulates the DNA-binding activity of the simian virus 40 T antigen. J Virol 1986;60:888–894.

89. DiMaio D, Neary K, Kaczmarek L, et al: Mutational analysis of bovine papillomavirus-type 1 transforming functions. In: Steinberg BM, Brandsma JL, Taichman LB, eds. Cancer cells. Cold Spring Harbor, NY: Cold Spring Harbor Laboratory, 1987;5:187–194.

90. Neary K, Horwitz BH, DiMaio D: Mutational analysis of the open reading frame E4 of bovine papillomavirus type 1. J Virol 1987;61:1248–1252.

91. Chow LT, Hirochika H, Nasseri M, et al: Human papillomavirus gene expression. In: Steinberg BM, Brandsma JL, Taichman LB, eds. Cancer Cells. Cold Spring Harbor, NY: Cold Spring Harbor Laboratory, 1987;5:55–72.

92. Chow LT, Reilly SS, Broker TR: Identification and mapping of human papillomavirus type 1 RNA transcripts recovered from plantar warts and infected epithelial cell culture. J Virol 1987;61:1913–1918.

93. Doorbar J, Campbell D, Grand RJA: Identification of the human papilloma virus-1a E4 gene products. EMBO J 1986;5:355–362.

94. DiMaio D, Guralski D, Schiller JT: Translation of open reading frame E5 of bovine papillomavirus is required for its transforming activity. PNAS 1986;83:1797–1801.

95. Schiller JT, Vass WC, Vousden KH, et al: The E5 open reading frame of bovine papillomavirus type 1 encodes a transforming gene. J Virol 1986;57:1–6.

96. Groff DE, Lancaster WD: Genetic analysis of the 3′ early region transformation and replication functions of bovine papillomavirus type 1. Virology 1986;150:221–230.

97. Rabson MS, Yang YC, Howley PM: A genetic analysis of bovine papillomavirus type-1 transformation and plasmid-maintenance functions. *In:* Botchan M, Grodzicker T, Sharp PA, eds. DNA tumor viruses: Control of gene expression and replication. Cancer cells. Cold Spring Harbor, NY: Cold Spring Harbor Laboratory, 1986;4:235–243.

98. Burkhardt, DiMaio D, Schlegel R: Genetic and biochemical definition of the bovine papillomavirus E5 transforming protein. EMBO J 1987;6:2381–2385.

99. Schlegel R, Wade-Glass M, Rabson MS, et al: The E5 transforming gene of bovine papillomavirus encodes a small hydrophobic polypeptide. Science 1986;233:464–467.

100. Horwitz BH, Brukhardt AL, Schlegel R, et al: 44-amino-acid E5 transforming protein of bovine papillomavirus requires a hydrOphobic core and specific carboxyl-terminal amino acids. Mol Cell Biol 1988;8:4071–4078.

101. Green M, Loewenstein PM: Demonstration that a chemically synthesized BPV1 onco-protein and its C-terminal domain function to induce cellular DNA synthesis. Cell 1987;51:795–802.

102. Prakash SS, Horwitz B, Zibello T, et al: Bovine papillomavirus E2 gene regulates expression of the viral E5 transforming gene. J Virol 1988;62:3608–3613.

103. Komly CA, Breitburd F, Croissant O, et al: The L2 open reading frame of human papillomavirus type 1a encodes a minor structural protein carrying type specific antigens. J Virol 1986;60:813–816.

104. Cowsert LM, Pilacinski WP, Jenson AB: Identification of the bovine papillomavirus L1 gene product using monoclonal antibodies. Virology 1988;165:613–615.

105. Pilacinski WP, Glassman DL, Glassman KF, et al: Cloning and expression in *Escherichia coli* of the bovine papillomavirus L1 and L2 open reading frames. Biotechnology 1984;1:356–360.

106. Pass F: Vaccines for latent viruses. J Am Acad Derm 1988;18:224–226.

107. Pilacinski WP, Glassman DL, Glassman KF, et al: Development of a recombinant vaccine against bovine papillomavirus infection in cattle. In: Howley PM, Broker TR, eds. Papillomaviruses: Molecular and clinical aspects. New York: Alan R. Liss, 1985:257–271.

108. Pilacinski WP, Glassman DL, Glassman KF, et al: Immunization against bovine papillomavirus infection. In: Evered D, Clark S, eds. CIBA Foundation Symposium. Chichester, UK: John Wiley and Sons, 1986;120:136–156.

109. Shope RE, Mangold R, McNamara LG, et al: An infectious cutaneous fibroma of the Virginia white-tailed deer (*Odocoileus virginianus*). J Exp Med 1958;108:797–802.

110. Jarrett W, McNeil P, Laird H, et al: Virus-induces papillomas of the alimentary tract of cattle. Int J Cancer 1980;22:323–328.

111. Lancaster WD, Olson C: Demonstration of two distinct classes of bovine papilloma virus. Virology 1978;89:371–379.

112. Pfister H, Linz U, Gissmann L, et al: Partial characterization of a new type of bovine papilloma virus. Virology 1979;96:1–8.

113. Campo MS, Moar MH, Laird HM, et al: A new papillmavirus associated with alimentary tract cancer in cattle. Nature 1980;286:180–182.

114. Campo MS, Moar MH, Jarrett WFH, et al: Molecular heterogeneity and lesion site specificity of cutaneous bovine papillomaviruses. Cancer Res 1981;113:323–335.

115. Fulton RE, Doane FW, Macpherson LW: The fine structure of equine papilloma and the equine papilloma virus. J Ultrastruct Mol Struc Res 1970;30:328–343.

116. Chambers VC, Evans CA: Canine oral papillomatosis. 1. Virus assay and observations of the various stages of the experimental infection. Cancer Res 1959;19:1188–1195.

117. Pfister H, Meszaros J: Partial characterization of a canine oral papillomavirus. Virology 1980;104:243–246.

118. Gibbs EPJ, Smale CJ, Lauman MJP: Warts in sheep. J Comp Pathol 1975;85:327–334.

119. Moreno-Lopez J, Petersson U, Dinter Z, et al: Characterization of a papilloma virus from the European Elk (EEPV). Virology 1981;113:589–595.

120. Tajima M, Gordon DE, Olson C: Electron microscopy of bovine papilloma and deer fibroma viruses. Am J Vet Res 1968;29:1185–1194.

121. Lina PHC, van Noord MJ, de Groot FG: Detection of virus in squamous papillomas of the wild bird species *Fringilla coelebs*. J Nat Cancer Inst 1973;50:567–571.

CHAPTER 3

The Human Papillomaviruses: Classification and Molecular Biology

Matthias Dürst, PhD

Papillomaviruses are members of the Papovaviridae family,[1] but because of a number of molecular and biologic features, they should effectively represent a distinct virus group of their own. There is no cross-reactivity either by nucleic acid hybridization or serology that would point to a common evolutionary trait between papillomaviruses and the other members of the family (mouse polyoma virus, simian virus 40, BK and JC virus). Indeed, the genome organization of papillomaviruses differs fundamentally from the other viruses. In the polyoma/SV40 group, transcription of genes for early and late functions diverge from a single control region along opposite strands of DNA, with early and late messages converging about halfway around the molecule.[2] In papillomaviruses, the complete genetic information is encoded on only one of the two DNA strands.[3]

Papillomaviruses infect all kinds of vertebrates, including amphibians, reptiles, birds, and a wide range of mammals.[4,5] The viruses are usually species specific and, in the case of human papillomaviruses (HPV), strictly epitheliotropic. Because of the lack of a suitable cell culture system for their propagation, a detailed characterization of individual virus isolates was only possible after molecular cloning of the respective genomes. Based on the degree of genomic cross-hybridization, some 57 different HPV types have been identified so far (Table 3–1).

In recent years, evidence has accumulated suggestive of a causative role of certain papillomavirus types in the pathogenesis of some human cancers. In addition to giving a brief overview on HPV classification, this chapter will review some of the clinical and experimental data that permit speculation on the molecular mechanisms involved in the development of malignant tumors, in particular of squamous cell carcinoma of the uterine cervix.

Clinical Practice of Gynecology: **2,** 29–41, 1989
© 1989 Elsevier Science Publishing Co., Inc.
655 Avenue of the Americas, New York, NY 10010

ISSN 1043-3198/89/$3.50

TABLE 3–1.

HPV Type	Associated Disease
1,2,4	Plantar and common warts
3,28,29	Flat warts
7	Common warts of meat and animal handlers
5,8,9,10,12,14,15,17,19,20, 21,22,23,24,25,36,37, 38,47,50	Flat warts, macules and pityriasis, versicolor-like lesions in *Epidermodysplasia verruciformis* (E.v.) patients, some types occasionally found in keratoacanthoma, solar keratosis and melanoma
53	No specific disease (cloned from cervical scraping)
6,11,42,43,44,54,55,57	Ano-genital condylomata acuminata, some types also found in laryngeal papilloma
6,11,16,18,30,31,33,34,35, 39,40,42,43,44,45,51,52, 56,57	Cervical intraepithelial neoplasia (CIN), vaginal intraepithelial neoplasia (VIN), penile intraepithelial neoplasia (PIN), bowenoid papulosis and genital Bowen's disease
6,11,16,18,31,33,35,39,45,51,52, 56	Cervical, vulvar, and penile cancer, perianal and anal cancer
13,32	Oral focal epithelial hyperplasia (Heck's disease)
26,27,49	Cutaneous warts from a patient with immune difficiency and from a renal transplant recipient
41,48	Disseminated warts, squamous cell carcinoma of the skin
46	E.v.-like lesions in a patient with Hodgkin's disease

References: HPV 1,[12,13] HPV 2,[13,14] HPV 3,[15,16] HPV 4,[13] HPV 5,[18,19] HPV 6,[26] HPV 7,[17] HPV 8,[15,20] HPV 9,[18] HPV 10,[15] HPV 11,[27] HPV 12,[15] HPV 13,[38] HPV 14,[21] HPV 15,[21] HPV 16,[33] HPV 17,[21] HPV 18,[34] HPV 19,[21,22] HPV 20,[21,22] HPV 21–24,[21] HPV 25,[22] HPV 26,[40] HPV 27,[41] HPV 28,29 (Favre, personal communication), HPV 30,[35] HPV 31,[36] HPV 32,[39] HPV 33,[28] HPV 34,[37] HPV 35,[29] HPV 36,[23] HPV 37,38,[24] HPV 39,[30] HPV 40 (deVilliers, personal communication), HPV 41,[42] HPV 42,[30] HPV 43,44 (Lorinez, personal communication), HPV 45,[31] HPV 46,[43] HPV 47,[25] HPV 48 (Gallahan and Müller, personal communication), HPV 49,50 (Favre, personal communication), HPV 51,[32] HPV 52 (Ito, personal communication), HPV 53 (Gallahan and Müller, personal communication), HPV 54 (Favre, personal communication), HPV 55 (Favre, personal communication), HPV 56 (Lorinez, personal communication), HPV 57 (deVilliers, personal communication). For review, see de Villiers E. M. Heterogeneity of the human papillomavirus group. J Virol 1989; 63 (in press).

CLASSIFICATION OF HUMAN PAPILLOMAVIRUSES

Because of the very restricted host range, the host name itself is part of papillomavirus nomenclature, ie, HPV for *h*uman *p*apilloma*v*irus. Unlike many other virus groups, classification is not based on serology. The reason for this is the lack of an in vitro system that would permit the propagation of virus in sufficient quantities for raising type specific antisera. Historically, papillomavirus antigen could only be obtained from clinical material, and this was further complicated by the considerable variation in productivity of individual virus types in vivo. By using whole virus particles from clinical lesions, type specific antisera were prepared for HPV 1–4 and some HPVs associated with patients suffering from a cutaneous disease known as epidermodysplasia verruciformis.[6,7] A common papillomavirus antigen can be detected by antisera raised against detergent disrupted human (HPV), cottontail rabbit (CRPV), or bovine (BPV) papillomaviruses.[8,9] Fortunately, the availability of virus antigen is no longer a limiting factor. DNA recombinant technology permits the production of any protein, provided its genetic information is known. With the aid of this technology, poly- and monoclonal antisera directed against various proteins of different HPV types may turn out to be of great value for future diagnostic purposes and possibly also for classification.

Therefore, papillomavirus classification is still based on the degree of genomic relatedness between the different isolates. Prerequisite for such a detailed analysis are molecular clones of the genomes in question.[10] By definition, a new type of papillomavirus has to show less than 50% cross-reactivity with any other HPV type as measured by reassociation kinetics under stringent conditions of hybridization.[10,11] With this technique, the rate of hybridization, ie, the formation of double-stranded DNA over a period of time, is determined. Stringent hybridization conditions are given if the reaction is incubated 18°C below the melting point (Tm) of the DNA. This point defines the temperature at which 50% of double-stranded molecules are denatured at any one time. If, under stringent conditions, cross-reactivity is very high, the genomes are considered as subtypes or variants. The DNA of many different papillomavirus types do not cross-hybridize under stringent conditions, even if they are of the same species. By lowering the stringency of hybridization to Tm − 40°C, all papillomavirus types hybridize with each other.

Besides the possible future influence of serology, the present classification scheme based on reassociation kinetics alone is likely to be modified further as more and more detailed information about the biology of these viruses becomes available.

CORRELATION BETWEEN GENOMIC RELATEDNESS OF PAPILLOMAVIRUSES AND CLINICAL PROPERTIES OF INDUCED LESIONS

Human papillomavirus types are classified according to the degree of reassociation of their genomes. It is surprising, however, that in some cases the cross-reactivity is smaller than expected, although the HPV types in question induce clinically indistinguishable lesions, ie, 25% cross-reactivity for HPV 6 and 11, which induce genital condyloma,[27] and only 1% cross-reactivity for HPV 9 and 20, typically found in flat lesions of epidermodysplasia verruciformis patients.[22] One likely explanation for this is that the similar biologic properties of the above types are not determined by the overall homology of their genomes but by short stretches of nucleotide homology comprising regulatory sequences, signals for mRNA processing, or even encoding particular surface epitopes, which may be required for infection. These relatively small regions would not significantly influence the outcome of reassociation kinetics, which is based on the cross-hybridization of the *entire* genome. Detailed nucleotide sequence comparisons and functional analysis appear to be more promising for uncovering similarities and differences between HPV types that may also correlate with their biologic properties. Evidence for this is given in the examples below.

Nucleotide sequence analysis of cDNA clones (derived from mRNA) obtained from HPV-positive cell lines and mRNA mapping data has shown splicing events in E6 open reading frames (ORF), which are peculiar for HPV 16 and 18 but not for HPV 6 and 11 (M Rohlfs, personal communication).[44–46] The spliced E6 mRNA encodes a putative protein, designated E6*, which differs from the unspliced version both in number and in sequence of the encoded amino-acids at its C-terminus. So far, the E6* protein was immunoprecipitated from a HPV 18 positive carcinoma but could not be detected in the carcinoma cell line HeLa.[47] The reason for this discrepancy is not clear, since the majority of E6 mRNAs in HeLa cells are of the spliced form. It is possible that translation of this particular transcript may not be efficient in tissue culture cells maintained in vitro and, thus, would remain undetected. As yet no function has been assigned to the HPV E6* protein. Because signals for mRNA splicing in the E6 ORF have also been found in HPV 31 and 33,[48] it is tempting to speculate that the E6* protein contributes to the oncogenic properties of some genital HPV types.

Certain genetic elements termed enhancers appear to play an important role in the host and tissue specificity of papillomaviruses. Together with the origin of replication and several promoters, enhancers have been mapped to the upstream regulatory region (URR) that is located downstream of the late and preceding the early region of the papillomavirus genome.

An enhancer can be composed of several components that may function more or less additively in stimulating transcription of linked genes.[49,50] The enhancer elements in the URR of papillomaviruses are not only recognized by virally encoded transacting factors[51,52] but also by tissue specific cellular factors.[53] Transcriptional activity of papillomaviruses in vivo is most likely governed by a complex interaction of these factors. The URR represents one of the most diverged regions between different papillomaviruses and, taken together with its role in transcription, may offer an explanation for the host- and tissue-specificity of these viruses. It was shown experimentally that tandem multiplication of the HPV 11 enhancer sequence dramatically increased its response to transactivation by the viral E2 gene product.[52] Indeed, a duplication found in HPV 6 subtype d[54] corresponds to the enhancer region identified in HPV 11. HPV 6 is usually associated with benign tumors but this particular isolate was recovered from a squamous cell tumor (Buschke-Löwenstein).

Another variant, HPV 6 VC, isolated from a invasive verrucous carcinoma, also carries a short insertion duplication in the same region.[55] Similarly, HPV 33, which is associated with cervical cancer,[28] contains a 78 bp tandem duplication in the URR.[48] In view of the results obtained with artificially assembled tandem multiplications of the enhancer element, a natural selection for enhancer duplications resulting in increased transcriptional activity may be involved in the higher tumorigenic potential of certain viruses.

LINKING HPV TO CANCER: CLINICAL AND EXPERIMENTAL EVIDENCE

Animal papillomaviruses, like HPV, are associated with a number of benign and neoplastic lesions. In contrast to those of the human viruses, the oncogenic properties of the animal viruses could readily be demonstrated in experimental in vivo systems. Shope-virus (CRPV) induced benign papillomas in domestic rabbits were shown to convert to malignancy at a high frequency.[56] This effect could be enhanced by the application of carcinogens.[57] Similarly, an interaction between a bovine papillomavirus type (BPV4) and the ingestion of bracken fern play a key role in the pathogenesis of squamous cell carcinoma of the esophagus in cattle.[58]

The association of papillomavirus and human cancers is particularly strong for cancers of the uterine cervix. There is considerable evidence that points to an infectious component in the development of this disease.[59–61] Papillomaviruses are considered the most likely transmissible agent for a number of reasons:

1. Papillomavirus infections of the genital tract are very common. Mass screening of asymptomatic women by means of filter in situ hybridization of cells from cervical smears showed evidence for HPV infection in 10–30% of cases.[62,63]

2. Cervical intraepithelial neoplasias (CIN), which are considered as putative precancers,[64] can be virus induced.[65–67] Recently, the viral etiology of these lesions could be proven in an experimental system that is based on the implantation of HPV-infected human normal squamous epithelium into nude mice. Subsequent examination of the tissue showed histopathologic changes characteristic of those observed in clinical lesions. The heterotransplanted tissue also permitted reisolation of infectious virus tested in another round of infection.[68]

3. Prospective studies show that virus-induced CIN lesions have the potential for progression.[69] In one study, the risk for progression of HPV-

16-induced CIN is significantly increased as compared to lesions containing HPV 6 and 11.[70]

4. More than 90% of cervical cancer biopsies contain the DNA of HPV 16, 18, 31, 33, 35, or 39—HPV 16 and 18 being the most frequent representatives.

The mere association of certain HPV types with malignant tumors, of course, is no proof for a causal relationship. The regular presence of viral DNA could also be attributed to the high affinity of a particular virus for a transformed cell. However, in the experiments discussed below, the oncogenic properties of some HPV types can be readily underlined.

The circular genome of papillomaviruses replicates as an extra-chromosomal plasmid in benign genital lesions.[71] In invasive cervical carcinoma and possibly also in some premalignant lesions, DNA sequences of HPV 16 and 18 are often found integrated in the cellular genome. Viral integration observed in these biopsies and cervical-carcinoma-derived cell lines shows a common pattern. The upstream viral region is preserved, but the downstream early region is deleted, disrupted, or inactivated,[44,72–75] and consistently leaves the potentially transforming E6 and E7 ORF of the viral genome intact. Despite passage in vitro for many years, the HPV positive cervical carcinoma cell lines not only continue to express the E6 and E7 region as mRNA, but their translation products have also been identified.[45,76–78] Since chromosomal instability in form of rearrangements and deletions are typical in the development of a cell line, the conservation of viral information and expression may be taken as evidence for their requirement in the maintenance of the transformed phenotype.

Direct evidence for the above assumption was obtained in experiments that permit modulation of viral mRNA in vitro. For this purpose, expression plasmids that, after stimulation of their hormone-inducible MMTV regulatory element, code for antisense (complementary) HPV 18 E6–E7 mRNA, were constructed and transfected into C4-I cells (containing endogenous HPV 18 DNA). In a number of stable cell clones, growth retardation, together with a reduced synthesis of E7 protein, was observed after hormone induction.[79]

In analogy, HPV specific transcription in somatic cell fusion hybrids (HeLa × normal human keratinocytes or fibroblasts) could be suppressed by the DNA methylation inhibitor 5′Azacytidine.[80] It is known that a large number of genes are transcriptionally silent in vitro because of hypermethylation.[81] Treating the cells with 5′Azacytidine resulted in a down regulation of HPV 18 transcription, which correlated directly with cessation of cell growth. Other reference genes, like c-myc, erb-B, β-actin, and ribosomal RNA remained unaffected. Since the 5′Azacytidine effect could be blocked by cycloheximide (a protein biosynthesis inhibitor), the most likely explanation for the above observations is the induction of a labile cellular protein that is silent in vitro but not in vivo (the tumorigenic phenotype of these hybrid lines is normally suppressed). It is postulated that HPV expression is directly or indirectly regulated by this protein.[80]

HPV 16 contains sequences capable of transforming cell cultures in vitro.[82–84] In order to localize the transforming genes within the HPV 16 genome, individual ORFs were linked to expression plasmids and were tested for their transforming capacity. Only plasmids containing the intact E7 coding region were found to induce morphological alteration and anchorage independent growth in 3Y1 cells (an established rat fibroblast cell line).[85] Similar observations were made for HPV 18.[86,87] Transformation of primary baby rat kidney cells (BRK), however, could only be achieved by the cooperating activity of the E6–E7 region of HPV 16 and an activated oncogene, EJ ras.[88] More pertinent to human tumorigenesis is the transformation of primary human cells in vitro. The natural targets for papillomavirus infection are the proliferating cells (keratinocytes) of the epidermis, which are confined to the basal membrane. During transit to the upper layers, the basal cell undergoes a program of irreversible differentiation. Viral DNA-replication and particle production is only permissible in cells of an advanced stage of differentiation and, therefore, can only take place in the upper layers of the skin. It was shown recently that HPV 16 DNA is able to immortalize human primary keratinocytes in vitro.[89,90] These cells normally have a finite life span in culture. In a most recent report, a quantitative keratinocyte assay is described that enabled the detection of HPV-induced cell proliferation irrespective of the viral type tested (HPV 6, 11, 16, 18), but an altered pattern of cellular differentiation for cells transfected with the potentially malignant HPV types.[91] The viral gene(s) responsible for these transformation phenomena have not yet been identified but are likely to be derived from the E6–E7 region. None of the HPV-immortalized human cell lines are tumorigenic in nude mice. This is consistent with the multistep process thought to be involved in the pathogenesis of genital cancer. Secondary events that are required for malignant conversion of these cell lines are presently being investigated.

POSSIBLE MECHANISMS INVOLVED IN THE PATHOGENESIS OF GENITAL CANCER

Although subclinical HPV infections occur at a high frequency, cancer develops in only a small proportion of infected individuals. This makes it evident that HPV may only be a necessary but not a sufficient event in the development of this disease. In addition, the long latency period (up to 30 years) between primary infection and the manifestation of cancer suggests the need for co-factors.

As described in the previous section, integration of the papillomavirus genome into the host DNA is frequently observed in cancer biopsies and also in some precancerous lesions. This event may be a prerequisite in the sequence of events leading to cancer. There also appears to be a preferred region within the virus genome that is disrupted during integration. As a consequence, it is only the 5' part of the early region of the genome (ORF E6–E7) that can be transcribed from the viral promoter. Viral genes downstream of the integration site (some of which are known to encode regulatory proteins) are thus uncoupled from the viral promoter element and are no longer active. An uncontrolled expression of the putative viral transforming genes E6–E7 may result. Integration could result from mutagenic events mediated by carcinogens. Major constituents of tobacco smoke have been identified in the vaginal fluids of smokers.[92] These mutagens may be further modified by specific bacterial infections or may also be generated in their own metabolic pathways. In response to carcinogens, the cellular repair system becomes activated, and, under these conditions, recombination events are favored.[93] This possible mechanism is consistent with studies that point to an increased relative risk for heavy smokers to develop cervical cancer.

However, it is unlikely that the integration event outlined above per se is sufficient for the induction of the malignant phenotype. This becomes particularly evident from cell fusion experiments of HeLa cells with normal human keratinocytes or fibroblasts. In the stable hybrid cell lines, the tumorigenic phenotype is suppressed,[94] despite the fact that the HPV 18 integration locus remained unaltered.[95] Experimental data shows that in these cell lines, HPV 18 transcription can be down-regulated in vitro by a cellular factor(s) that is derived from the normal cell counterpart.[80] Very rarely, some of the fusion cells have again acquired the tumorigenic phenotype. This alteration was always accompanied by the loss of specific genetic information from the normal cell counterpart.[96] In the tumorigenic revertants, HPV 18 transcription can no longer be down-regulated.[80] This is in line with a model that postulates the existence of cellular genes that control the expression of the persisting viral genome.[97,98] In vivo, this intracellular surveillance mechanism must be tightly linked to the differentiation state of the cell. Viral expression is negatively regulated in the basal cell that provides the only pool of mitotically active epidermal cells. In cells committed to terminal differentiation, the block is released and ensures production of progeny virus.

In other studies, it is suggested that the activation of cellular oncogenes may be an additional event at least in the progression of cervical carcinoma.[99] Amplification of the c-myc and c-H-ras genes was observed in more than 50% of tumors analyzed, preferentially in those corresponding to stages 2–4 of malignant progression. High levels of c-myc RNA were not only found in carcinoma but were also found in HeLa, C4-I, and CaSki cells. In HeLa cells, HPV 18 DNA is integrated in close proximity of the c-myc locus,[100,101] and the high steady-state-level of myc transcripts may be due to cis-activation by HPV-18-enhancing elements.

In summary, unregulated expression of HPV early genes caused by the loss of cellular control function is considered one of the key factors in the pathogenesis of cervical cancer. However, other factors, such as impaired immune function and hormonal status, are known to increase the relative risk for developing HPV-associated cancer and, therefore, must also be considered in the overall disease process.

ACKNOWLEDGMENT

I am grateful to Drs. H. zur Hausen and L. Gissmann for stimulating discussion, to E.-M. de Villiers for her help in compiling an up-to-date list of all human papillomaviruses, and to Dan Gallahan for critical reading of the manuscript.

REFERENCES

1. Matthews REF: Classification and nomenclature of viruses. Intervirology 1982;17:1.
2. Griffin BE: Structure and genomic organization of SV40 and polyoma virus. In: Tooze J (ed). DNA tumor viruses. Cold Spring Harbor. 1980;61.
3. Engel LW, Heilman CA, Howley PM: Transcriptional organization of bovine papillomavirus type 1. J Virol 1983;47:516.
4. Pfister H: Biology and biochemistry of papillomaviruses. Rev Physiol Biochem Pharmacol 1984;99:111.
5. Sundberg JP: Papillomavirus infections in animals. In: Syrjänen K, Gissmann L, Koss L (eds). Papillomaviruses and human disease. Springer-Verlag. 1987;40.
6. Orth G, Favre M, Breitburd F, et al: Epidermodysplasia verruciformis: a model for the role of papillomaviruses in human cancer. In: Essex M, Todaro G, zur Hausen H (eds). Viruses in naturally occuring cancers. Cold Spring Harbor. 1980;259.
7. Jablonska S, Orth G, Lutzner MA: Immunopathology of papillomavirus-induced tumors in different tissues. Springer Semin Immunopathol 1982;5:33.
8. Orth G, Breitburd F, Favre M: Evidence for antigenic determinants shared by the structural polypeptides of (Shope) rabbit papillomavirus and human papillomavirus type 1. Virology 1978;91:243.
9. Jenson AB, Rosenthal JD, Olson C, et al: Immunologic relatedness of papillomaviruses from different species. JNCI 1980;64:495.
10. Gissmann L, Schwarz E: Cloning of papillomavirus DNA. In: Becker Y (ed). Recombinant DNA research and viruses. Martinus Nijhoff; Boston: 1985;173.
11. Coggin JR Jr, zur Hausen H: Workshop on papillomaviruses and cancer. Cancer Res 1979;39:545.
12. Danos O, Katinka M, Yaniv M: Molecular cloning, refined physical map and heterogeneity and methylation sites of papilloma virus type 1a DNA. Eur J Biochem 1980;109:457.
13. Heilman CA, Law MF, Israel MA, et al: Cloning of human papilloma virus genomic DNAs and analysis of homologous polynucleotide sequences. J Virol 1980;36:395.
14. Fuchs PG, Pfister H: Cloning and characterization of papillomavirus type 2c DNA. Intervirology 1984;22:177.
15. Kremsdorf D, Jablonska S, Favre M, et al: Human papillomaviruses associated with epidermodysplasia verruciformis. II. Molecular cloning and biochemical characterization of human papillomavirus 3a, 8, 10, and 12 genomes. J Virol 1983;48:340.
16. Ostrow RS, Zachow K, Watts S, et al: Characterization of two HV-3 related papillomaviruses form common warts which are distinct clinically from flat warts or epidermodysplasia verruciformis. J Invest Dermatol 1983;80:436.
17. Oltersdorf T, Campo MS, Favre M, et al: Molecular cloning and characterization of human papillomavirus type 7 DNA. Virology 1986;149:247.

18. Kremsdorf D, Jablonska S, Favre M, et al: Biochemical characterization of two types of human papillomaviruses associated with epidermodysplasia verruciformis. J Virol 1982;43:436.

19. Pfister H, Gassenmaier A, Nürnberger F, et al: Human papilloma virus 5-DNA in a carcinoma of an epidermodysplasia verruciformis patient infected with various human papilloma virus types. Cancer Res 1983;43:1436.

20. Pfister H, Nürnberger F, Gissmann L, et al: Characterization of a human papillomavirus from epidermodysplasia verruciformis lesions of a patient from Upper-Volta. Int J Cancer 1981;27:645.

21. Kremsdorf D, Favre M, Jablonska S, et al: Molecular cloning and biochemical characterization of the genomes of nine newly recognized human papillomavirus types associated with epidermodysplasia verruciformis. J Virol 1984;52:1013.

22. Gassenmaier A, Lammel M, Pfister H: Molecular cloning and characterization of the DNAs of human papillomaviruses 19, 20, and 25 from a patient with epidermodysplasia verruciformis. J Virol 1984;52:1019.

23. Kawashima M, Favre M, Jablonska S, et al: Characterization of a new type of human papillomavirus (HPV) related to HPV 5 from a case of actinic keratosis. Virology 1986;154:389.

24. Scheurlen W, Gissmann L, Gross G, et al: Molecular cloning of two new HPV types (HPV 37 and HPV 38) from a keratoacanthoma and a malignant melanoma. Int J Cancer 1986;37:505.

25. Adachi A, Yasue H, Ohashi M, et al: A novel type of human papilloma virus DNA from the lesions of epidermodysplasia verruciformis. Jpn J Cancer Res 1986;77:978.

26. de Villiers E-M, Gissmann L, zur Hausen H: Molecular cloning of viral DNA from human genital warts. J Virol 1981;40:932.

27. Gissmann L, Diehl V, Schultz-Coulon HJ, et al: Molecular cloning and characterization of human papilloma virus DNA derived from a laryngeal papilloma. J Virol 1982;44:393.

28. Beaudenon S, Kremsdorf D, Croissant O, et al: A novel type of human papillomavirus associated with genital neoplasias. Nature 1986;321:246.

29. Lörincz AT, Quinn AP, Lancaster WD, et al: A new type of papillomavirus associated with cancer of the uterine cervix. Virology 1987;159:187.

30. Beaudenon S, Kremsdorf D, Obalek S, et al: Plurality of genital human papillomaviruses: characterization of two new types with distinct biological properties. Virology 1987;161:374.

31. Nagashfar ZS, Rosenshein NB, Lorincz AT, et al: Characterization of human papillomavirus type 45, a new type 18-related virus of the genital tract. J Gen Virol 1987;68:3073.

32. Nuovo GJ, Crum CP, de Villiers E-M, et al: Isolation of a novel human papillomavirus HPV-51 from a cervical condyloma. J Virol 1988;62:1452.

33. Dürst M, Gissmann L, Ikenberg H, et al: A papillomavirus DNA from a cervical carcinoma and its prevalence in cancer biopsy samples from different geographic regions. Proc Natl Acad Sci 1983;80:3812.

34. Boshart M, Gissmann L, Ikenberg H, et al: A new type of papillomavirus DNA and its presence in genital cancer biopsies and in cell lines derived from cervical cancer. EMBO J 1984;3:1151.

35. Kahn T, Schwarz E, Ikenberg H, et al: Molecular cloning and characterization of the DNA of a new human papillomavirus (HPV 30) from a laryngeal carcinoma. Int J Cancer 1986;37:61.

36. Lörincz AT, Lancaster WD, Temple GF: Cloning and characterization of the DNA of a new human papillomavirus from a woman with dysplasia of the uterine cervix. J Virol 1986;58:225.

37. Kawashima M, Jablonska S, Favre M, et al: Characterization of a new type of human papillomavirus found in a lesion of Bowen's disease of the skin. J Virol 1986;57:688.
38. Pfister H, Hettich I, Runne U, et al: Characterization of human papillomavirus type 13 from focal epithelial hyperplasia Heck lesions. J Virol 1983;47:363.
39. Beaudenon S, Praetorius F, Kremsdorf F, et al: A new type of oral focal epithelias hyperplasia. J Invest Dermatol 1987;88:130.
40. Ostrow R, Zachow KR, Thompson O, et al: Molecular cloning and characterization of a unique type of human papillomavirus from an immune deficient patient. J Invest Dermatol 1984;82:362.
41. Ostrow RS, Zachow KR, Shaver MK, Faras AJ. Human papillomavirus type 27: detection of a novel human papillomavirus in common warts of a renal transplant recipient. J Virol 1989;63(in press).
42. Grimmel M, de Villiers E-M, Neumann Ch, et al: Characterization of a new human papillomavirus (HPV 41) from disseminated warts and detection of its DNA in some skin carcinomas. Int J Cancer 1988;41:5.
43. Gross G, Ellinger K, Roussaki A, et al: Epidermodysplasia verruciformis in a patient with Hodgkin's disease: Characterization of a new papillomavirus type and interferon treatment. J Invest Dermatol 1988;91:43.
44. Schneider-Gädicke A, Schwarz E: Different human cervical carcinoma cell lines show similar transcription patterns of human papillomavirus type 18 early genes. EMBO J 1986;5:2285.
45. Smotkin D, Wettstein FO: Transcription of human papillomavirus type 16 early genes in a cervical cancer and a cancer-derived cell line and identification of the E7 protein. Proc Natl Acad Sci 1986;83:4680.
46. Chow LT, Nasseri M, Wolinsky SM, et al: Human papillomavirus types 6 and 11 mRNAs from genital condylomata acuminata. J Virol 1987;61:2581.
47. Schneider-Gädicke A, Kaul S, Schwarz E, et al: Identification of the human papillomavirus type 18 E6* and E6 protein in nuclear fractions from human cervical carcinoma cells grown in the nude mouse or in vitro. Cancer Res 1988;48:2969.
48. Cole ST, Streeck RE: Genome organization and nucleotide sequence of human papillomavirus type 33, which is associated with cervical cancer. J Virol 1986;58:991.
49. Sen R, Baltimore D: Multiple nuclear factors interact with the immunoglobulin enhancer sequences. Cell 1986;46:705.
50. Schirm S, Jiricny J, Schaffner W: The SV40 enhancer can be dissected into multiple segments, each with a different cell type specificity. Genes Dev 1987;1:65.
51. Spalholz BA, Yang YC, Howley PM: Transactivation of a bovine papillomavirus transcriptional regulatory element by the E2 gene product. Cell 1985;42:183.
52. Hirochika H, Broker TR, Chow LT: Enhancers and trans-acting E2 transcriptional factor of papillomaviruses. J Virol 1987;61:2599.
53. Cripe TP, Haugen TH, Turk JP, et al: Transcriptional regulation of the human papillomavirus 16 E6-E7 promoter by a keratinocyte-dependent enhancer, and by viral E2 trans-activator and repressor gene products: implications for cervical carcinogenesis. EMBO J 1987;6:3745.
54. Boshart M, zur Hausen H: Human papillomaviruses (HPV) in Buschke-Löwenstein tumors: Physical state of the DNA and identification of a tandem duplication in the non-coding region of a HPV 6 subtype. J Virol 1986;58:963.
55. Rando RF, Sedlacek TV, Hunt J, et al: Verrucous carcinoma of the vulva associated with an unusual type 6 papillomavirus. Obstet Gynecol 1986;67i:70.
56. Rous P, Beard JW: The progression to carcinoma of virus-induced rabbit papilloma (Shope). J Exp Med 1935;62:523.
57. Rous P, Friedewald WF: The effect of chemical carcinogens on virus-induced rabbit carcinomas. J Exp Med 1944;79:511.

58. Jarrett WFH, McNeil PE, Grimshaw WTR, et al: High incidence area of cattle cancer with a possible interaction between an environmental carcinogen and a papillomavirus. Nature 1978;274:215.

59. Rotkin ID: A comparison review of key epidemiological studies in cervical cancer related to current searches for transmissible agents. Cancer Res 1973;33:1353.

60. Kessler II: Human cervical cancer as a veneral disease. Cancer Res 1976;36:783.

61. Koss LG: Pathogenesis of carcinoma of the uterine cervix. In: Dallenbach-Hellweg G (ed). Cervical cancer. Springer-Verlag. 1981.

62. de Villiers E-M, Wagner D, Schneider A, et al: Human papillomavirus infections with and without abnormal cervical cytology. Lancet 1987;ii:703.

63. Schneider A, Hotz M, Gissmann L: Increased prevalence of human papillomaviruses in the lower genital tract of pregnant women. Int J Cancer 1987;40:198.

64. Richart RM: The natural history of cervical intraepithelial neoplasia. Clin Obstet Gynecol 1967;10:784.

65. Meisels A, Fortin R: Condylomatous lesions of the cervix and vagina. Cytologic patterns. Acta Cytol 1976;20:505.

66. Purola E, Savia E: Cytology of gynecologic condyloma acuminatum. Acta Cytol 1977;21:26.

67. Laverty CR, Russel P, Hills E, et al: The significance of noncondyloma wart virus infection of the cervical transformation zone. A review with discussion of two illustrative cases. Acta Cytol 1978;22:195.

68. Kreider J, Howett M, Wolfe SA, et al: Morphological transformation in vivo of human uterine cervix with papillomavirus from condylomata acuminata. Nature 1985;317:639.

69. Koss LG: Carcinogenesis in the uterine cervix and human papillomavirus infection. In: Syrjänen K, Gissmann L, Koss LG (eds). Papillomaviruses and human disease. Springer-Verlag. 1987;235.

70. Campion MJ, McCance DJ, Cuzick J, et al: Progressive potential of mild cervical atypia: Prospective cytological, colposcopic, and virological study. Lancet 1986;i:237.

71. Dürst M, Kleinheinz A, Hotz M, et al: The physical state of human papillomavirus type 16 DNA in benign and malignant genital tumours. J Gen Virol 1985;66:1515.

72. Schwarz E, Freese UK, Gissmann L, et al: Structure and transcription of human papillomavirus sequences in cervical carcinoma cells. Nature 1985;314:111.

73. El Awady MK, Kaplan JB, O'Brien SJ, et al: Molecular analysis of integrated human papillomavirus 16 sequences in the cervical cancer cell line SiHa. Virology 1987;159:389.

74. Schneider-Maunoury S, Croissant O, Orth G: Integration of human papillomavirus type 16 DNA sequences: a possible early event in the progression of genital tumors. J Virology 1987;61:3295.

75. Baker CC, Phelps WC, Lindgren V, et al: Structural and transcriptional analysis of human papillomavirus type 16 sequences in cervical carcinoma cell lines. J Virol 1987;61:962.

76. Seedorf K, Oltersdorf T, Krämmer G, et al: Identification of early proteins of the human papilloma viruses type 16 (HPV16) and type 18 (HPV18) in cervical carcinoma cells. EMBO J 1987;6:139.

77. Androphy EJ, Hubbert NL, Schiller JT, et al: Identification of the HPV 16 E6 protein from transformed mouse cells and human carcinoma cell lines. EMBO J 1987;6:989.

78. Banks L, Spence P, Androphy E, et al: Identification of human papillomavirus type 18 E6 polypeptide in cells derived from human cervical carcinoma. J Gen Virol 1987;68:1351.

79. von Knebel-Doeberitz M, Oltersdorf T, Schwarz E, et al: Correlation of modified human papillomavirus early gene expression with altered growth properties in C4-I cervical carcinoma cells. Cancer Res 1988;48:3780.

80. Rösl F, Dürst M, zur Hausen H: Selective suppression of human papillomavirus transcription in non-tumourigenic cells by 5-azacytidine. EMBO J 1988;7:132.

81. Dörfler W: DNA methylation and its functional significance: studies on the adenovirus system. Curr Top Microbiol Immunol 1984;108:79.

82. Yasumoto S, Burkhardt A, Doninger J, et al: Human papillomavirus type 16 DNA-induced malignant transformation of NIH 3T3 cells. J Virol 1986;57:572.

83. Tsunokawa Y, Takebe N, Kasamatsu T, et al: Transforming activity of human papillomavirus type 16 DNA sequences in a cervical cancer. Proc Natl Acad Sci 1986;83:2200.

84. Matlashewski G, Osborn K, Murray A, et al: Transformation of mouse fibroblasts with human papillomavirus type 16 DNA using a heterologous promotor. In: Steinberg BM, Brandsma JL, Taichman LB (eds). Cancer cells 5: Papillomaviruses. Cold Spring Harbor. 1987;195.

85. Kanda T, Furuno A, Yoshiike K: Human papillomavirus type 16 open reading frame E7 encodes a transforming gene for rat 3Y1 cells. J Virol 1988;62:610.

86. Bedell MA, Jones KH, Laimins LA: The E6-E7 region of human papillomavirus type 18 is sufficient for transformation of NIH 3T3 and rat cells. J Virol 1987;61:3635.

87. Watanabe S, Yoshiike K: Transformation of rat 3Y1 cells by human papillomavirus type 18 DNA. Int J Cancer, 1988;44:896.

88. Matlashewski G, Schneider J, Banks L, et al: Human papillomavirus type 16 cooperates with activated ras in transforming primary cells. EMBO J 1987;6:1741.

89. Pirisi L, Yasumoto S, Feller M, et al: Transformation of human fibroblasts and keratinocytes with human papillomavirus type 16 DNA. J Virol 1987;61:1061.

90. Dürst M, Dzarlieva-Petrusevska RT, Boukamp P, et al: Molecular and cytogenetic analysis of immortalized human primary keratinocytes obtained after transfection with human papillomavirus type 16 DNA. Oncogene 1987;1:251.

91. Schlegel R, Phelps WC, Zhang Y-L, et al: Quantitative keratinocyte assay detects two biological activities of human papillomavirus DNA and identifies viral types associated with carcinoma. EMBO J 1988;7:3181.

92. Hoffmann D, Hecht SS, Haley NJ, et al: Tumorigenic agents in tobacco products and their uptake by chewers, smokers and nonsmokers. J Cell Biochem 1985;(suppl)9C;33.

93. Sarasin A: SOS response in mammalian cells. Cancer Invest 1985;3:163.

94. Stanbridge EJ: Suppression of malignancy in human cells. Nature 1976;260:17.

95. Schwarz E, Schneider-Gädicke A, zur Hausen H: Human papillomavirus type 18 transcription in cervical carcinoma cell lines and in human cell hybrids. In: Cancer cells: Papillomaviruses. Cold Spring Harbor. 1987;47.

96. Stanbridge EJ, Der CD, Doersen CJ, et al: Human cell hybrids: analysis of transformation and tumorigenicity. Science 1982;215:252.

97. zur Hausen H: The role of viruses in human tumors. Adv Cancer Res 1980;33:77.

98. zur Hausen H: Intracellular surveillance of persisting viral infections: Human genital cancer results from deficient cellular control of papillomavirus gene expression. Lancet 1986;ii:489.

99. Riou GF, Barrois M, Dutronquay V, et al: Presence of papillomavirus sequences, amplification of c-myc and c-Ha-ras oncogenes and enhanced expression of c-myc in carcinomas of the uterine cervix. In: Howley PM, Broker TR (eds). Papillomaviruses: Molecular and clinical aspects. New York; Alan R Liss. 1985;47.

100. Dürst M, Croce CM, Gissmann L, et al: Papillomavirus sequences integrate near cellular oncogenes in some cervical carcinomas. Proc Natl Acad Sci 1987;84:1070.

101. Mincheva A, Gissmann L, zur Hausen H: Chromosomal integration sites of human papillomavirus DNA in three cervical cancer cell lines mapped by in situ hybridization. Med Microbiol Immunol (Berl) 1987;176:245.

Clinical Spectrum of Genital HPV Infection in the Female. I. Cervix and Vagina

Michel Roy, MD, FRCS

It is well accepted today that human papilloma virus (HPV) is the agent responsible for condyloma acuminata[1] as well as intraepithelial lesions referred to as sub-clinical papilloma, flat condyloma, intraepithelial neoplasia, and even invasive cancers[2].

Different types of HPV seem to be responsible for different lesions, ie, HPV-6 and 11, for benign condyloma and HPV-16, 18, 33, and others recently described, for premalignant and malignant lesions.[2] Because we know the type of HPV only after a clinical evaluation and sampling (by scraping or biopsy), it is important to review the clinical spectrum of HPV infection from benign condyloma acuminatum to invasive cancer.

Some authors[3,4] have discussed the clinical appearance of HPV lesions, mostly their colposcopic features. They used a different terminology, so comparing results is nearly impossible, and discussing the accuracy of clinical diagnosis is very difficult. In this article, we will use the nomenclature proposed at the tenth meeting of the International Society for the Study of Vulvar Disease in Australia in 1987 (Table 4–1). This terminology is close to the one used in the original article on colposcopic description of HPV lesions by Meisels et al.[5] This does not introduce a new colposcopic nomenclature. We still use the one accepted by the ISCCP: white epithelium, punctation, mosaic, irregular vessels, adding only few terms like *spikes, asperities,* and *micropapillae.*

CLINICAL LESIONS

The Cervix

Condyloma Acuminatum

Condyloma acuminatum is the least frequent HPV lesion observed on the cervix.[6] Most of the time it is seen with the naked eye and appears as a

Clinical Practice of Gynecology: **2,** 42–58, 1989
© 1989 Elsevier Science Publishing Co., Inc.
655 Avenue of the Americas, New York, NY 10010

TABLE 4–1. HPV Nomenclature

Clinical
    Papillary
        Condyloma acuminatum
        Diffuse papillomatosis*
    Papular*

Subclinical
    Flat
    Spiked
    Diffuse micropapillomatosis

*Mostly vulvar lesions.

raised pink or grayish localized growth (Figure 4–1). When keratinized, they appear as "leucoplakia" (Figure 4–2).

Careful examination of the ectocervix and the vagina will usually demonstrate multiple identical lesions. It will rarely be alone in the transformation zone (TZ). Sometimes it covers it entirely. Then a directed biopsy should be done in order to rule out a papillary invasive cancer of the cervix. On the cervix, we should never treat a raised papillary lesion without a histopathologic evaluation. Excisional biopsy is probably the best treatment for a small condyloma acuminatum of the cervix. It has the advantage of being simple and giving an accurate histopathologic diagnosis.

Invasive Cancer

Except for its early invasive forms or its endocervical localization, cancer of the cervix is seen with the naked eye. It shows different pictures: necrosis, ulceration, or papillary growth (Figure 4–3). This last form is most important, because it happens in younger patients and can look like condyloma acuminatum. Furthermore, the symptomatology can be identical: postcoital bleeding and discharge.

Early invasive cancers will usually need colposcopy to be recognized.

Hyperkeratosis

Lesions with keratinization look white before the application of acetic acid (Figure 4–2). They used to be called leucoplakia, but today we prefer to refer to this entity as hyperkeratosis. They are induced by HPV in most cases, except when a cervical prolapse is present. Here again, a biopsy is indicated because intraepithelial neoplasia or invasive cancer can be keratinized and appears as leucoplakia.

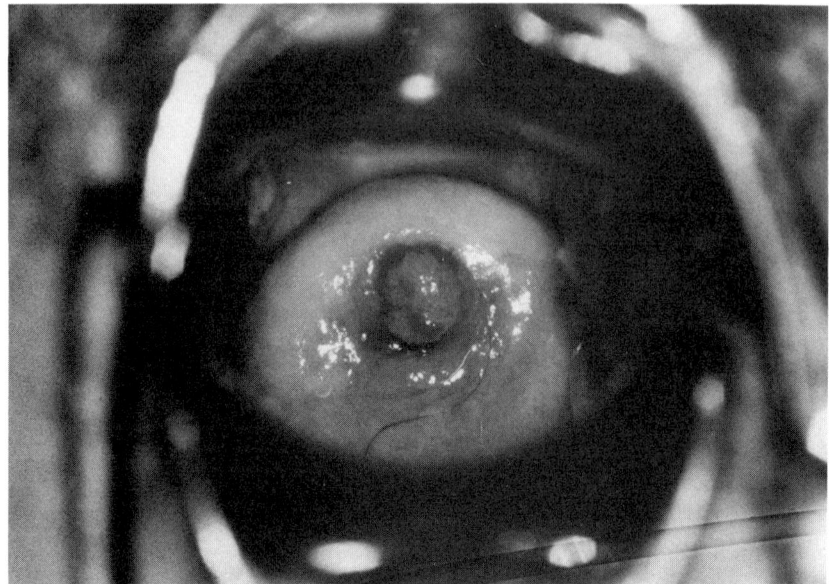

FIGURE 4–1 A condyloma acuminatum seen as a raised lesion of the anterior lip of the cervix.

FIGURE 4–2 The whole cervix is covered by a keratinized condyloma.

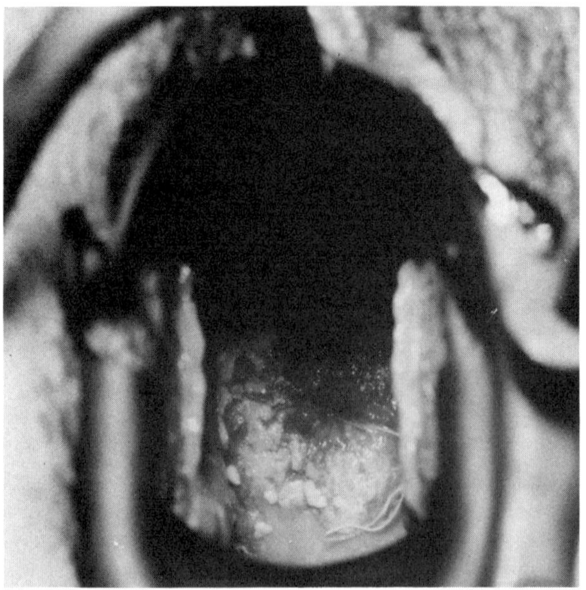

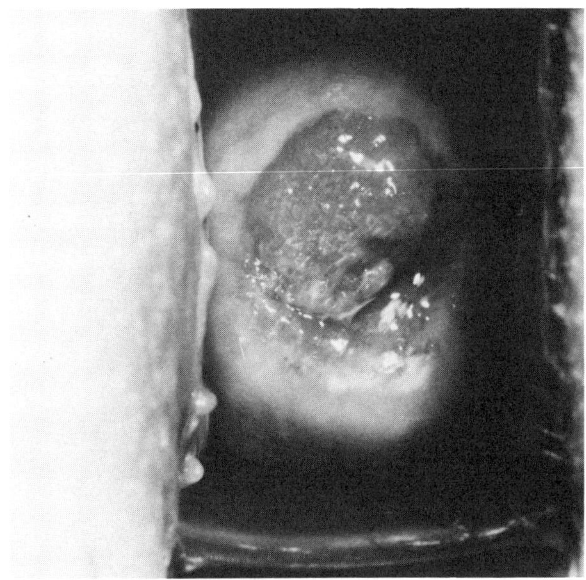

FIGURE 4–3 A papillary lesion seen on the cervix of a 30-year-old patient. Biopsy showed invasive cancer.

FIGURE 4–4 Multiple condyloma acuminata seen on the vaginal wall. Note that the cervix is covered by a keratotic condyloma.

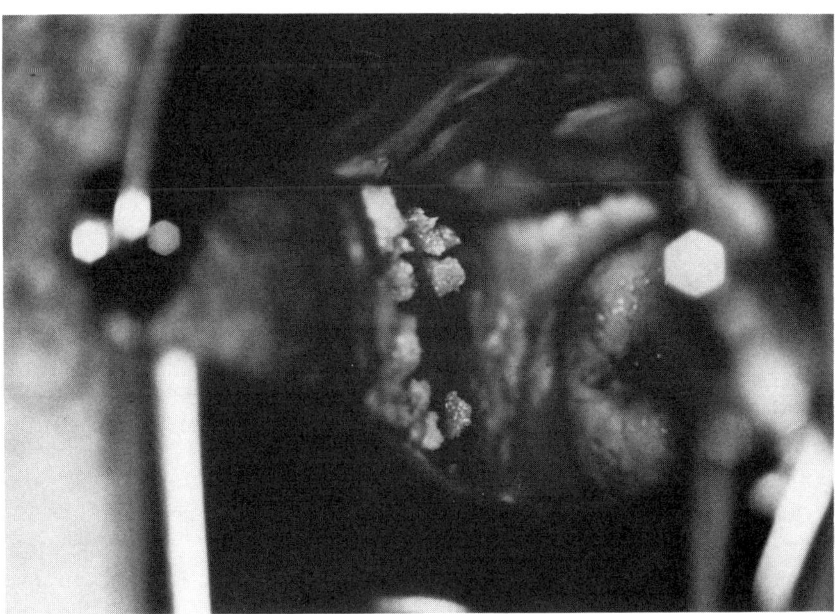

The Vagina

Condyloma acuminata of the vagina are usually multiple (Figure 4–4), and they are pretty typical: exophytic and papillary. Invasive cancer of the vagina is rare, but when a single papillary lesion is seen and bleeds easily, a biopsy should be done.

A rare form of invasive cancer of the vagina needs special attention. It almost covers the entire vaginal surface and is papillary (Figure 4–5). But, being very superficial, the invasion can be seen only with difficulty on a histopathologic specimen. Colposcopy is then very helpful in directing the biopsies to abnormal vessels areas.

SUBCLINICAL LESIONS

The Cervix

Small Condyloma Acuminata

Even if condyloma acuminatum is a clinical lesion, it is sometimes so small that it can be detected only with the help of a colposcope. It can be confused with an eversion of the cervix, or a cervical polyp.

With the colposcope, a condyloma acuminatum appears as a raised, irregular, acetowhite lesion, with fingerlike projections. Small vessels are visible when there is no keratinization (Figure 4–6). Columnar epithelium of an ectropion or of a cervical polyp does not become white after the application of acetic acid, and they are regular in size and shape. They rarely show long fingerlike projections (Figure 4–7), but rather a typical grapelike structure. Adenocarcinoma needs to be ruled out when columnar tissue is papillary.

Spiked Condyloma

When the surface of an acetowhite lesion is irregular and covered by budding fingerlike projections, spikes, or asperities (Figure 4–8), it is called a spiked condyloma.[5] The spike represents an elongation of the stroma toward the surface and is centered by a vessel (Figure 4–9). It can be in the transformation zone or on the ectocervix and is typical of a HPV infection. It is the most frequent form of HPV-induced lesion on the cervix, but it can show severe atypia on histology. Therefore, a directed biopsy should be done to determine the severity of the lesion. Sometimes the spikes are less formed; the surface then shows micropapillae without capillary, or only granulations (Figure 4–10).

One type of a spiked lesion needs special consideration, because it is quite typical of a high-grade intraepithelial neoplasia. The asperities are

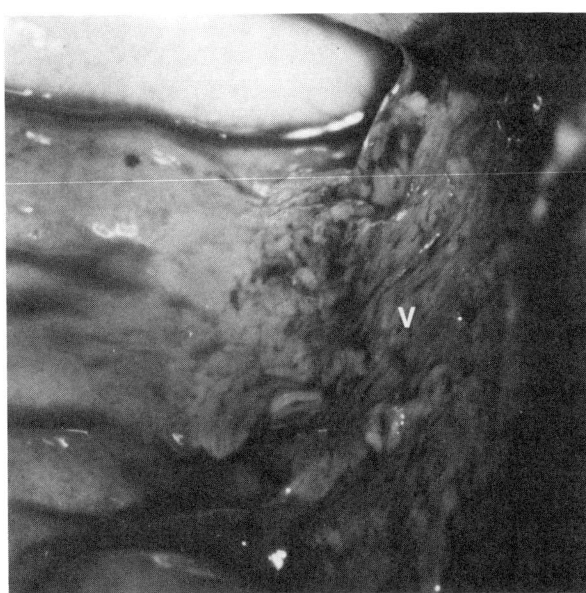

FIGURE 4–5 A colpophotograph showing an irregular surface, superficial vessels (V) covering the entire vaginal wall. Multiple biopsies were necessary to confirm invasion of the stroma. (×13)

FIGURE 4–6 A colpophotograph of a small condyloma acuminatum of the cervix. Note the fingerlike projections. (×13)

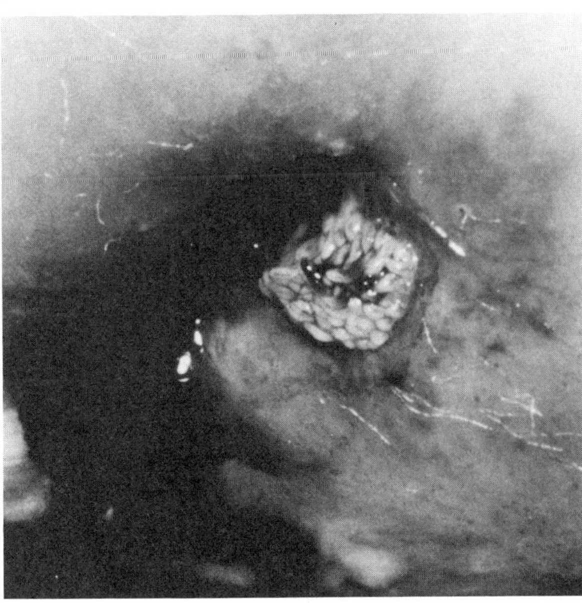

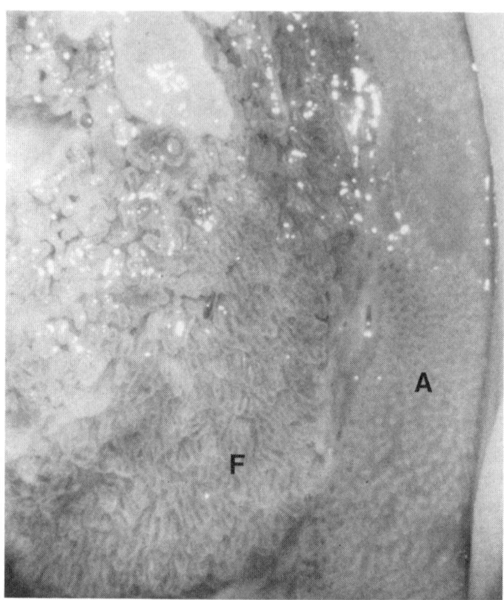

FIGURE 4–7 Columnar epithelium seen as regular fingerlike projections (F). Note the diffuse asperities (A) of the ectocervix. (×13)

FIGURE 4–8 The anterior lip of the cervix is covered with small asperities centered by a vessel. (×13)

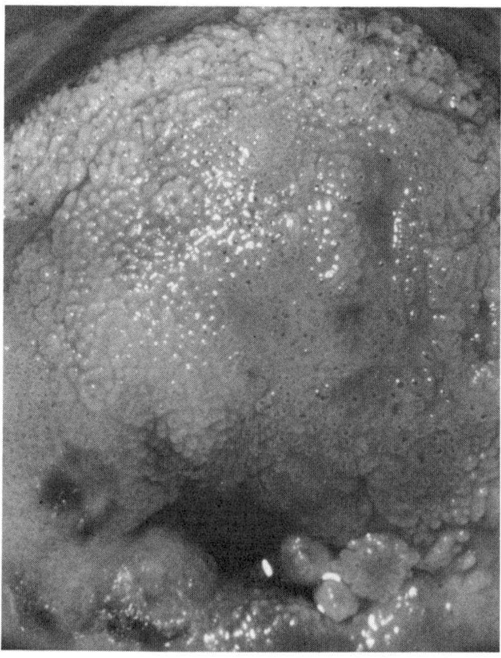

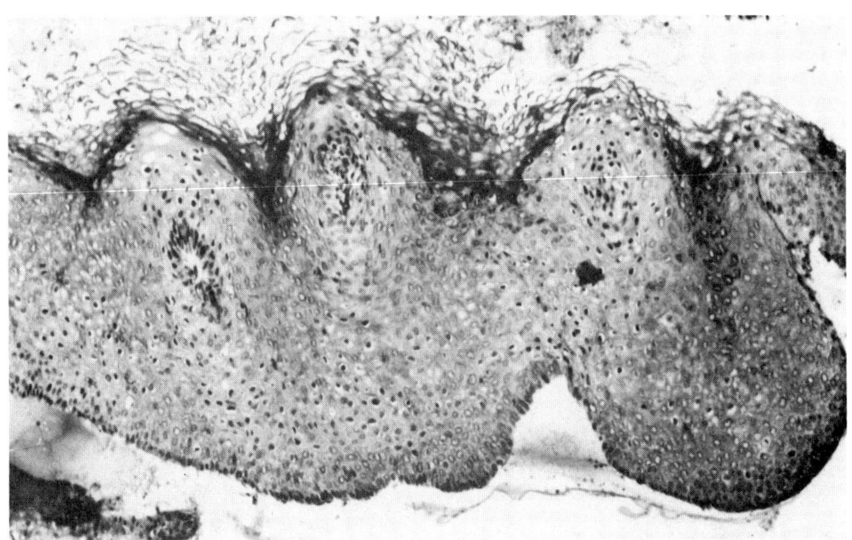

FIGURE 4–9 Histopathology of a "spiked condyloma" (by permission, Roy M, et al, Clin Obstet Gynecol 1983;26:4, 957).

FIGURE 4–10 The surface shows only spikes without vessels. ($\times$ 13)

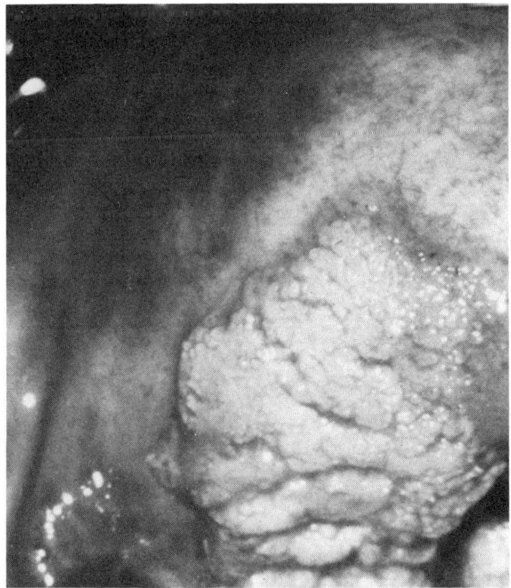

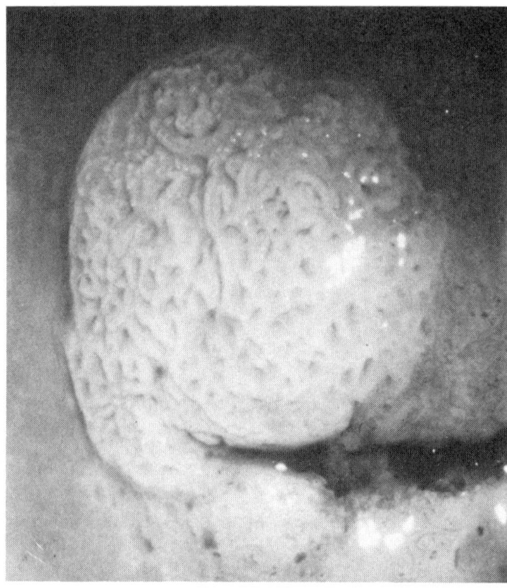

FIGURE 4–11 The anterior lip shows a sulcus-brain pattern of acetowhite lesion, spikes arranged in circonvolutions. ($\times$13)

FIGURE 4–12 Histopathology of Figure 4–11, showing CIN with some koilocytes near the surface (courtesy of Dr. Bernard Têtu, Hôtel-Dieu de Québec).

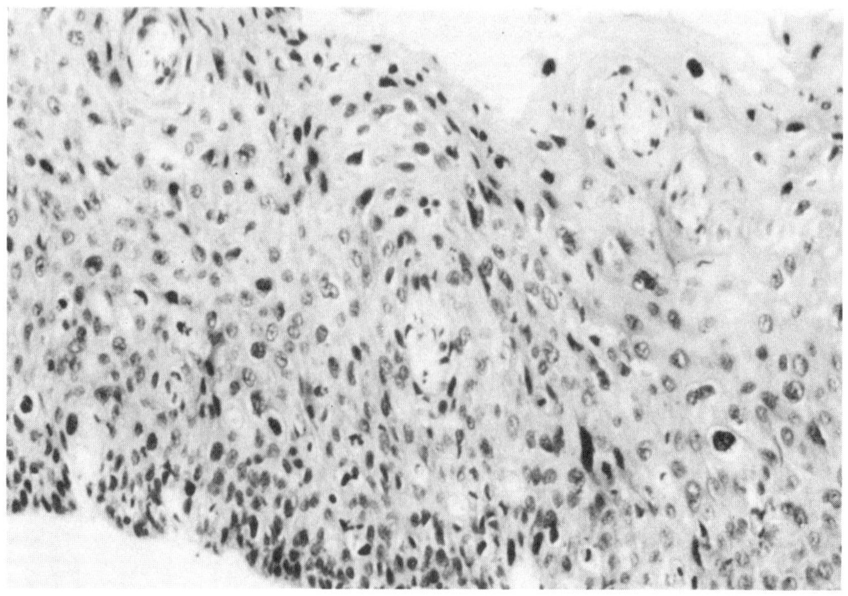

arranged in a sulcus-brain pattern (Figure 4–11), called "circonvolutions" by Morin[7] or "micro-convolutions" by Coppleson.[8] The lesion shows a thick, white epithelium covered many times with hyperkeratosis. On histopathology, there is koilocytosis, typical of HPV in the superficial layers of the epithelium, and lack of differentiation and atypia, typical of intraepithelial neoplasia, in the lower half (Figure 4–12). Coppleson,[8] on the other hand, refers to that pattern as typical of benign condyloma, and Reid[9] in his index records micropapilloferous surface changes as nonsignificant, without special reference to the sulcus-brain pattern. Our experience tends to support Morin's opinion that in most of the cases, it is a *high-grade intraepithelial neoplasia*. Furthermore, Bouchard[10] suggests that the failure rate of cryotherapy or laser vaporization of sulcus-brain pattern HPV lesions is significantly higher than benign HPV or intraepithelial neoplasia.

Differential diagnosis of spiked condyloma has to be made not only with benign HPV and intraepithelial neoplasia, but also with superficial invasive cancer, whose surface can show the same micropapillae (Figure 4–13). Usually, though, they are not as regular in shape and form as benign spiked condyloma (see Figure 4–8).

Flat Condyloma

Here we define *flat condyloma* as an acetowhite lesion whose surface has no irregularity (Figure 4–14). We think it is important to differentiate the flat ones from the others, because most of the severe intraepithelial neoplasia are found in the "flat" group. On the other hand, metaplasia appears as a flat white lesion, whose borders are feathery, compared with HPV lesion, which shows a raised flat surface with sharp borders, more like CIN.

Other Signs

When hyperkeratosis is present, HPV is likely, but intraepithelial neoplasia (CIN) can be found also. Diffuse micropapillae or asperities can be seen on the ectocervix, but will be discussed in the vaginal lesions.

CIN

As stated above, CIN is a histopathologic diagnosis and cannot be differentiated from benign HPV lesions by colposcopy. In fact, on the cervix we can find a high-grade intraepithelial neoplasia in flat surfaces as well as granular or spiked lesions as demonstrated by Follen et al.[11] CIN appears whiter, denser, and thicker (Figure 4–15) than do low-grade HPV lesions. Its borders are usually sharper, its mosaic and punctation coarser, but only biopsies can give an accurate diagnosis.

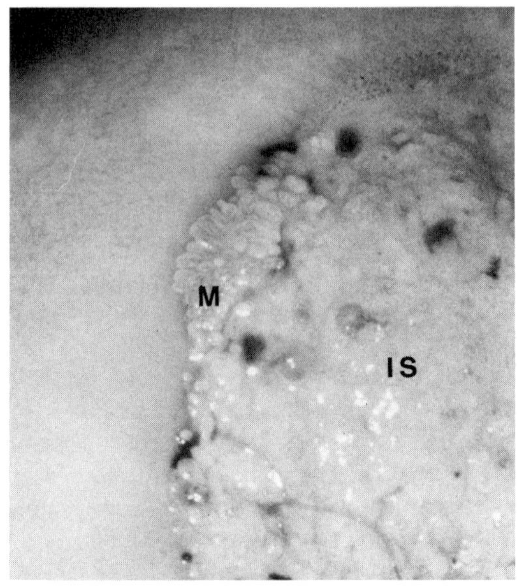

FIGURE 4-13 The transformation zone is covered by an irregular surface (IS). Note the micropapillae (M) at 10 o'clock. ($\times$13)

FIGURE 4-14 A colpophotograph showing a flat acetowhite lesion of low grade appearance on the posterior lip. Biopsy showed a benign HPV. ($\times$13)

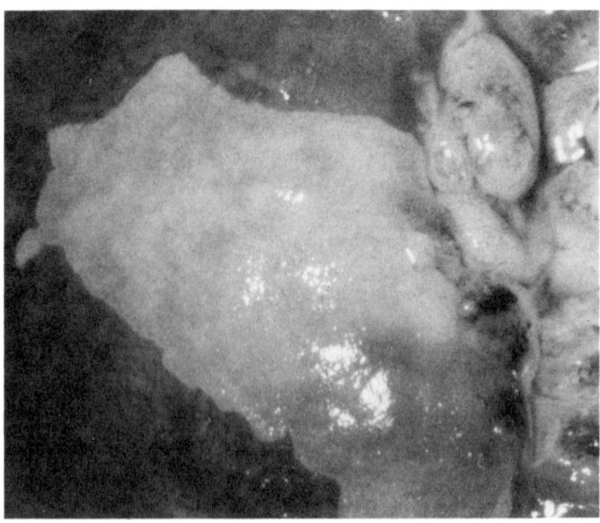

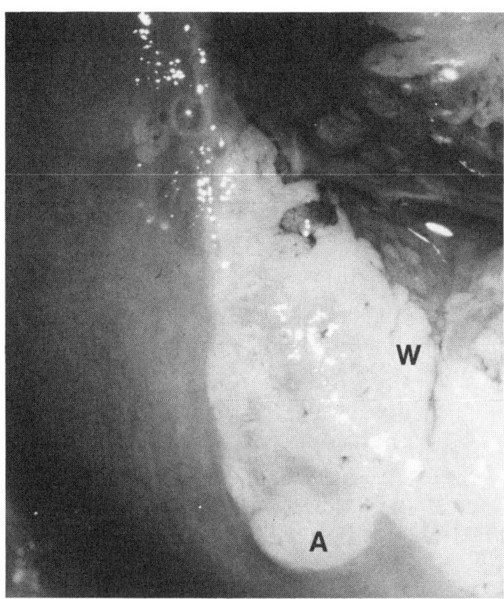

FIGURE 4–15 A localized dense acetowhite lesion (W) with sharp borders is seen on the posterior lip, at the SC junction. Note asperities (A) at the original junction. A high-grade CIN was diagnosed on biopsy. (× 13)

FIGURE 4–16 A flat acetowhite (W) lesion on the lateral wall of the vagina. Note two different lesions with asperities (A). VAIN was diagnosed on the biopsy of the flat lesion. (× 13)

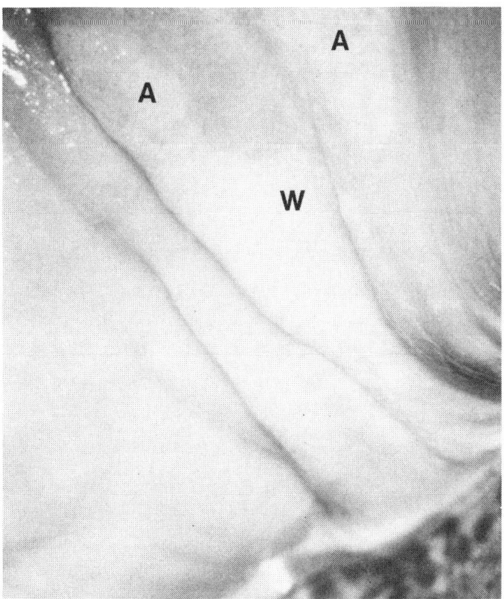

The Vagina

The lesions described for the cervix are the same affecting the vagina.

The prediction by colposcopic examination is somewhat easier. Totally flat acetowhite lesions (Figure 4–16) are usually a vaginal intraepithelial neoplasia (VAIN). Rarely will benign HPV appear as a perfectly flat lesion. They are rather granular and show surface asperities in the forms of a spiked condyloma (Figure 4–17). But, as on the cervix, spiked condyloma can harbor severe atypia and then is considered as VAIN. Therefore, directed biopsies are mandatory.

Diffuse micropapillomatosis, also referred to as condylomatous vaginitis, or reverse colpitis, shows on colposcopy a surface with very small asperities or spikes called micropapillae (Figure 4–18). There is no acetowhite background. The micropapillae can be localized in defined areas or cover the whole vagina and the cervix. Sometimes it is the only abnormal finding with the colposcope after an abnormal Pap smear.[12] Other times, it coexists with other HPV lesions, intraepithelial neoplasia, or invasive cancer.

SYMPTOMATOLOGY

Most of HPV lesions are asymptomatic. Condyloma acuminata can produce an abnormal discharge or contact bleeding, but subclinical lesions do not, except the diffuse micropapillomatosis. Then the patient can complain of dryness or roughness of the vagina. In fact, even the naked-eye examination can show a "sand paper" appearance of condylomatous vaginitis (Figure 4–19).

THE ROLE OF COLPOSCOPY

Colposcopic examination is mandatory in the evaluation of a patient with an abnormal Pap smear. Most of the time, when condyloma is detected with cervico-vaginal cytology, colposcopically directed biopsies confirm the diagnosis of benign HPV in around 70% of cases, but in 20% a high-grade CIN is found (Table 4–2). Therefore, the finding of HPV on a cervico-vaginal smear is a clear indication for colposcopy.

But authors do not agree with the value of colposcopic patterns to accurately diagnose condyloma. Directed biopsies have to be made. According to Reid,[9] a colposcopist can be 97% confident, if his proposed index is used. We think that many of the criteria evaluated in the index are very subjective and hard to transfer from one another. Barrasso[13] and Kirkup[14] showed very well that prediction of the severity of the lesion could not be done accurately by colposcopy: benign HPV and CIN appearing in the same form independently.

The situation has been well summarized by Walker,[15] who suggests

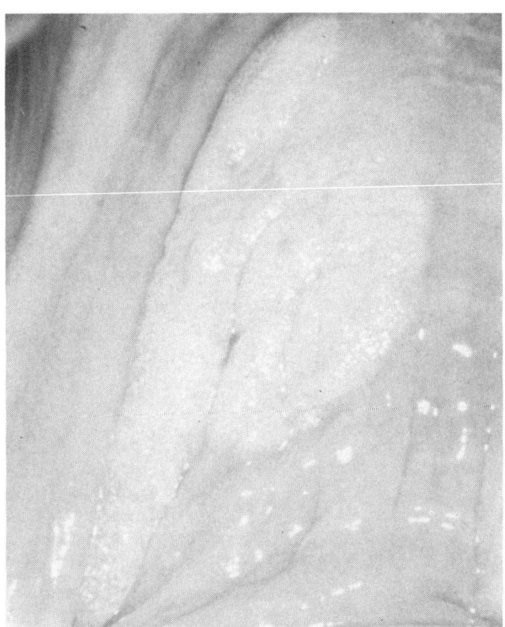

FIGURE 4–17 A colpophotograph of a raised acetowhite lesion of the vagina with spikes on the surface. (×13)

FIGURE 4–18 The vaginal mucosa is covered by micropapillae. (×13)

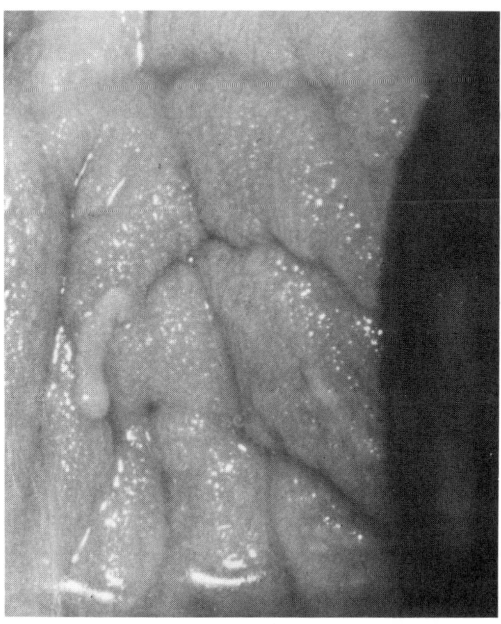

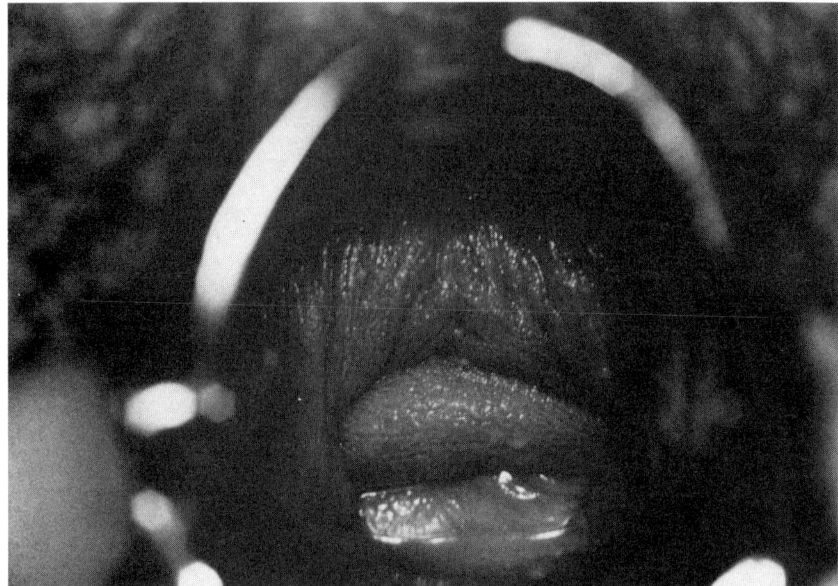

FIGURE 4–19 Naked eye appearance of Figure 4–18. The vaginal mucosa appears dry and granular (by permission, Roy M, et al, Clin Obstet Gynecol 1981:4:470.

that certain patterns are definitely associated with HPV infection (papillary surface), but the presence of severe atypia in the tissue does not necessarily give a typical colposcopic pattern. Conversely, those lesions can have only koilocytosis on histopathology. Directed biopsies are mandatory.

In North America and Australia, colposcopy has been used selectively for the evaluation of the abnormal Pap smear, while in Europe, it was used extensively as a screening procedure. While cytology has become the screening method, colposcopy was more selective. But with the more widely used hybridization techniques (Vira Pap), colposcopy might have more indications than the abnormal Pap smear and become a screening

TABLE 4–2. HPV–CIN

Histologic Diagnosis	No. of Patients*	%
Benign HPV	145	69.0
HPV + CIN	13 ⎫	6.2 ⎫
CIN II-III	27 ⎬ 40	12.9 ⎬ 19.1
No lesion seen	25	11.9
Total	210	100

*Referred to colposcopy clinic for HPV alone on Pap smear. HPV, human papilloma virus; CIN, intraepithelial neoplasia.

procedure in HPV. In fact, Schneider[16] showed that in a retrospective study of HPV-DNA hybridization group, 70% would have been detected by colposcopy, while cytology would have detected only 20%.

With the more widely used Vira Pap, which shows an incidence of HPV carriers in 12% of asymptomatic women,[17] against 2–4% by Pap smear,[4,18] colposcopic evaluation will become very useful, not only in research, but in clinical work as well. The management of HPV carriers is not established yet, but the colposcopic findings of HPV lesions will help in discussing the indications of appropriate therapy with patients.

This is why a meaningful nomenclature should be accepted by everyone involved in that field. Comparing one's results is possible only if wording is the same.

REFERENCES

1. Almeida JD, Oriel JD, Stannard LM: Characterization of the virus found in human genital warts. Microbios 1969;3:225–232.
2. Dürst M, Gissman L, Ikenberg H, et al: A papilloma virus DNA from a cervical carcinoma and its prevalence in cancer biopsy samples from different geographic regions. Proc Natl Acad Sci USA 1983;80:3812–3815.
3. Roy M, Fortier M, Meisels A: Colposcopy of cervical condyloma acuminatum. Obstet Gynecol Survey 1979;34:11,853.
4. Reid R, Laverty CR, Coppleson M, et al: Non condylomatous cervical wart virus infection. Obstet Gynecol 1980;55:476.
5. Meisels A, Fortin R, Roy M: Condylomatous lesions of the cervix. II. Cytologic, colposcopic and histopathologic study. Acta Cytol 1977;21:279.
6. Roy M, Morin C, Casas-Cordero C, Meisels A: Human papilloma virus and cervical lesions. Clin Obstet Gynecol 1983;26:949.
7. Morin C, Bouchard C, Fortier M, et al: A colposcopic lesion of the uterine cervix frequently associated with papilloma virus type 16 as detected by in situ and southern blot hybridization: A cytohistological correlation study. Int J Cancer: 1988;41:531–536.
8. Coppleson M: Colposcopic features of papillomaviral infection and premalignancy in the female lower genital tract. Obstet Gynecol Cl North Am· 1987;14:471–494.
9. Reid R, Scalzi P: Genital warts and cervical cancer VII. An improved colposcopic index for differentiating benign papillomaviral infections from high-grade cervical intraepithelial neoplasia. Am J Obstet Gynecol 1985;153:611–618.
10. Bouchard C: personal communication.
11. Follen MM, Levine RU, Carillo E, et al: Colposcopic correlates of cervical papillomavirus infection. Am J Obstet Gynecol 1987;157:809.
12. Roy M, Meisels A, Fortier M, et al: Vaginal condylomata: a human papillomavirus infection. Clin Obstet Gynecol 1981;24:461–483.
13. Barrasso R, Coupez F, Ionesco M, et al: Human papilloma viruses and cervical intraepithelial neoplasia: the role of colposcopy. Gynecol Oncol 1987;27:197–207.
14. Kirkup W, Evans AS, Brough AK, et al: Cervical intraepithelial neoplasia and "warty" atypia. A study of colposcopic, histological and cytological characteristics. Br J Obstet Gynecol 1982;89:571–577.
15. Walker PG, Singer A, Dyson JL, et al: Colposcopy in the diagnosis of papillomavirus infection of the uterine cervix. Br J Obstet Gynecol 1983;90:1082–1086.
16. Schneider A, Sterzink K, Buck G, DeVilliers EM: Colposcopy is superior to cytology for

the detection of early genital human papillomavirus infection. Obstet Gynecol 1988;71:236–241.

17. Schneider A, Kraus H, Schuhmann R, et al: Papillomavirus infection of the lower genital tract: Detection of viral DNA in gynecological swabs. Int J Cancer 1985;35:443.

18. Meisels A, Fortin R: Condylomatous lesions of the cervix and vagina. I. Cytologic patterns. Acta Cytol 1976;20:505.

Clinical Spectrum of Genital HPV Infection in the Female. II. Vulva, Perineum, and Anus

Christine Bergeron, MD, PhD and Alex Ferenczy, MD

INTRODUCTION

The external anogenital skin is the seat of approximately one-third of all clinically visible human papillomavirus (HPV) infections in the female.[1] The most frequent sites of involvement are those that are susceptible to microtrauma during intercourse, ie, the introitus and perianal and intraanal mucus membranes. These alterations are consistent with experimental observations suggesting that the cells that are infected first by HPV are those of the basal layer.[2] In recent years, the prevalence of anogenital HPV infections have increased dramatically in "sexually liberated" societies worldwide; in the United States in 1982 alone, there were 2,000,000 clinically visible genital warts reported in men and women.[3] External anogenital HPV infections may be contracted also by means other than sexual intercourse, presumably by autoinoculation of common skin warts[4] and during delivery.[5] Human papillomavirus infections in the form of condylomata acuminata may be produced by transfection experiments in the nude mice,[6] and fomites such as surgical gloves, biopsy forceps, cryoprobe tips,[7] and undergarments[8] contain HPV DNA. However, the major means of viral transmission is suspected to occur during sexual events.[9] The clinical significance of undetected/untreated external anogenital HPV infections are the following: 1) perpetuation of disease to sexual partners, particularly with HPV-6-rich lesions; 2) transmission of viruses to neonates by infected mothers; and 3) risk of developing invasive squamous cell carcinoma.[10–15] The sexual contact rates of HPV-infected partners range between 60% and 85%.[16,17] Types 6 and 11 are found in recurrent laryngeal papillomata in neonates and infants, 50% of whom were born of mothers with anogenital warts.[18,19] Oncogenic HPV 16 and 18 and related viruses are found in invasive carcinoma and their precursors of the vulva-perineal-anal skin.[10–15] Between 15% and 28%

Clinical Practice of Gynecology: **2,** 59–72, 1989
© 1989 Elsevier Science Publishing Co., Inc.
655 Avenue of the Americas, New York, NY 10010

ISSN 1043-3198/89/$3.50

TABLE 5–1. Anogenital HPV Infection by Clinical/Colposcopic Presentation*

		%
Macropapillary (acuminate)	35	35
Micropapillary (papular)	10	10
Acetowhite (macular)	55	55
TOTAL:	100	100

*Referral patient population.

of vulvar carcinomas are associated with or preceded by condylomatous lesions.[20–22] Of import are the clinical and colposcopic observations of multicentric HPV infections of the lower-female-genital tract. Indeed, about 50% of women with vulvar and perianal condylomata acuminata have been found to have either flat condyloma of the cervix or cervical intraepithelial neoplasia (CIN).[23,24]

In view of the clinical significance of external anogenital HPV infections, it is pertinent to review their clinical and subclinical presentation in relation to their management.

CLINICAL AND COLPOSCOPIC PRESENTATION

Condylomata

Macropapillary (Acuminate) Condylomata

They represent 35% of HPV-induced lesions in the lower external anogenital tract (Table 5–1). They are small-to-voluminous (chiefly during pregnancy) benign warty lesions, often multiple, and are confined to the surface of the external anogenital skin or mucous membranes (Figure 5–1). They involve mainly the labia majora and minora but also are relatively frequent in the clitoral, mons pubis, and groin regions. Most often they are asymptomatic, however; pruritis and, less frequently, burning may be associated symptoms. They are found either by the patient herself and/or her clinician. By colposcopy, the papillae are seen to contain fine double-capillary loops. Acuminate condylomata should be distinguished from other raised lesions such as molluscum contagiosum, intradermal nevi, seborrheic keratosis (women aged 35 years and older), condylomata lata, granuloma inguinale, hidroadenoma papilliferum, hidradenitis suppurativa, and carcinoma, including the verrucous type.[25,26] Ordinary condylomata acuminata usually are not biopsied by the expert. The novice, however, should biopsy all condylomatous lesions, including the ordinary variant until expertise in clinical and colposcopic impression has been achieved.

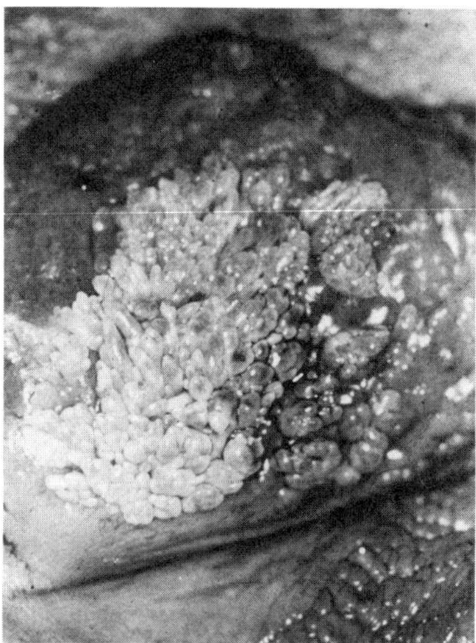

FIGURE 5–1 Macropapillary condylomata acuminata: Extensive, coalescent papillary projections involving the vulvar skin.

Micropapillary (Papular) Condylomata

These are the diminutive variants of ordinary condylomata acuminata. They are multiple, slightly raised lesions occasionally grouped together, and they are better appreciated with the colposcope. Following the application of 5% acetic acid, the lesions are white with irregular spiky surface (asperities) or have fine, hairy, blunt-ended papillae (Figure 5–2A). Papular condylomata are most often found on the labia minora; however, isolated lesions may be seen in any other hairy and nonhairy skin of the vulvar and perianal skin as well as in the anal canal. They should be distinguished from bilateral and symmetrical, tiny fingerlike projections that are also found in the inner surface of labia minora in many patients (Figure 5–2B). These lesions are micropapillomatosis labialis (MPL). Following the application of 5% acetic acid, the projections may appear white because of surface parakeratosis. Each projection contains a double-looped capillary. The vast majority of patients with MPL are young, less than 35 years old, and a significant number have recurrent candidiasis, *Trichomonas* vaginitis, Gardnerella vaginitis, and *Chlamydia trachomatis.* Pruritus, burning, and dyspareunia may be encountered in patients with MPL. An earlier report indicated that the condition was HPV-induced, because HPV antigen was found in some patients with MPL by immunoperoxidase technique.[27] However, recent correlative studies with dot blot hybridization demonstrated HPV DNA only in less than 6% of the cases. Furthermore, this rate was not statistically different than the control population with a more vulvar skin.[28] The results reported

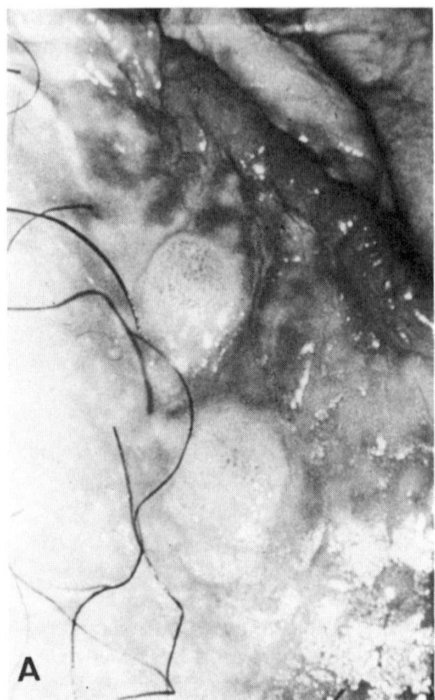
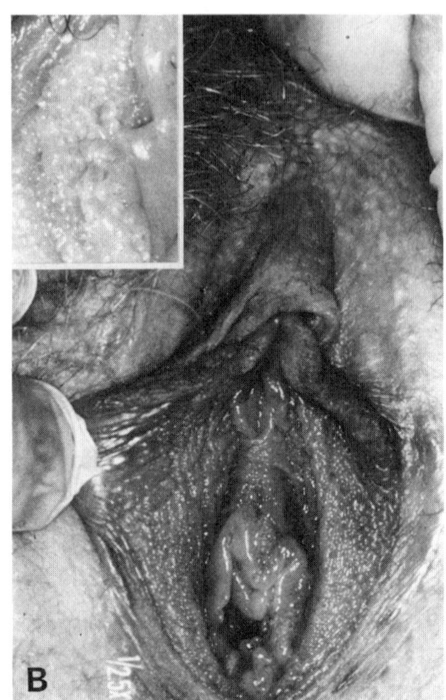

FIGURE 5–2 Papular condylomata: A) Slightly raised acetowhite lesions with punctate surface. B) Micropapillomatosis labialis composed of multiple tiny papillary projections of the inner labial epithelium. **Inset:** Higher magnification of labial micropapillomatosis.

earlier are believed to be a reflection of HPV contamination from cervical HPV infections that are relatively frequent in patients with MPL. Thus, it appears that MPL is a nonspecific exaggeration (hypertrophy) of the labial squamous epithelium in response to various irritative stimuli, chiefly chronic cervico-vaginitis. It is the opinion of the authors that asymptomatic MPL should not be treated. In our experience, most patients with symptomatic MPL are relieved by intravaginal and topical application of mycostatin ovules and creams, respectively. Conservative treatment-resistant patients with MPL may test positive for HPV, and, if symptomatic, they should be treated accordingly. Treatment modalities include topical application of 5% 5-fluoracil (5-FU) cream (Efudex), 50% trichloracetic acid, and superficial laser vaporization.

Acetowhite Flat (Macular) Condyloma

Since the use of the colposcope on the external anogenital skin, it became apparent that this area of the lower-female-genital tract is also the seat of HPV infections of the flat variant. In fact, in the experience of the authors and that of others,[29] at least 50% of all HPV infections of the female external

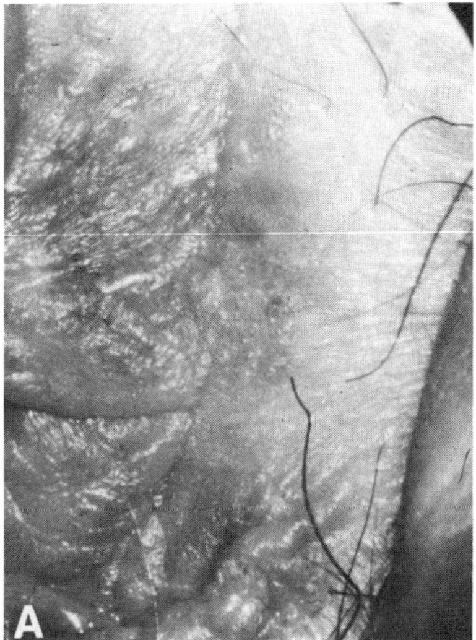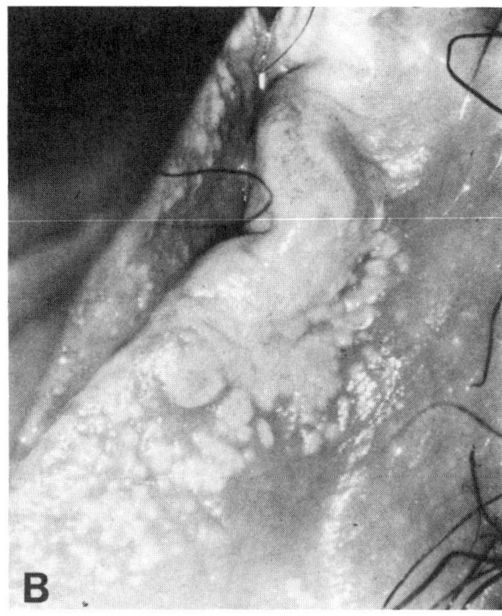

FIGURE 5–3 Flat (macular) condylomata: A) Labial epithelium prior to application of acetic acid contains no obvious alterations. B) After application of acetic acid, multiple coalescent, flat, and "flaky" lesions appear on the labia minora. Histology contained epithelial acanthosis and parakeratosis with few superficial koilocytes consistent with HPV infection of the vulva.

anogenital skin are of the macular type (Table 1). They present either as isolated, well-demarcated, acetowhite, focal lesions, or most commonly as confluent, "flaky" white epithelium (Figure 5–3). The latter is seen chiefly on the external aspect of the labia minora, the perianal skin, and the vestibular skin and less often on the labia majora. Histologically, vulvar flat condylomata (plana) contain acanthosis and surface parakeratosis, and lack abnormal mitotic figures. Koilocytosis, the best morphologic marker of HPV infection may be absent, however. In a large number of patients, acetowhite lesions with or without pruritis/burning of the vulva and perianal skin are not HPV-related. Candidiasis, folliculitis, contact dermatitis, psoriasis, and other allergic reactions may present with positive acetic acid reaction. Clinical inquiry and/or expert histologic examination usually grant accurate diagnosis.

Human papillomavirus infections of all morphologic types may extend into the urethra. Fortunately, the vast majority (98%) are confined to the fossa navicularis, within 1 cm of the external orifice of the urethra. The most common presentation of urethral HPV infections occurs in the form of acuminate condylomata, although in 5% of the cases, acetowhite flat lesions are observed. The distal urethra may be examined with the aid of the colposcope, gently dilating the meatus using an endocervical speculum. Prior to colposcopic examination, a cotton-tip applicator soaked in 5%

acetic acid is applied to the urothelium. In cases of extensive intraurethral condylomatosis, the limit of which cannot be assessed with the colposcope, a consultation with a urologist for urethroscopy and cystoscopy is recommended.

Neoplasia

Vulvar intraepithelial neoplasia (VIN) is the unifying term for preinvasive carcinoma of the vulvar skin. It includes the traditional names such as Bowen's disease, Bowenoid papulosis, Bowenoid dysplasia, erythroplasia of Querat, and carcinoma simplex.[30] When the anus or the perineum is involved, the lesions are called perianal intraepithelial neoplasia (PAIN) or perineal intraepithelial neoplasias (PEIN), respectively. In the past 10 years, VIN has increased in incidence and definitely has become a disease of young women with a mean age of 28–30 years.[31-34] Vulvar intraepithelial neoplasia is considered to be related to HPV infection, particularly type 16. Most VINs are associated with vulvar condylomata, and 60% of the cases with cervical intraepithelial neoplasia (CIN).[23,24] Recent observations using calibrated (microscaled) microscope on over 300 histologic sections taken from 62 VINs showed that hair follicle and sebaceous gland involvement occurs in 32% and 21% of the cases, respectively, and the depth of involvement rarely exceeds 2 mm and 1 mm in the follicles and sebaceous glands, respectively.[35] Vulvar intraepithelial neoplasia that develops during pregnancy and in prepubertal children may regress after delivery and puberty, respectively.[36-38] Most lesions persist and/or expand in nongestational women, however, and, if untreated, they may progress to carcinoma, especially in older patients. The often-quoted 6–10% progression rates in postmenopausal women and those who are immunosuppressed[31,32,39-43] are misleading, because the majority of these women have received multiple treatments or diagnostic biopsies for their disease. The latter often are therapeutic as well as diagnostic. A relatively low carcinoma progression rate is observed with the pigmented variant of VIN (Bowenoid papulosis).[39,44,45] Such lesions are found to have integrated HPV 16 in both the invasive foci and the adjacent intraepithelial neoplasia.[39] When invasion develops, it is often multifocal in fields of VIN, and the area of the greater risk is the perianal skin (Figure 5–4). Nearly all (99%) premenopausal patients with VIN are heavy smokers (20 cigarettes or more per day) and tend to have minor-to-severe personality disorders, particularly exaggerated anxiety to psychologic or physical stimuli (personal observations). Vulvar intraepithelial neoplasia is multifocal (Figure 5–4) and multicentric in premenopausal women[32-34,39-41,46] whereas in the postmenopausal women, it tends to be unifocal (Figure 5–5) and unicentric.[32-34,39,41,46] About 85% of VIN are located in the nonhairy part of the vulva, chiefly the labia minora and posterior fourchette, and 15% are located in the hairy part.[35,47,48]

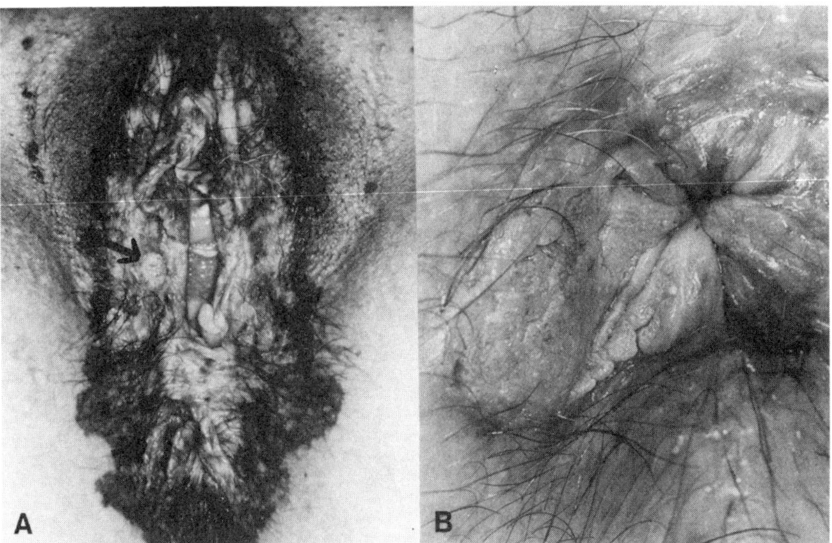

FIGURE 5–4 Vulvar intraepithelial neoplasia (VIN): A) Extensive multifocal pigmented papular lesions involving the entire vulvar and perianal regions typical of Bowenoid papulosis. The right labium major (long arrow) and the right perianal region (short arrow) contain histologically verified invasive squamous cell carcinomas. B) Detailed view of invasive carcinoma of the right perianal region. (Reprinted by permission from ref 39).

FIGURE 5–5 Vulvar intraepithelial neoplasia (VIN): Colposcopic view of flat acetowhite lesion of the left labia minora, which, on histology, contained intraepithelial neoplasia.

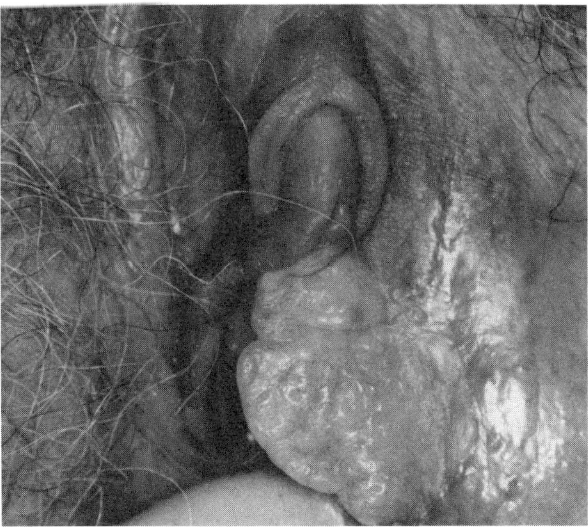

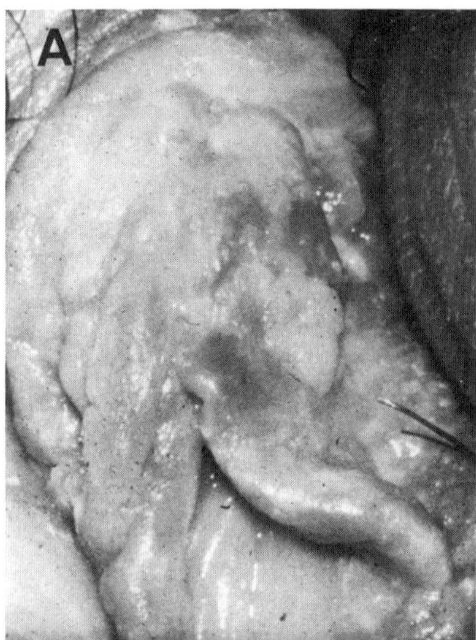
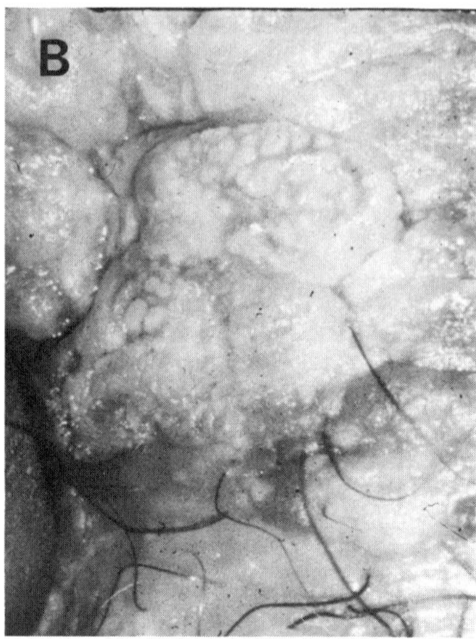

FIGURE 5–6 Vulvar intraepithelial neoplasia (VIN): A) Slightly raised, white, multifocal lesions with hyperkeratotic surface involving the clitoral hood. B) Detail of "white" VIN with cerebriform surface.

Many forms of clinical presentation are assumed by VIN. It may be pink, white (Figure 5–6) or red (Figure 5–7), or still pigmented (Figure 5–4). The latter (also referred to as Bowenoid papulosis in the dermatology literature) is by far the most common form, occurring in two-thirds of premenopausal women with VIN. The anal skin and squamous mucosa of the anal canal are the most frequently involved secondary sites.[31,49] Most patients (60%) are asymptomatic, although some complain of pruritis. Colposcopy of VIN is only appropriate for the nonkeratinized type with clinically red or pigmented surface. Many times, such lesions become white following the application of 3–5% acetic solution and have coarsely granular punctate and occasionally mosaic surface patterns by colposcopy (Figure 5–5). Colposcopy is also useful to detect and include small satellite lesions into the treatment field and for examination of the intraanal limit of PAIN. It is essentially noncontributory for keratinized VIN. The thick keratin layer prevents visualization of predictive colposcopic patterns. As a result, all keratinized lesions should be biopsied thoroughly to rule out possible underlying invasive carcinoma. Biopsies also should be obtained from nonkeratinized, red-surfaced VIN. In cases of extensive VIN, the application of 1% Toluidine blue solution on the lesional tissue may help to select the area of greatest nuclear density and significance.[50] In such areas, toluidine blue stain will be retained by nuclei. The operator must be careful, however,

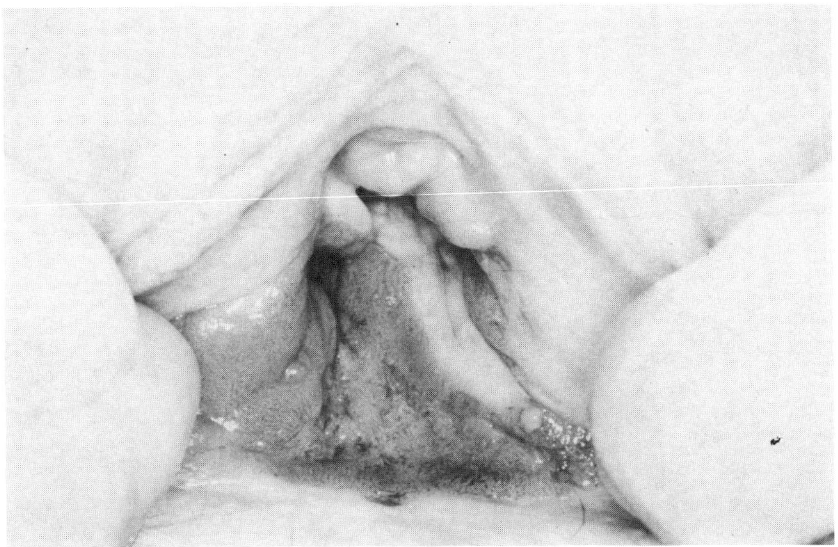

FIGURE 5–7 Vulvar intraepithelial neoplasia (VIN): The lesion presents with red surface and has punctation pattern. It involves the vestibular and hymenal epithelium and extends into the lower two-thirds of the vagina. It was associated with cervical intraepithelial neoplasia.

to select only those toluidine blue positive areas that are intact and devoid of excoriation. The latter produce false-positive staining reaction because of accumulated nuclear DNA-rich chronic inflammatory exudate on the surface of denuded dermis. The differential diagnoses include confluent flat or papular condylomata (resembling "white" VIN), melanoma (pigmented VIN), and Paget's disease (red or white VIN). The latter is found in elderly, postmenopausal Caucasian women, often has an eczematoid appearance, and is associated in 50% of the cases with longstanding pruritis.[25,26] Histologic examination of the aforementioned lesions provides for their precise diagnosis.

The clinical presentation of classical invasive squamous carcinoma may vary from exophytic and papillomatous to an endophytic, ulcerated, hard mass located on the labia minora or majora, and, rarely, the clitoris.[25] The tumor is usually solitary, especially in postmenopausal patients. Less than 10% of patients have multifocal distribution including the perianal skin[25] (Figure 5–4). In a significant number of postmenopausal patients with vulvar cancer, malignancy develops in skin that contains epithelial hyperplasia (hyperplastic dystrophy) and/or lichens sclerosus. The pathogenic relationship between vulvar dystrophies and carcinoma is not clear. However, chronic irritation and inflammation associated with the former may be associated with the production of carcinogenic agents.[51] Colposcopically, in-

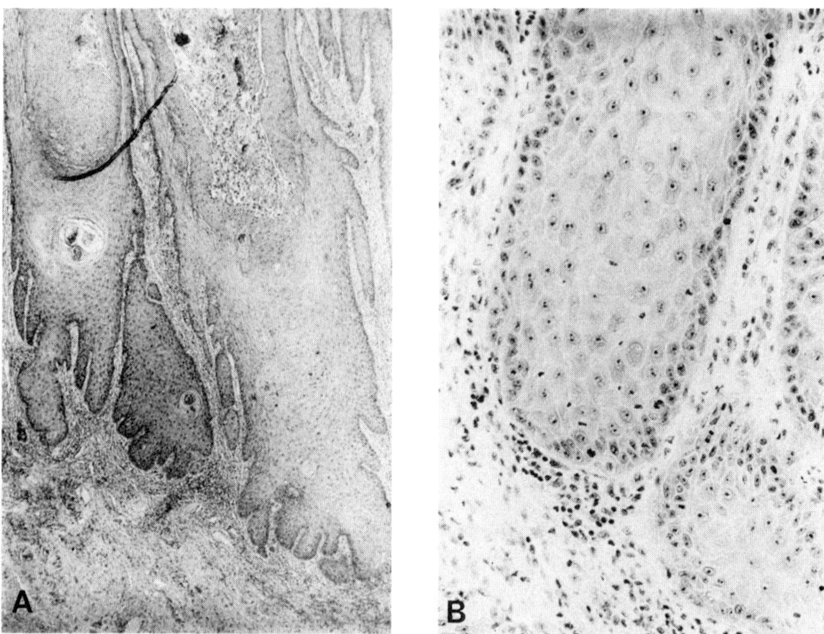

FIGURE 5–8 Very well-differentiated, verrucous squamous cell carcinoma of vulva: A) Histology of deep dermal extension of prominent, club-shaped rete ridges. B) Note lack of significant cytologic atypia typical of this rare lesion.

vasive carcinoma often has a necrotic surface with abnormal vascular pattern made of highly irregular tortuous vessels with horizontal T-shaped branching.

A rare variant of invasive squamous cell carcinoma of the anogenital skin is the so-called verrucous carcinoma, also known as the giant condyloma of Buschke-Loewenstein.[52–57] Such lesions involve large areas, are sessile and confluent, and form cauliflowerlike tumors. This lesion is slow-growing, ulcerates frequently in deeper tissue, causes fistulous tracks, but does not produce metastases. It has been described not only in the vulva but also in the perineum and buttocks, and it may even infiltrate the rectal wall. Wide surgical excision is often the only rational approach. It is often unrecognized by the clinician and biopsied only after many attempts of eradication with topical chemical treatment, especially in postmenopausal patients. On microscopy, it infiltrates deeply the dermis with club-shaped pushing margins (Figure 5–8) and contains HPV 6b and rarely 11.[58] The episomal physical state of HPV in verrucous carcinoma is consistent with its indolent clinical course. External radiotherapy, however, may be followed by cellular dedifferentiation and metastasis.[54–58] As a result, wide surgical excision seems to be the best treatment approach.[55,57]

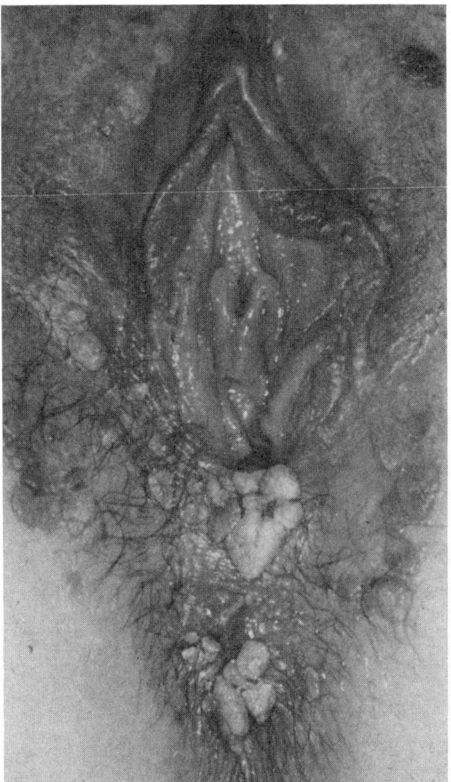

FIGURE 5–9 Condylomata acuminata: Multiple lesions involve the skin of the vulva (multifocal disease) and anus (multicentric disease).

Multicentric Disease

Condylomata of the external genital skin are almost always multifocal, and a significant number of patients have HPV-related lesions (multicentric diseases) elsewhere in the lower anogenital tract as well[9] (Figure 5–9). As mentioned earlier, over 50% of patients with vulvar condylomata acuminata are found with flat condylomata of the cervix and 35% with cervical intraepithelial neoplasia.[9,23,24] Conversely, about 60% of patients with cervical condylomata have similar disease on the vulva, chiefly the flat condylomata variant (unpublished observations). Vulvar intraepithelial neoplasia, PAIN, and invasive carcinoma of the vulva and/or the anus are often associated with or preceeded by condylomata acuminata,[20–22, 39,59] and the multicentric nature of VIN in premenopausal women (over 60% having CIN as well) has been extensively documented.[24,29,60,61] Failure to examine the entire anogenital tract may not only miss coexistent lesions but may also allow perpetuation of viral transmission and, in some cases, progression to carcinoma. As a result, all patients with HPV infection of the vulva should benefit from a thorough colposcopic examination of the entire lower-female-genital tract. In cases of perianal and urethral condylomata, the anal canal and urethra should be examined with the colposcope. In all patients with external anogenital condylomata or intraepithelial neoplasia, cervical colposcopy is mandatory even though the Pap test is negative. Indeed, Pap tests may be associated with false negative results.[62]

REFERENCES

1. Roy M, Meisels A, Fortier M, et al: Vaginal condylomata: A human papillomavirus infection. Clin Obstet Gynecol 1981;24:461–483.
2. Fletcher S, Norval M: On the nature of the deep cellular disturbances in human papillomavirus infection of the squamous cervical epithelium. Lancet 1983;ii:546–549.
3. Centers for disease control condyloma acuminatum, United States 1966–1981. MMWR 1983;23:306–308.
4. Fleming KA, Venning V, Evans M: DNA typing of genital warts and diagnosis of sexual abuse of children. Lancet 1987_:454.
5. Shah K, Kashima HK, Polk F, et al: Rarity of cesarean delivery in cases of juvenile respiratory papillomatosis. Obstet Gynecol 1986;68:795–799.
6. Kreider J, Howett MK, Stoler MH, et al: Susceptibility of various tissues to transformation in vivo with HPV type 11. Int J Cancer 1987;39:459–468.
7. Ferenczy A, Bergeron C, Richart RM: HPV DNA in fomites used for the management of patients with genital HPV infections. Obstet Gynecol, in press.
8. Bergeron C, Ferenczy A, Richart RM: Underwear: Contamination by human papilloma viruses. Am J Obstet Gynecol, in press.
9. Oriel JD: Natural history of genital warts. Br J Vener Dis 1971;47:1–3.
10. Zur Hausen H, Schneider A: The role of papillomaviruses in human anogenital cancer. In: Howley P, Jalzmann NP, eds. The papilloma viruses. New York: Plenum Press, 1985:245–259.
11. Durst M, Gissmann L, Ikenberg H, et al: A papillomavirus DNA from a cervical carcinoma and its prevalence in cancer biopsies from different geographic regions. Proc Natl Acad Sci USA 1983;80:3812–3815.
12. Zachow KR, Ostrow RS, Bender M, et al: Detection of human papillomavirus DNA in anogenital neoplasias. Nature 1982;300:771–772.
13. Ikenberg H, Gissmann L, Gross G, et al: Human papillomavirus type 16-related DNA in genital Bowen's disease and in bowenoid papulosis. Int J Cancer 1983;32:563–565.
14. Gupta J, Pilotti S, Rilke F, et al: Association of human papillomavirus type 16 with neoplastic lesions of the vulva and other genital sites by in situ hybridization. Am J Pathol 1987;127:206–215.
15. Palmer JG, Shepherd NA, Jass JR, et al: Human papillomavirus type 16 DNA in anal squamous cell carcinoma. Lancet 1987;ii:42.
16. Campion MJ, Singer A, McCance DJ, et al: Subclinical penile human papilloma virus infection in consorts of women with cervical neoplasia: A clue to the high risk male. Colpo Gynecol Laser Surg 1987;3:11–22.
17. Barasso R, De Brux J, Croissant O, et al: High prevalence of papilloma virus-associated penile intraepithelial neoplasia in sexual partners of women with cervical intraepithelial neoplasia. New Engl J Med 1987;317:916–923.
18. Quick CA, Watts SL, Krzyzek RA, et al: Relationship between condylomata and laryngeal papillomata. Ann Otol 1980;89:469–471.
19. Cook T, Cohen AM, Brunschwig JP, et al: Laryngeal papilloma: Etiologic and therapeutic considerations. Ann Otol 1973;82:649–654.

20. Shafeek MA, Osman ME, Hussein MA: Carcinoma of the vulva arising in condylomata acuminata. Obstet Gynecol 1979;54:120–123.
21. Schmauz R, Owor R: Epidemiology of malignant degeneration of condyloma acuminata in Uganda. Pathol Res Pract 1980;170:91.
22. Daling JR, Weiss NS, Hislop TG, et al: Sexual practices, sexually transmitted diseases and the incidence of anal cancer. New Engl J Med 1987;317:973–977.
23. Walker PG, Colley NY, Grubb C, et al: Abnormalities of the uterine cervix in women with vulvar warts. Br J Vener Dis 1983;59:120–123.
24. Bergeron C, Ferenczy A, Shah KV, et al: Multicentric human papillomavirus infections of the female genital tract: Correlation of viral types with abnormal mitotic figures, colposcopic presentation and location. Obstet Gynecol 1987;69:736–742.
25. Friedrich EG: Vulvar disease. Philadelphia: WB Saunders, 1983.
26. Wilkinson EJ, Friedrich EG: Diseases of the vulva. In: Kurman R, ed. Blaustein's pathology of the female genital tract. 3rd ed. New York: Springer Verlag, 1987:36–96.
27. Growdon WA, Fu YS, Lebherz TB, et al: Pruritic vulvar squamous papillomatosis: Evidence for human papillomavirus etiology. Obstet Gynecol 1985;66:564–568.
28. Bergeron C, Ferenczy A, Richart RM: Micropapillomatosis labialis appears unrelated to HPV, in preparation.
29. Reid R, Greenberg M, Bennett-Jenson A, et al: Sexually transmitted papillomaviral infections. I. The anatomic distribution and pathologic grade of neoplastic lesions associated with different viral types. Am J Obstet Gynecol 1987;156:212–222.
30. Report of the ISSVD Terminology Committee: Proc VIII World Congress, Stockholm, Sweden. J Reprod Med 1986;31:973.
31. Friedrich EG, Wilkinson EJ, Fu YS: Carcinoma in situ of the vulva: A continuing challenge. Am J Obstet Gynecol 1980;136:830–838.
32. Buscema J, Woodruff JD, Parmely TH, et al: Carcinoma in situ of the vulva. Obstet Gynecol 1980;55:225–230.
33. Bernstein SG, Kovacs BR, Townsend DE, et al: Vulvar carcinoma in situ. Obstet Gynecol 1983;61:304–307.
34. Benedet JL, Murphy KJ: Squamous carcinoma in situ of the vulva. Gynecol Oncol 1982;14:213–219.
35. Shatz P, Bergeron C, Wilkinson E, et al: Vulvar intraepithclial neoplasia with emphasis on skin appendage involvement. Obstet Gynecol, in press.
36. Friedrich EG: Reversible vulvar atypia. Obstet Gynecol 1972;39:173–81.
37. Hilliard GD, Massey FM, O'Toole RV: Vulvar neoplasia in the young. Am J Obstet Gynecol 1979;135:185–188.
38. Skinner MS, Sternberg WII, Ichinose H, et al: Spontaneous regression of bowenoid atypia of the vulva. Obstet Gynecol 1973;42:40–46.
39. Bergeron C, Naghashfar Z, Canaan C, et al: Human papillomavirus type 16 in intraepithelial neoplasia (Bowenoid papulosis) and coexistent invasive carcinoma of the vulva. Int J Gynecol Pathol 1987;6:1–11.
40. Japaze H, Garcia-Bummel R, Woodruff JD: Primary vulvar neoplasia. A review of in situ and invasive carcinoma 1935–1972. Obstet Gynecol 1977;49:404–411.
41. Jones RW, McLean MR: Carcinoma in situ of the vulva: a review of 31 treated and five untreated cases. Obstet Gynecol 1986;68:499–503.
42. Rasthkar G, Okagaki T, Twiggs LB, et al: Early invasive and in situ carcinoma of the vulva. Clinical, histologic and electron microscopic study with particular reference to viral association. Am J Obstet Gynecol 1982;143:814–820.
43. Pilotti S, Delle Torre G, Rilke F, et al: Immunohistochemical and ultrastructural evidence of papillomavirus infection associated with in situ and microinvasive squamous cell carcinoma of the vulva. Am J Surg Pathol 1984;8:751–761.
44. Wade TR, Kopf AW, Ackerman AB: Bowenoid papulosis of the genitalia. Arch Dermatol 1979;115:306–308.

45. Ulbright TM, Stehman FB, Roth LM, et al: Bowenoid dysplasia of the vulva. Cancer 1982;50:2910–2919.
46. Powell LC, Dinh TV, Rajaraman S: Carcinoma in situ of the vulva: A clinicopathologic study of 50 cases. J Reprod Med 1986;31:808–814.
47. Mene A, Buckley CH: Involvement of the vulvar skin appendages by intraepithelial neoplasia. Br J Obstet Gynecol 1985;92:634–638.
48. Wright VC, Davies E: Laser surgery for vulvar intraepithelial neoplasia: principles and results. Am J Obstet Gynecol 1987;156:374–378.
49. Kaplan AL, Kaufman RH, Briken RA: Intraepithelial carcinoma of the vulva with extension to the anal canal. Obstet Gynecol 1981;58:368–371.
50. Collins CG, Hansen LH, Theriot E: A clinical stain for use in selecting biopsy sites in patients with vulvar disease. Obstet Gynecol 1966;28:158–163.
51. Zur Hausen H: Papillomaviruses in human cancer. Cancer 1987;59:1692–1696.
52. Partridge EE, Murad T, Shingleton HM, et al: Verrucous lesions of the female genitalia. I. Giant condylomata. Am J Obstet Gynecol 1980;137:412–418.
53. Bogomoletz, Potet F, Molas G: Condylomata acuminata, giant condyloma acuminatum (Busche-Loewenstein tumor) and verrucous squamous carcinoma of the perianal and anorectal region. A continuous precancerous spectrum. Histopathology 1985;9:1155–1169.
54. Powell LC, Franklin EW, Nickerson JF: Verrucous carcinoma of the female genital tract. Gynecol Oncol 1978;6:565–573.
55. Lucas WE, Benirschke K, Lebherz TB: Verrucous carcinoma of the female genital tract. Am J Obstet Gynecol 1974;119:435–440.
56. Partridge EE, Murad T, Shingleton HM, et al: Verrucous lesions of the female genitalia. II. Verrucous carcinoma. Am J Obstet Gynecol 1980 137:419–424.
57. Japaze H, Van Dinh T, Woodruff JD: Verrucous carcinoma of the vulva. Study of 24 cases. Obstet Gynecol 1982;60:462–466.
58. Rando RF, Groff DE, Chirikjian JG, et al: Isolation and characterization of a novel human papillomavirus type 6 DNA from an invasive vulvar carcinoma. J Virol 1986;57:353–356.
59. Gillat DA, Teasdale C: Squamous cell carcinoma of the anus arising within condylomata acuminata. Eur J Surg Oncol 1985;11:369–371.
60. Bornstein J, Kaufman H, Adam E, et al: Multicentric intraepithelial neoplasia involving the vulva. Cancer 1988;62:1601–1604.
61. Hammond IG, Monaghan JM: Multicentric carcinoma of the female lower genital tract. Br J Obstet Gynecol 1983;20:557–561.
62. Schneider A, Sawada E, Gissman L, et al: Human papillomaviruses in women with a history of abnormal Papanicolaou smears and in their male partners. Obstet Gynecol 1987;69:554–562.

CHAPTER 6

Clinical, Colposcopic, and Histologic Spectrum of Male Human Papillomavirus-associated Genital Lesions

Renzo Barrasso, MD, and Stephania Jablonska, MD

Condylomata acuminata were known to the ancient Greeks, who already surmised their sexual transmission. These lesions were associated with a viral cytopathic effect in 1968[1] and with the presence of human papillomaviruses in 1981.[2]

The identification of deoxyribonucleic acid (DNA) of human papillomaviruses (HPV) in genital intraepithelial and invasive neoplasia in women and in men[3-8] has given new interest to the epidemiologic data linking cervical cancer to a sexually transmitted agent.[9,10] Consequently, screening of the male partner of women with cervical disease has been proposed,[11] thus leading to the description of several new male HPV-associated lesions and, mostly, to the discovery of flat subclinical lesions detected by the aid of a colposcope after application of 5% acetic acid.[12]

In this chapter, we present a review of the literature and our observations on the morphologic spectrum of male HPV-associated genital lesions, as well as data on the sexual transmission of genital HPVs.

CONDYLOMATA ACUMINATA

These warts are exophytic protuberances with lobated or irregular surface, pink-reddish or white-grayish depending mainly on the location. Their number varies from a few to 50 or more lesions, and the sizes from 0.2 to 1.0 cm, but, if numerous, they become confluent involving large areas of genitalia (Figure 6–1). These lesions correspond to the hyperplastic type of genital warts in the classification by Oriel.[13]

The lesions are prevalent on the inner aspect of the prepuce, at the frenum and coronal sulcus; less frequently, they are located on the shaft, the glans, and within the urinary meatus.[14] Condylomas in the urinary meatus and terminal urethra often show a bright red color. Extension of warts to

Clinical Practice of Gynecology: **2,** 73–101, 1989
© 1989 Elsevier Science Publishing Co., Inc.
655 Avenue of the Americas, New York, NY 10010

ISSN 1043-3198/89/$3.50

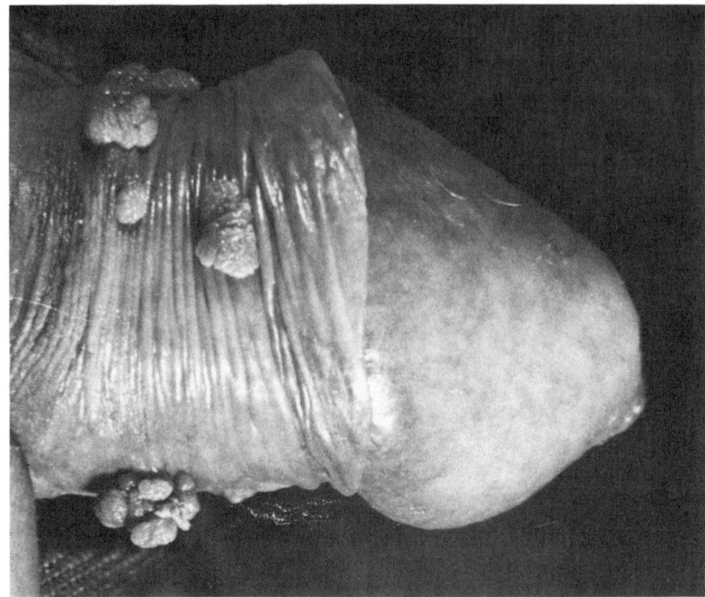

FIGURE 6–1 Condylomata acuminata: pedunculated cauliflowerlike excrescences, located on inner and outer surface of the prepuce.

the proximal urethra has been described,[15] although it seems to be a rare event.[7] Still more rare are warts extending into the bladder.[16] Condylomata acuminata in circumcised men, although less frequent,[13] show the same gross appearance.

Condylomata extending to the surrounding area include the following: perineal, inguinal, anal, and pubertal, which have a somewhat different gross appearance, forming a papillary growth or papilloma. The anal condylomas have all characteristics of classic condylomata acuminata, and their location is perianal, anal and above the dental line.[17]

Condylomata acuminata have to be distinguished from other papillomatous lesions in this area. On the penis, a condition that may simulate warts has been described as pearly papules[18] or hirsutoid papillomas. Parallel rows of discrete acuminate structures distributed circumferentially around the coronal sulcus may resemble filiform warts. Histologically, these are hypertrophic papillae covered by a normal epithelium. The colposcopic magnification allows their distinction from condylomata acuminata, since their surfaces are mostly smooth and dome-shaped, and they do not show the typical vascular pattern presented by mucosal condylomata.

The condylomata lata of secondary syphilis should be distinguished from condylomata acuminata. Although condylomata lata are broader and flatter,[19] the differentiation may be difficult in some cases. The serologic

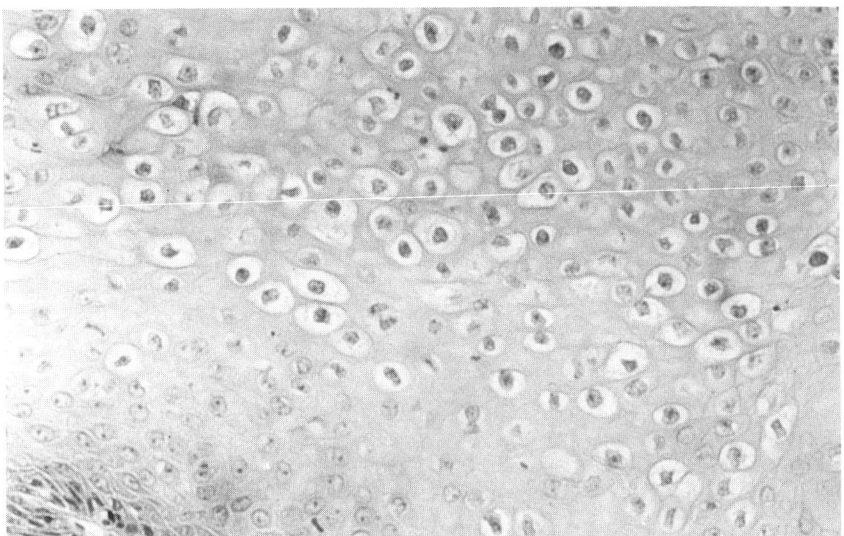

FIGURE 6–2 Widespread koilocytosis in the acanthotic epidermal overgrowth (H+E, × 450).

tests for syphilis and the microscopic detection of spirochetes in the lesions are decisive for the diagnosis.

The differentiation of condylomata acuminata from genital malignancies is of importance. Some lesions of Bowen's disease and some cancers at the early stages may resemble genital warts. In older patients and in warts resistant to treatment, biopsy is recommended.[19]

Histology

The characteristic feature is epidermal proliferation with variously pronounced hyper- and parakeratosis. In most cases, in the upper layers of the epidermis, there is an evident perinuclear vacuolization with usually slight koilocytotic atypia. In some cases, koilocytosis is very abundant, present almost throughout the whole epidermis (Figure 6–2). The normal mitotic figures are numerous and not infrequently scattered throughout the epidermis. In the corium there are usually abundant inflammatory infiltrations and newly formed vessels, seen also within the elongated papillae, in spikes or papillary excrescences.

Virology

Human papillomavirus 6 and 11 are detected in 70–95% of condylomata acuminata, independent of the location, extent, and duration of lesion.[2,20,21]

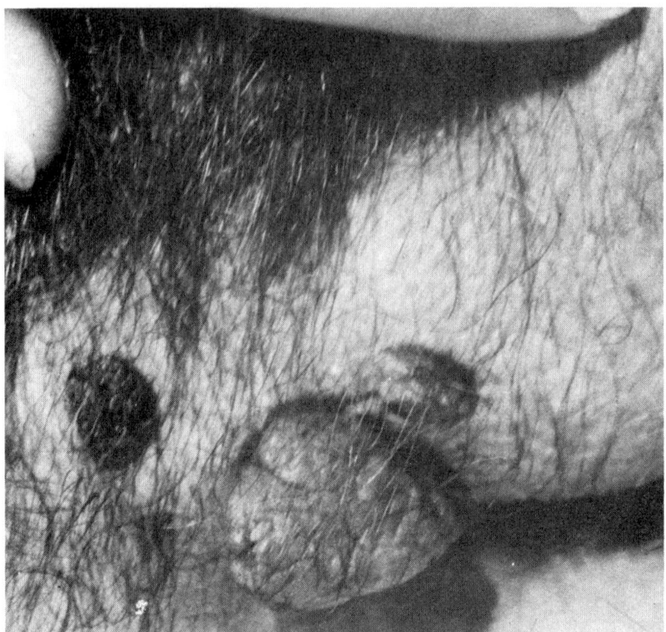

FIGURE 6–3 Extensive brownish or heavily pigmented papillomas located in dry regions.

In our series, only eight of 131 condylomata acuminata contained other HPV types (HPV 18 in two cases, HPV 16 in one case, and as yet uncharacterized HPV types in five cases).

GENITAL PAPILLOMAS

These proliferative lesions have more hyperkeratotic and papillomatous surface and are larger (from 0.8 to several centimeters). They lack the surface irregularities typical of condylomata acuminata. Usually pedunculated and darker than the surrounding skin, they may be brownish or even blackish. They are preferentially located on the skin: the shaft, the scrotum, inguinal, perineal, and pubertal areas (Figure 6–3). In this group we include cutaneous wartlike lesions, defined by Oriel[13] as the verruca vulgaris type of genital warts (Figure 6–4). Papillomas rarely coexist with other HPV-associated genital lesions. Their duration is much longer than that of condylomata acuminata, and their resistance to podophylline treatment has been reported.[13]

Histology

The histologic features are those of papilloma, with pronounced epidermal proliferation, elongation of rete pegs, hyperkeratosis, and usually increased

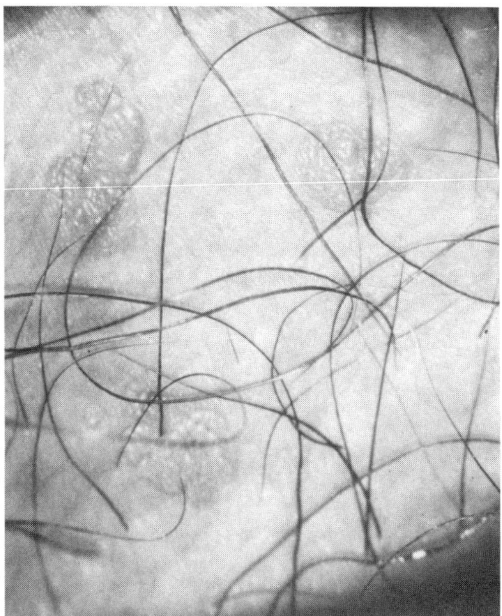

FIGURE 6–4 Colposcopy: cutaneous wartlike papules of penile skin. The DNA of an as-yet-uncharacterized HPV type was present (× 12).

melanin accumulation in the basal cell layer. If hyperkeratosis is very extensive, leading to the formation of hyperkeratotic kists, they may be a similarity to seborrhoic warts (Figure 6–5). Koilocytosis is discrete or absent. Some lesions show histologic features closely resembling those of cutaneous warts.

Virology

Pigmented papillomas mostly contain HPV 6 or 11. In our series, however, potentially oncogenic HPV have been found in absence of histologic atypia in three out of 23 lesions. Interestingly, one out of three female partners had shown cervical carcinoma in situ. As yet uncharacterized HPVs may occasionally be found in genital papillomas. Although papillomas do not differ significantly from condylomata acuminata in their association with HPV types, if associated with potentially oncogenic HPV types, because of more prolonged duration, they present a somewhat higher risk of malignant conversion, especially for cervical lesions of the sexual partners. Wartlike lesions localized on skin may contain cutaneous HPV types or HPV 6. The clinical differentiation of lesions is impossible. They may also contain as-yet-uncharacterized HPVs (three of eight cases in our series).

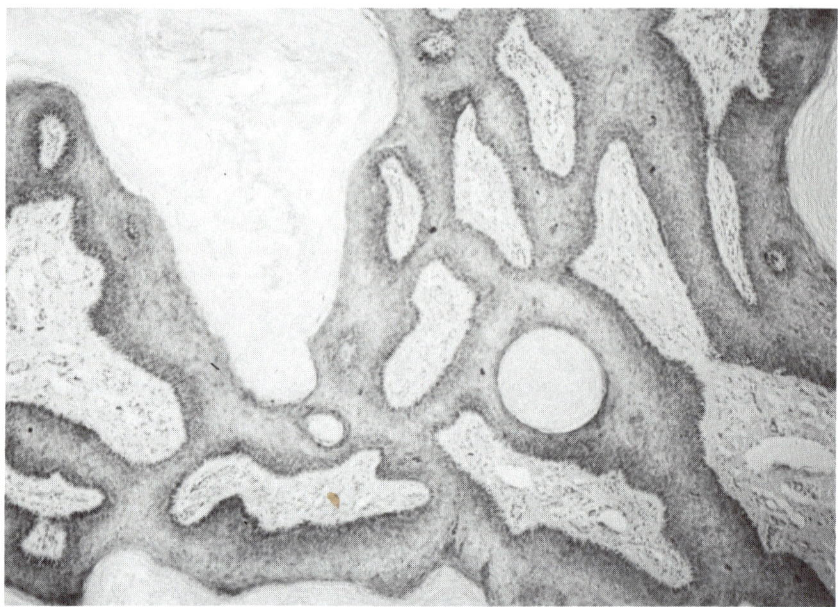

FIGURE 6–5 Histology of a pigmented papilloma. There is marked hyperkeratosis, acanthosis, and proliferation of rete pegs composed mainly of basaloid-cells. The interwoven tracts of epithelial cells surround islands of connective tissue and horn cysts. Melanin accumulation in the basal cell-layer (H + E, × 80).

NONPIGMENTED PAPULES

These lesions are clearly outlined, variably elevated but not pedunculated, with a round (Figure 6–6) or dome-shaped (Figure 6–7), slightly hyperkeratotic or smooth surface. Most of them correspond to the sessile type of genital warts described by Oriel.[13] Their size mostly vary from 0.3 to 0.8 cm, and their number from a few lesions to 20–40. The color is that of normal skin, grayish, pinkish or, not infrequently, slightly brownish when located on the penile skin. The lesions are preferentially located on the shaft. Some resemble plane warts of the skin, while some are nodular (Figure 6–8). Some slightly elevated papular lesions are similar to psoriatic papules and lichen planus. Nonpigmented papules are easily distinguished from the umbilicated papules pathognomonic of molluscum contagiosum. With the colposcope, punctate vessels are regularly seen at their top, as described by Levine, unless the lesion is dark. The colposcopic detection of punctate vessels allows the identification of small, early lesions or recurrences after treatment (Figure 6–9) and their distinction from normal skin folds, mostly in circumcised men (Figure 6–10).

When located on mucosa, nonpigmented papules are translucent. They show a clear vascular punctuation on the top,[12] which allows their distinc-

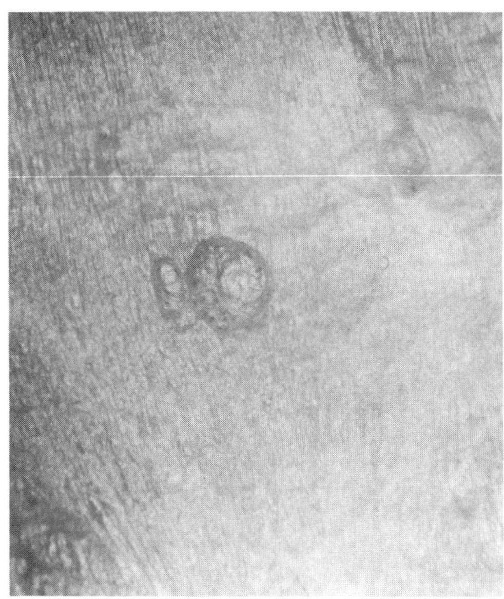

FIGURE 6–6 Colposcopy: small nonpigmented papules with round, slightly hyperkeratotic surface. Histology: condyloma. Virology: HPV 6 ($\times$ 12).

FIGURE 6–7 Small dome-shaped papules with smooth surface on the shaft of the penis, displaying gross features of plane warts.

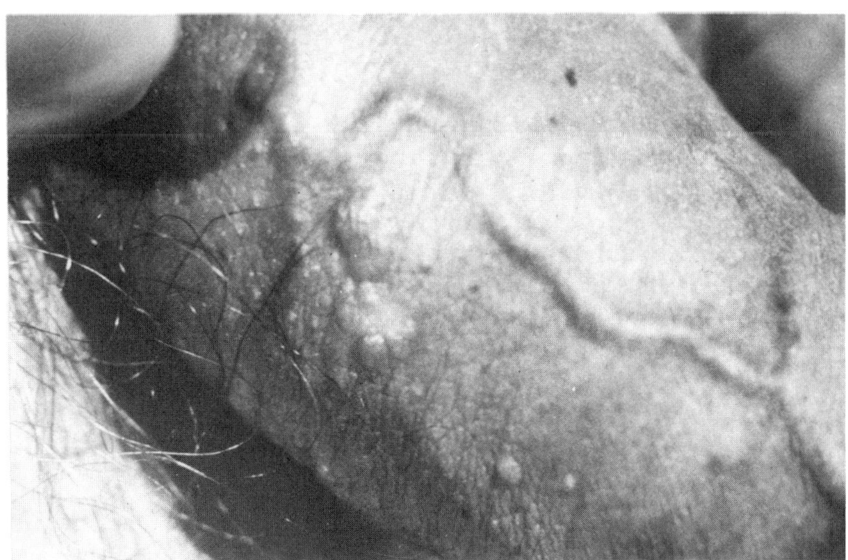

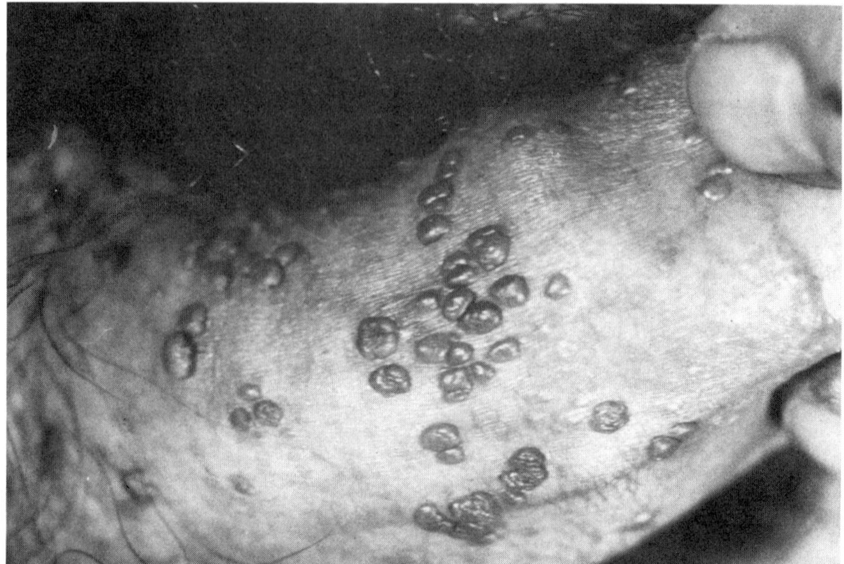

FIGURE 6–8 Papules with smooth glistening surface and central depression.

tion from small pearly papules. Often small, they may be undetected without the aid of the colposcope. The application of 5% acetic acid produces a strong, well-demarcated reaction, as shown by Levine in the urethral meatus,[11] by Rosenberg in the preputial cavity,[22] and by Sedlacek on the glans.[23] The white reaction usually preserves the punctate vessels (Figure 6–11).

Histology

The histology of these lesions differs by the absence of marked epidermal proliferation. In most lesions the dermoepidermal border is flattened; in the upper layers of the epidermis, there is a variously abundant koilocytosis (Figure 6–12) and, almost constantly, a discrete parakeratosis. The mitotic figures are scarce, and dyskeratosis is absent. In the subepithelial stroma, the dilated capillaries are usually not surrounded by inflammatory infiltrates. There are no signs of dysplasia, or only slight dysplastic changes. Slightly elevated papules may show an endophytic pattern. Translucent acetowhite papules show the same histologic features, although koilocytosis is usually scarce or absent (Figures 6–13, 6–14).

Virology

Nonpigmented papules of the penile skin mostly contain the same HPVs as evidenced in genital condylomas. Translucent acetowhite papules represent

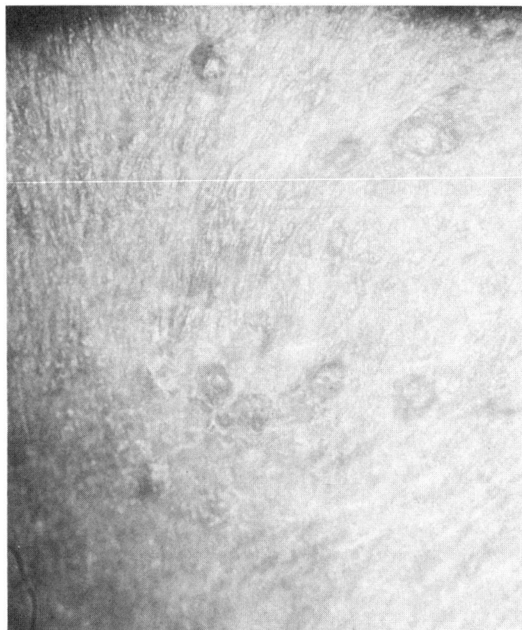

FIGURE 6–9 Colposcopy: small nonpigmented papules of penile skin. Colposcopy allows the detection of vascular punctuation on the top of some papules. Histology: condyloma. Virology: HPV 11 ($\times$ 12).

a more heterogeneous HPV reservoir than condylomata acuminata or non-pigmented cutaneous penile papules: in our series, only two out of nine such lesions contained HPV 6 or 11, HPV 42 was found in three cases, as yet uncharacterized HPV in two cases, and two lesions were negative. Potentially oncogenic HPVs were not identified.

PIGMENTED PAPULES

The term *bowenoid papulosis* was coined for clinically inconspicuous papular lesions of the genitalia, displaying histologic features of Bowen's atypia[24] (for review see refs 25 and 26).

The papules are usually small, several millimeters in diameter, often flat at the skin level, reddish or slightly brownish, with a smooth, glistening surface (Figure 6–15). Their number varies from single lesions to about 30. They are localized on the glans, the foreskin, and the shaft; in the latter location, they are often somewhat pigmented. In two patients, we have seen coalescent lesions involving almost the whole glans and partially the shaft. When they are reddish and localized on the mucosa, they show a strong reaction to the application of acetic acid (Figure 6–16). Punctate vessels

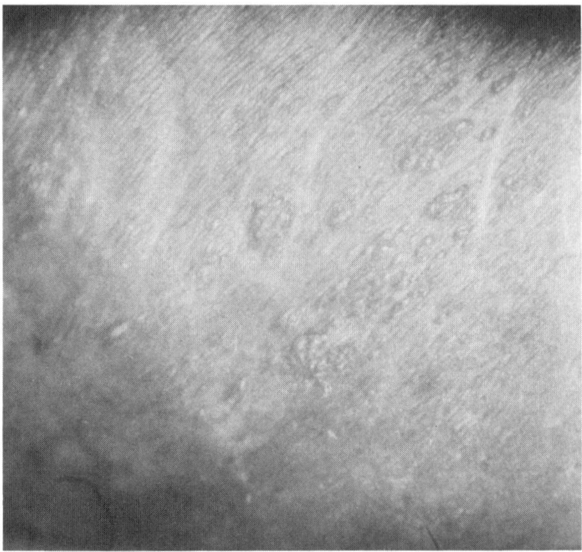

FIGURE 6–10 Colposcopy: normal skin folds, lacking surface vascular punctuation (× 12).

are detected with the use of the colposcope before and after the acetic acid application. Red, acetowhite, or white keratinized papular areas (Figure 6–17) may also be detected at the healing site after treatment of condylomata acuminata: In these cases, biopsies may show features of intraepithelial neoplasia, and HPV DNA of the oncogenic types may be detected (R Barrasso and G Orth, unpublished data). These features appear to represent a different morphologic expression of the same HPV infection but also of the reinfection of the healing tissue with different HPV types, or of reactivation of latent infection. The latest hypothesis is also supported by the finding of HPV-16-associated lesions at the epithelial site in which HPV-6-associated condylomata acuminata were previously treated (A Langenberg, personal communication; R Barrasso and G Orth, unpublished data).

The clinical distinction of bowenoid papules from papular condylomas is sometimes difficult or even impossible (Figure 6–18). In our series, 17 lesions clinically defined as bowenoid papules were revealed to be histologic condylomas, mostly HPV 6 associated. However, in our opinion, all pigmented or reddish penile papules should be considered as potential bowenoid papules and biopsied before treatment.

Histology

The histology of bowenoid papulosis shows epidermal proliferation with numerous, partially abnormal mitotic figures and atypical pleomorphic cells

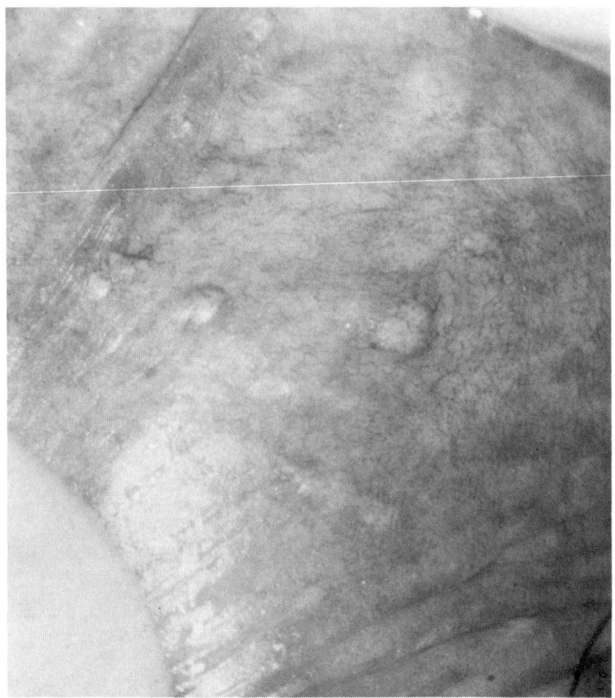

FIGURE 6–11 Colposcopy: small translucent papules of the prepuce, featuring surface vascular punctuation, whitening after application of acetic acid. Histology: papilloma without koilocytosis. Virology: HPV 42 (× 12).

with hyperchromatic and clumped nuclei, and pronounced dyskeratosis (Figure 6–19). In the corium, there are slight inflammatory infiltrates and dilated capillaries, by preserved dermal–epidermal border. Thus, the histologic picture is of the type of penile intraepithelial neoplasia (PIN) grade III or Bowen's carcinoma in situ.

Virology

In cases of pigmented papules in men, there is a clear prevalence of HPV 16.[6,25–27] The other potentially oncogenic HPV types may also be detected.[29] We have seen only one case associated with HPV 6 (double infection by an as-yet-uncharacterized type) and one case associated with HPV 42. Double infection is not a rare event.

MACULES

Macules have been defined[12] as well-demarcated flat areas showing a white reaction after acetic acid application and containing capillary loops. They

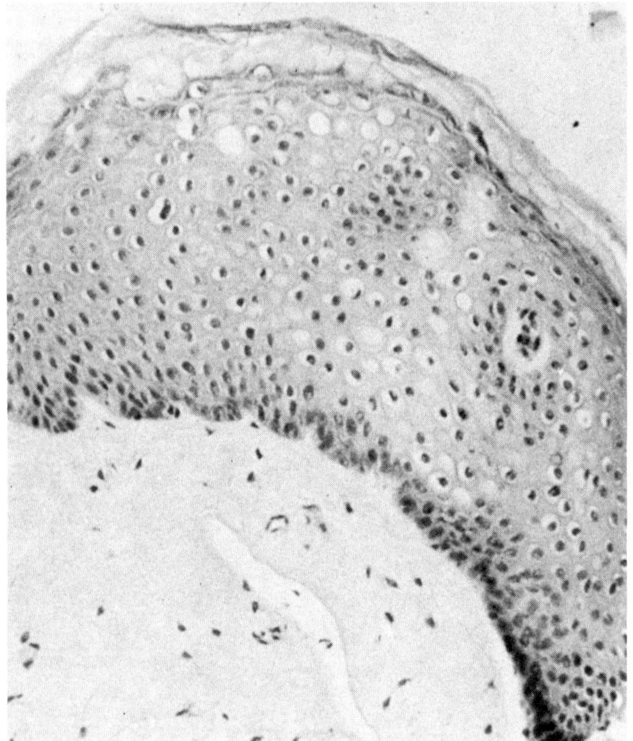

FIGURE 6–12 Histology of penile papules in Figure 6–7 with flattened dermale-pidermal border and koilocytosis in the upper layers (H + E, × 200).

correspond to pink or reddish areas with capillary loops detected by the colposcope (Figures 6–20, 6–21) or to areas of epithelial surfaces that had been normal on colposcopy before the test (Figures 6–22, 6–23). Well-demarcated white areas not showing capillary loops at the colposcopy and ill-delimited acetowhite areas should not be considered as macules (Figures 6–24, 6–25).

Their size may vary from 0.1 to 10 mm, rarely more, and their number from one to ten, sometimes more. One or several groups of small lesions are often observed. They are usually found on the prepuce, gland, or, occasionally, in the uretral meatus. They are rarely detected on the penile skin. Macules may be the only feature, or they may be associated with condylomata acuminata or papules. They may even occur around clinically identifiable lesions, thus showing the extent of viral infection. Moreover, their appearence at a site where previous condylomas have been treated and healed is suggestive of the persistence of HPV infection. In our series, one patient submitted to colposcopy, since his wife presented cervical

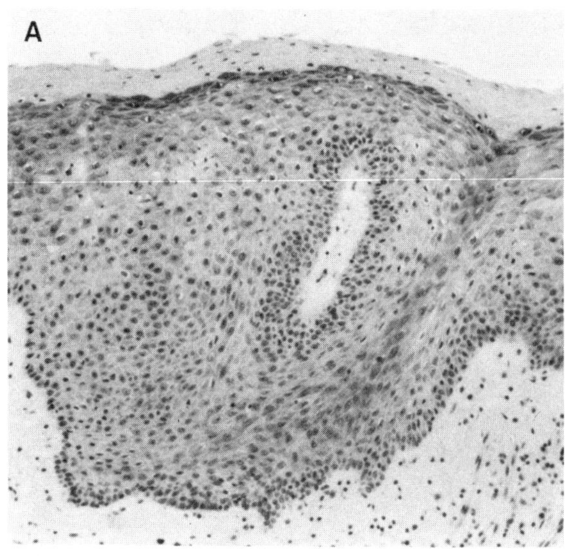

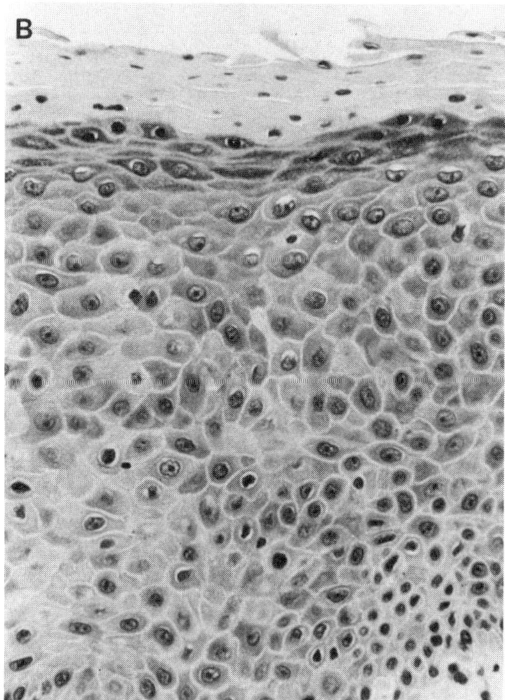

FIGURE 6–13 Histology of penile acetowhite papules in Figure 6–11: papillomatous changes with marked parakeratosis (H+E, × 200 [A], × 450 [B]).

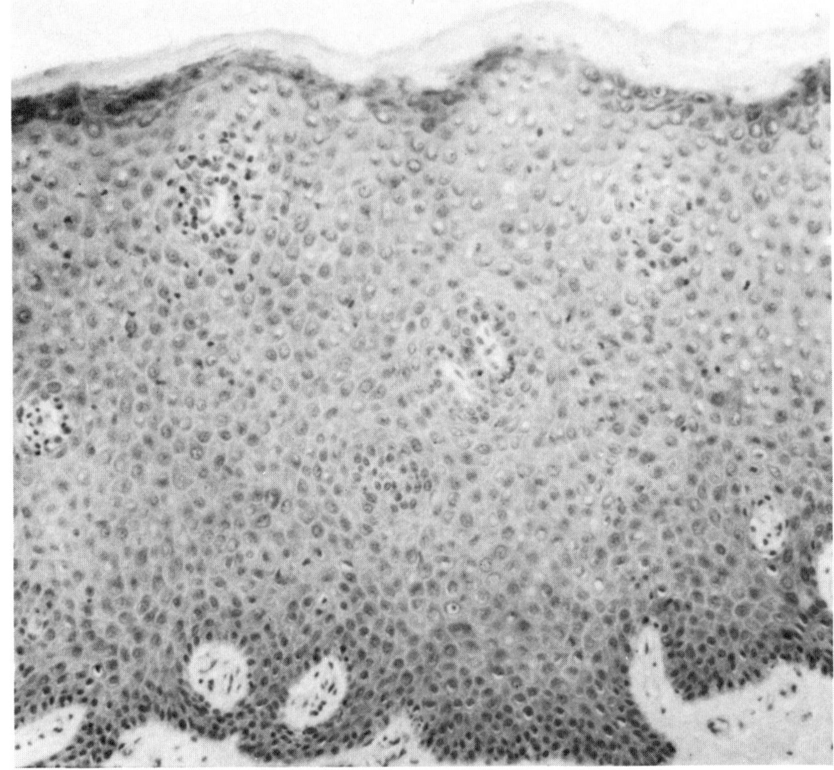

FIGURE 6–14 Histology of penile acetowhite papules showing papillomatous changes with discrete focal parakeratosis. Virology: as yet uncharacterized HPV type (H + E, × 200).

intraepithelial neoplasia (CIN) III and showed a macule at the clinically normal site where a condyloma was treated 8 years earlier.

However, macules do not always correspond to HPV infection. About 50% of such areas show minimal or no HPV-related histologic changes,[7] and not more than 40% of lesions with minimal histologic changes contained detectable HPV DNA in a previous study.[7] There is no clinical or colposcopic criterion that allows a distinction between HPV-positive and negative macules.

We stress that penile macules must be distinguished from diffuse and ill-defined aceto-whitening and from well-delimited white areas devoid of capillary loops. Such areas may correspond to various infections as herpes virus, traumatic abrasion (Figure 6–24), candidiasis (Figure 6–25), nonspecific irritation, or healing after treatment. A clinical distinction is often possible since these conditions usually regress after local treatment.

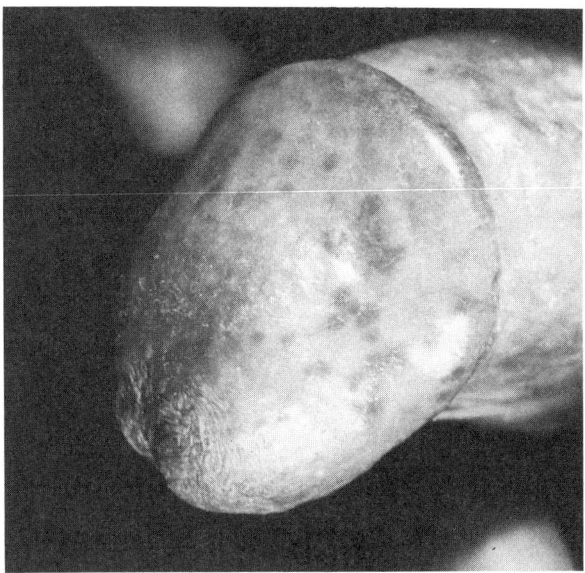

FIGURE 6–15 Bowenoid papules on the glans: small, rounded, somewhat raised, and slightly pinkish.

Histology

Histology of macules may show features ranging from minimal histologic changes to high-grade intraepithelial neoplasia. In our experience, macules on a previously normal epithelium mostly consist of endophytic papillomas (Figure 6–22) or, less frequently, of flat lesions displaying only minimal histologic changes, ie, parakeratosis and acanthosis. They rarely show features of condyloma. Macules appearing on a previously red area mostly show features of intraepithelial neoplasia (Figures 6–20, 6–21)

Virology

All genital HPV types may be identified in penile macules.[7,30,31] HPV 6 and 11 are mostly associated with the few macules showing histologic features of condyloma, while potentially oncogenic HPVs are associated with about 70% of erythematous macules, like the pigmented papules, showing histologic features of intraepithelial neoplasia. Thus, the latter need to be biopsied before treatment. HPV 42 is by far the most prevalent MPV type in nonerythematous macules showing histologic features of endophytic papilloma without koilocytosis (70% of positive lesions in our series). As-yet-uncharacterized types are also found in such lesions. In situ hybridization on HPV-42-associated endophytic papillomas is mostly positive, the signal

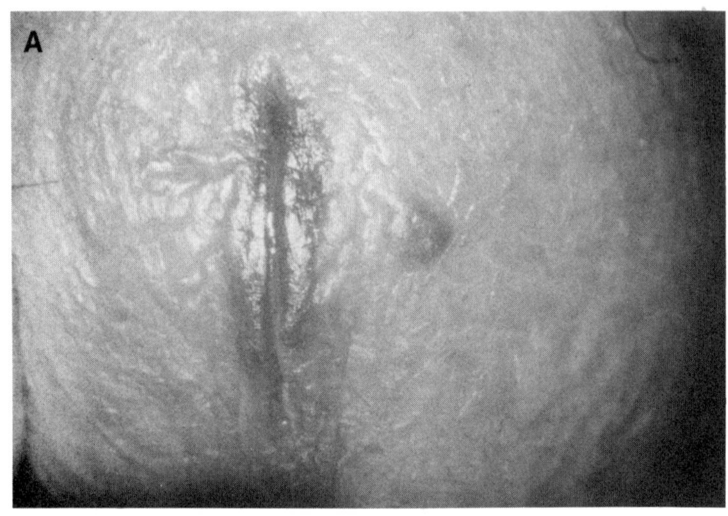

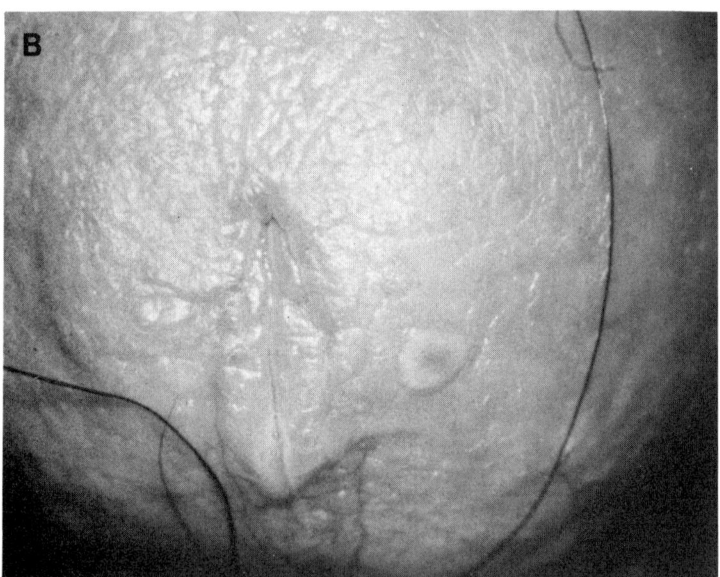

FIGURE 6–16 Colposcopy: A) red papule of the glans, which B) markedly reacts to the acetic acid test. Histology: penile intraepithelial neoplasia. Virology: HPV 16 ($\times$ 12).

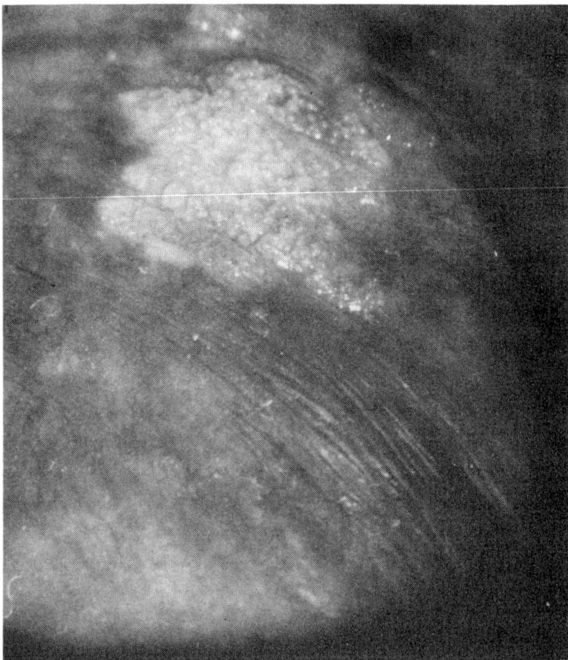

FIGURE 6–17 Colposcopy: white papular area of the prepuce, after laser treatment for condylomata acuminata. Histology: penile intraepithelial neoplasia. Virology: HPV 16. The female partner presented HPV-16-assciated cervical intraepithelial neoplasia. The couple did not use condoms after the male laser treatment for condylomata ($\times$ 12).

being stronger at the surface of lesions (O Croissant et al, in preparation). This suggests that endophytic papilloma without koilocytosis is a new HPV-associated lesion, in which virus might replicate. The infectious potential of these lesions suggests that they need to be treated.

Virtually all acetowhite areas that do not correspond to our description of macules show minimal (parakeratosis, acanthosis) or nonspecific histologic changes and are HPV-negative.

In conclusion, for clinical purposes, we stress that colposcopy and histology allow the identification of subclinical HPV-associated lesions among acetowhite areas. Macules showing histologic features of endophytic papilloma, condyloma, or intraepithelial neoplasia need to be treated. Acetowhite areas showing other histologic features should not be considered as HPV-associated lesions. If HPV DNA is evidenced by blot hybridization or by more sensitive techniques (polymerase chain reaction) in specimens from such areas, a positive in situ hybridization is needed to distinguish HPV-associated lesions from epithelial areas containing latent HPV infection (M Stoler, personal communication).

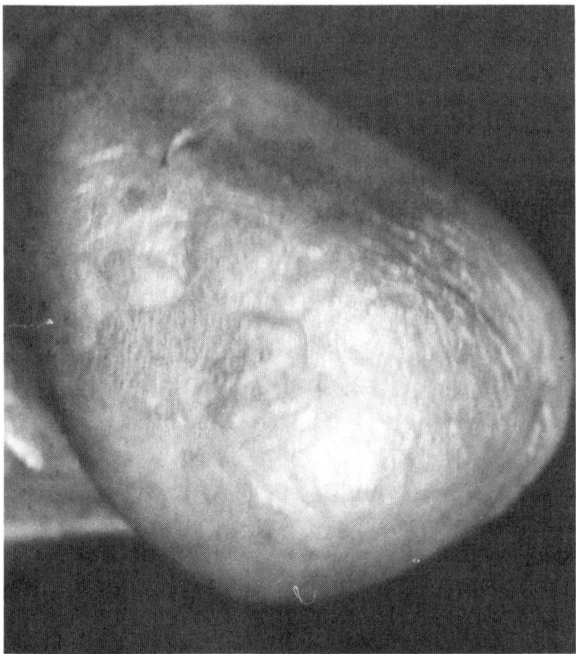

FIGURE 6–18 Pseudobowenoid papules. Flat papules were found to be associated with HPV 6. The clinical appearance is the same as that of bowenoid papulosis.

At the actual state of knowledge, destructive treatment of acetowhite epithelial areas not showing histologic features of endophytic papilloma, condyloma, or intraepithelial neoplasia, even in the case of HPV-positive blot hybridization, is not justified.

GENITAL BOWEN'S CARCINOMA

The Bowen's cancer in situ, erythroplasia of Queyrat, a well-demarcated, flat, solitary lesion located on the glans (Figure 6–26) occurs in elderly patients, and this might be due to a decreased immunity in old age.[32,33] The changes may last more than 10 years but may also show transition into invasive carcinoma in about 10% of the cases (Figure 6–27).[34] The noninvasive and invasive Bowen's carcinomas are associated with the same types of HPVs as bowenoid papulosis, and the greatest risk factor for developing invasive cancer in the patients infected with potentially oncogenic HPVs appears to be the age of the patients, as found also by Crum et al[35] for vulvar intraepithelial neoplasia (VIN), as well as the susceptibility of the tissue to the specific HPV infection and the immune state of the patient.

In our series, two of four biopsies from noninvasive Bowen's carcinoma

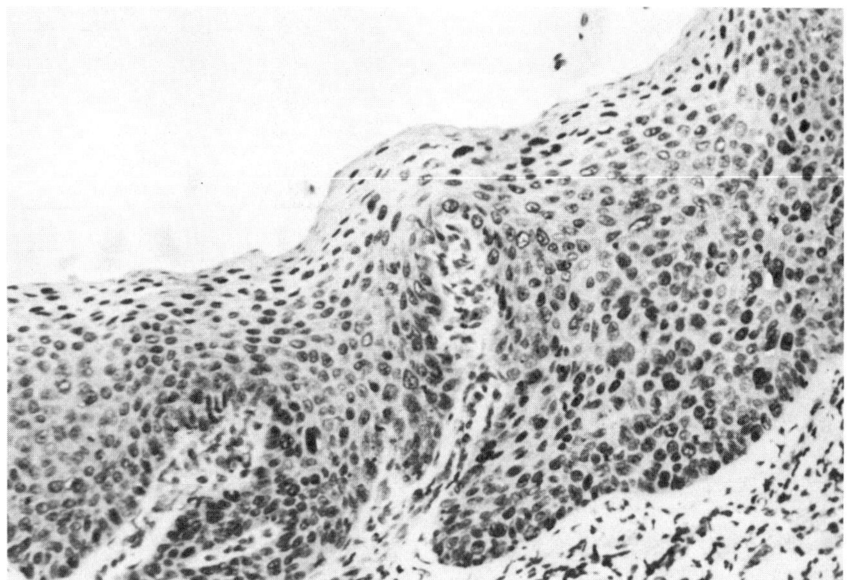

FIGURE 6–19 Histology of bowenoid papules: penile intraepithelial neoplasia grade III, with numerous abnormal mitoses and dyskeratotic and pleomorphic cells (H+E, × 200).

contained HPV DNA type 33, and two were negative. Four of ten biopsies from invasive Bowen's disease contained HPV DNA (type 16 in three cases, an as yet undetermined type in one case), and six were negative. The same types of HPV were detected in our series in females with genital Bowen's disease.

VERRUCOUS CARCINOMA

This is a slowly growing, locally destructive carcinoma with relatively benign histologic features, developing from long-lasting, proliferating gigantic condylomas.[36–38] The development of a squamous-cell carcinoma from a penile verrucous carcinoma occurs either spontaneously or after excision and relapse.[39,40] However, the metastases are very rare.[41] Histology is characterized by broad, expanding rete ridges, well-differentiated squamous epithelium with pronounced hyperkeratosis, and an increased number of mitoses. However, the dermalepidermal border remains intact until the lesion transforms into squamous-cell carcinoma.

The virological studies have disclosed an association of verrucous carcinoma with some subtypes of HPV 6.[21,42–44] A new HPV, tentatively named HPV 54 (G Orth, S Jablonska, et al, in preparation), was characterized from one typical case in a 40-year-old man with condylomata of the penis since

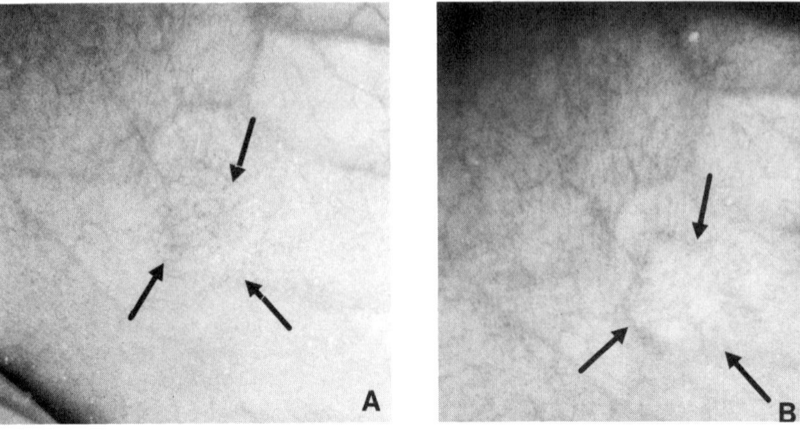

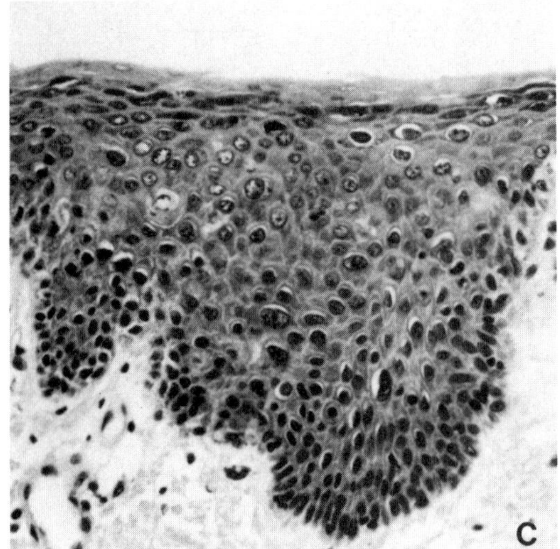

FIGURE 6–20 Colposcopy: A) erythematous area showing B) a discrete white reaction after the acetic acid test. Histology C): penile intraepithelial neoplasia, featuring mild diskariosis. Virology: HPV 16 ($\times$ 12).

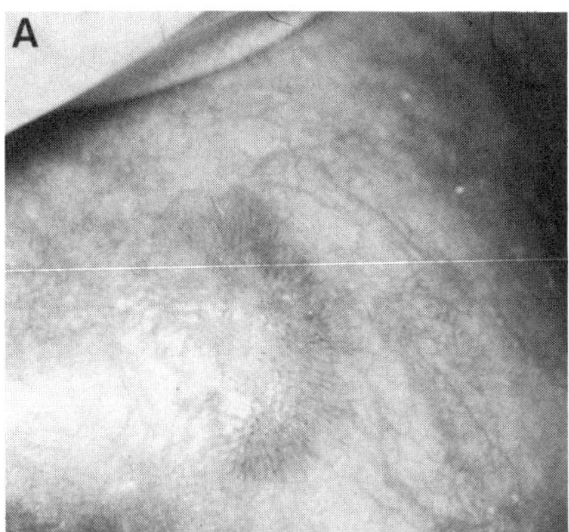
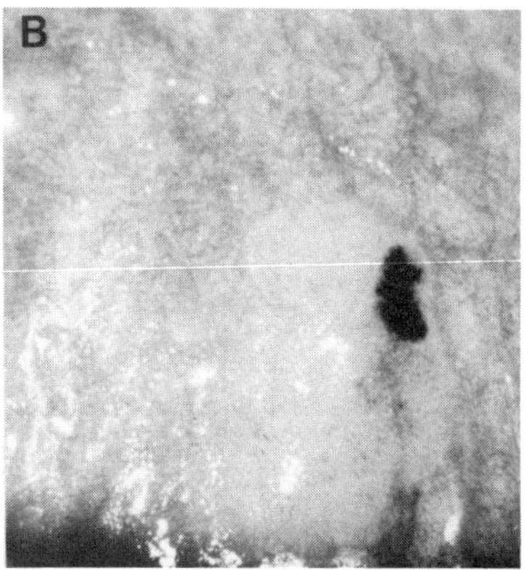
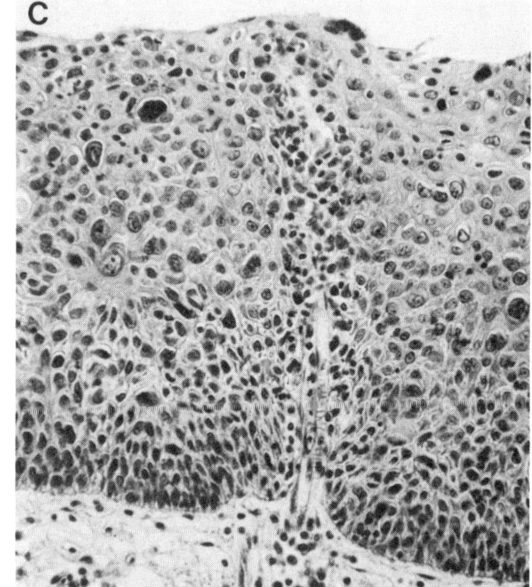

FIGURE 6–21 Colposcopy: A) erythematous area showing B) a marked reaction after the acetic acid test. Histology: C) penile intraepithelial neoplasia. Virology: as-yet-uncharacterized HPV type ($\times$ 12).

age 23, which became gigantic and locally invasive, of Buschke-Lowenstein type, at age 40. Of importance is that this patient died of laryngeal carcinoma, which developed from papilloma 9 years after surgery for verrucous carcinoma of the penis. The histology of penile lesions preserved benign features in spite of an almost complete destruction of genitalia. Laryngeal carcinoma had a structure of carcinoma planoepitheliale keratodes.

The anal lesions of verrucous carcinoma have the same features as

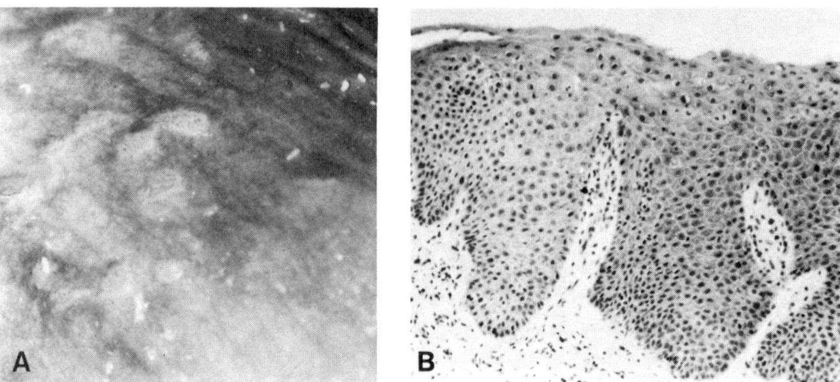

FIGURE 6–22 A) Colposcopy: well-delimited white areas showing surface vascular punctuation appearing after acetic acid test on a previously normal epithelium. B) Histology: endophytic papilloma, lacking koilocytosis. Virology: HPV 42 (× 12).

those in the penile area. In one case studied by us, the condylomatous lesions had been present for 15 years before malignant transformation, and they were associated with HPV 6 as a unique virus, found also in a metastatic tumor that developed after irradiation of the primary verrucous carcinoma. In another case, verrucous anal carcinoma was found to be associated with

FIGURE 6–23 Colposcopy: small, well-delimited white area after acetic acid test. Histology: endophytic papilloma, lacking koilocytosis. Virology: HPV 42 (× 12).

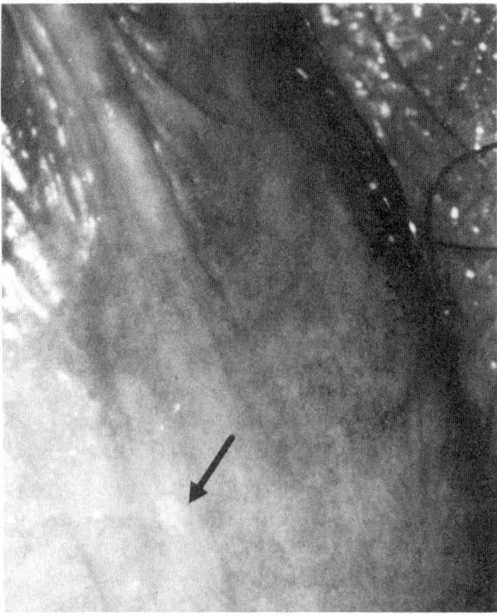

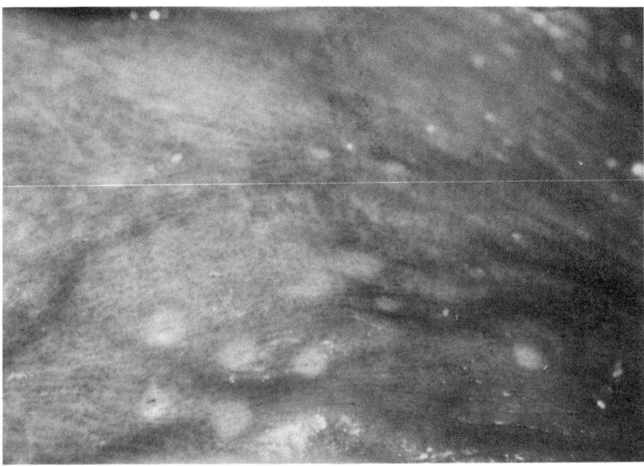

FIGURE 6–24 Colposcopy: several small abrasions of the prepucial mucosa, whitening after the acetic acid test. Lesions lack the surface vascular punctuation. Histology: inflammatory. Virology: negative ($\times$ 12).

HPV 33. Human papillomavirus-16-related DNA sequences were also found in five of six verrucous carcinomas of the larynx.[45]

Pseudoepitheliomatous micaceous and keratotic balanitis are, in essence, unusual clinical varieties of verrucous carcinoma of the penis, differing by gross manifestation but with similar histologic features and

FIGURE 6–25 Colposcopy: diffuse and ill-delimited white reaction of the glans mucosa after the acetic acid test. Bacteriology: Candidiasis. Virology: negative. Normal after local treatment ($\times$ 12).

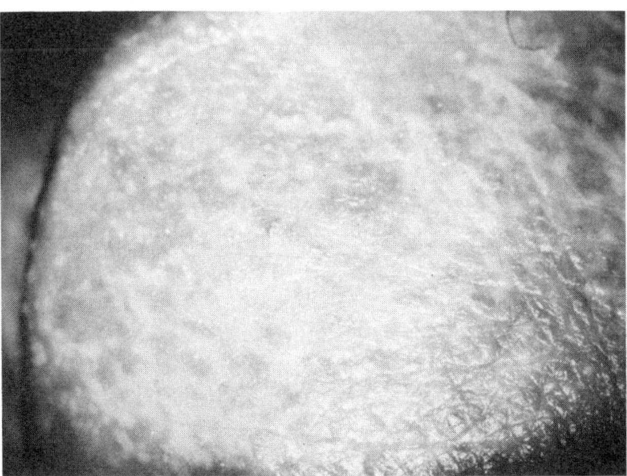

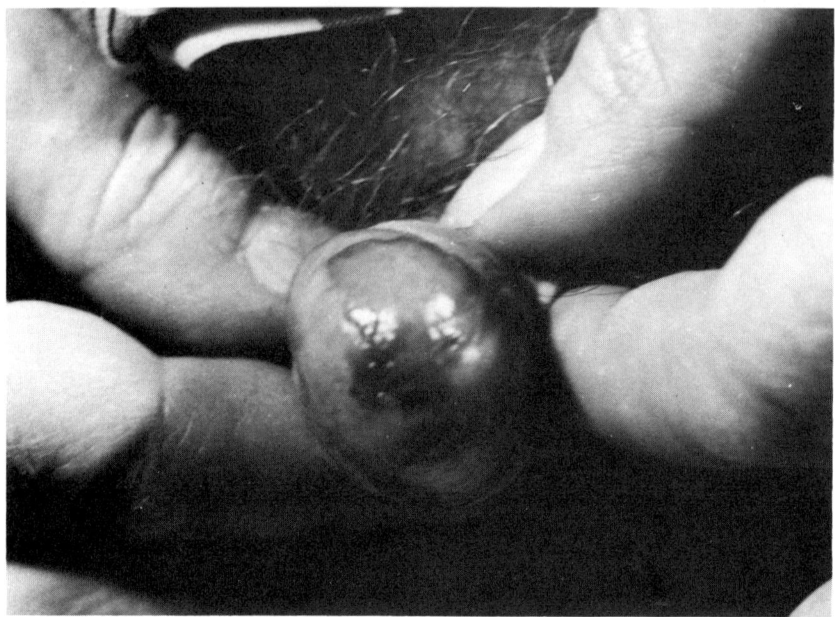

FIGURE 6–26 Erythroplasia of Queyrat. A single, dull-red patch on the glans of sharp, irregular outline, showing little infiltration.

oncogenic potential, ie, possible transformation into a squamous-cell carcinoma.[46] Virological association has not yet been studied.

THE SEXUAL TRANSMISSION

The sexual transmission of genital warts has been known since the age of the ancient Greeks and Romans (for review, see ref 13). Epidemiologic studies on sexual contacts of individuals with warts suggest an infectious rate of at least 65%.[13,47] A prospective study on virgin women partners of individuals with disease showed 100% transmission.[13]

The association of cervical flat condylomata with HPV infection[48] and the detection of HPV DNA 16 in cervical[3] and vulvar[6] precancers, that have linked papillomaviruses already known to be responsible for genital warts, to the possible development of cervical cancer, strengthens the hypothesis of the venereal origin of cervical cancer and of the existence of a male reservoir of a venereal factor potentially oncogenic for the uterine cervix.

The biologic link among HPV-associated lesions of external genitalia and cervical precancers was confirmed by the detection of cervical condyloma or intraepithelial neoplasia in 76% of female partners of men with genital warts.[49] Cervical intraepithelial neoplasia was also found in partners

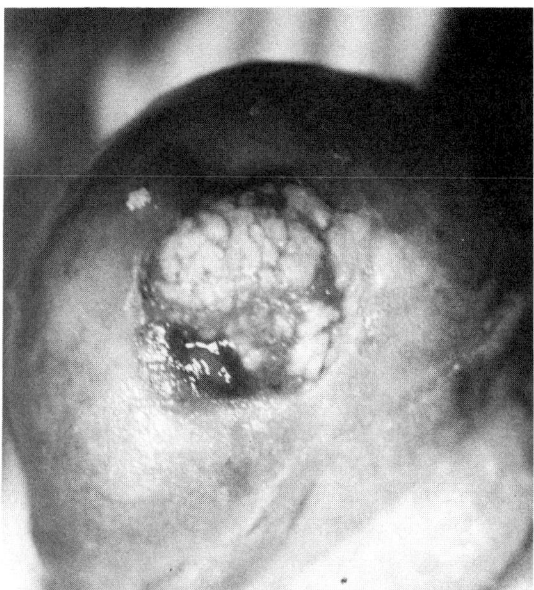

FIGURE 6–27 Invasive penile carcinoma. A raised, verrucous, fungoid tumor, which developed from noninvasive Bowen's disease of a relatively low-grade of malignancy.

of men with bowenoid papulosis[25] and in women with vulvar intraepithelial or invasive neoplasia.

All these epidemiologic, clinical, and virologic findings have justified the introduction of the screening of the asymptomatic male partners of women with cervical HPV-associated lesions. However, only after the use of the colposcope[11] and of the acetic acid test[23] was proposed for this screening, 53–80% of male partners of women with cervical flat condyloma or intraepithelial neoplasia were shown to present easily detectable or discrete genital lesions that mostly displayed histologic features of HPV infection.[11,23,50] The use of the acetic acid test also allowed the detection of subclinical lesions, which appeared only after the application of the test,[12] and that may show features of intraepithelial neoplasia[12] and contain potentially oncogenic HPVs.[7,30,31]

When histologic features in regular partners have been correlated, about one-third of male partners of women with CIN have been shown to present PIN.[7] Nine percent of partners of women with CIN III presented PIN III,[31] while about 40% of partners of women with cervical flat condyloma have been shown to present penile condyloma, and only 2% intraepithelial neoplasia.[7] However, a 36% frequency of CIN in female partners of men with genital lesions defined as warts has also been reported.[49]

When the presence of HPV infection has been virologically studied by genital scrapings in women with disease and in their regular partners, one-third[26] to one-half[51] of couples have been shown to harbor the same HPV type. Correlative clinical, histologic, and virological studies have revealed that condylomata acuminata of external genitalia, when present in both partners, mostly contain the same HPV type (6,11),[52] as well as concomitant CIN and PIN (HPV 16 or 33) (G Orth, R Barrasso, et al, in preparation). However, virologic correlation is poor in partners showing other presumably HPV-associated lesions, ie, cervical flat condyloma and papules and macules of external genitalia with histologic features of condyloma, papilloma, or minimal changes. Partners may be infected by different HPV types; double infection in one or both partners is a frequent event, as well as the lack of HPV DNA identification in one or both partners. Prolonged incubation time, acquired immunity, and spontaneous regression could explain some of those discrepancies, thus underlying the difficulties of the study of the sexual transmission of genital HPVs.

On the other hand, in situ hybridization has shown the presence of viral DNA in superficial cells from colposcopically detected and histologically endophytic lesions presenting papillomatosis without koilocytosis (O Croissant, personal communication). Thus, in our opinion, those lesions should be considered potentially infectious and, as a consequence, treated.

Studies on the application of uretral cytology to screen males has produced unsatisfactory results,[11,53] and the significance of the identification of viral DNA in penile scrapings from men with colposcopically and histologically normal tissue[54,55] remains to be elucidated.

In conclusion, there is a strong association of various penile lesions with the diversity of specific papillomaviruses. The HPV typing, as related to the gross, colposcopic, and histologic features, is of basic importance for diagnosing and preventing malignant conversion. Moreover, the finding of the same potentially oncogenic HPV in concomitant CIN and VIN,[25] VIN and PIN,[26] and CIN and PIN (G Orth, R Barrasso, et al, in preparation) provides evidence for the oncogenic potential and the sexual transmission of those viruses, as well as the need for a systematic male partner screening and treatment. For this purpose, the detection of genital lesions with the aid of the acetic acid test and of the colposcope actually seems to be the most effective method.

ACKNOWLEDGMENTS

We are indebted to Gerard Orth for all the virologic studies reported in this chapter, for personal communications, and for his advice and encouragement during this undertaking. We are very grateful to Odile Croissant for personal communications and fruitful discussions.

REFERENCES

1. Dunn AEG, Ogilvie MM: Intranuclear virus particles in human genital wart tissue: Observations on the ultrastructure of the epidermal layer. J Ultrastruct Res 1968;22:282.

2. De Villiers EM, Gissmann L, zur Hausen H: Molecular cloning of viral DNA from human genital warts. J Virol 1981;40:932.
3. Durst M, Gissmann L, Ikenberg H, et al: A papillomavirus DNA from a cervical carcinoma and its prevalence in cancer biopsy samples from different geographic regions. Proc Natl Acad Sci USA 1983;80:3812.
4. Crum CP, Mitao M, Levine RU, et al: Cervical papillomaviruses segregate within morphologically distinct precancerous lesions. J Virol 1985;54:675.
5. Boshart M, Gissmann L, Ikenberg H: A new type of papillomavirus DNA, its presence in genital cancer biopsies and in cell lines derived from cervical cancer. EMBO J 1984;3:1151.
6. Ikenberg H, Gissmann L, Gross G, et al: Human papillomavirus type 16-related DNA in genital Bowen's disease and in bowenoid papulosis. Int J Cancer 1983;32:563.
7. Barrasso R, de Brux J, Croissant O, et al: High prevalence of papillomavirus-associated penile intraepithelial neoplasia in sexual partners of women with cervical intraepithelial neoplasia. New Engl J Med 1987;317:916.
8. McCance DJ, Kalache A, Ashdown K, et al: Human papillomavirus types 16 and 18 in carcinomas of the penis from Brazil. Int J Cancer 1986;37:55.
9. Rotkin ID: A comparison review of key epidemiological studies in cervical cancer related to current searches for transmissible agents. Cancer Res 1973;33:1353.
10. Kessler II: Venereal factors in human cervical cancer: evidence for marital clusters. Cancer 1977;39:1912.
11. Levine RU, Crum CP, Herman E, et al: Cervical papillomavirus infection and intraepithelial neoplasia: A study of the male sexual partner. Obstet Gynecol 1984;64:16.
12. Barrasso R, Guillemotonia A, Catalan F, et al: Lésions génitales masculines à Papillomavirus: intérêt de la colposcopie. Ann Dermatol 1986;113:787.
13. Oriel JD: Natural history of genital warts. Br J Vener Dis 1971;47:1.
14. von Krogh G, Syrjänen SM, Syrjänen KJ: Advantage of human papillomaviruses typing in the clinical evaluation of genitoanal warts. Experience with in situ deoxyribonucleic acid hybridization technique applied on paraffine sections. J Am Acad Dermatol 1988;18:495.
15. Gartman E: Intraurethral verruca acuminata in men. J Urol 1956;75:717.
16. Pettersson S: Condyloma acuminatum of the bladder. J Urol 1976;115:535.
17. Rüdlinger R, Grob R, Buchmann P, et al: Anogenital warts of the condyloma acuminatum type in HIV-positive patients. Dermatologica 1988;176:277.
18. Johnson BL, Baxter DL: Pearly penile papules. Arch Dermatol 1964;90:166.
19. Oriel JD: Genital warts. In: Holmes KK, Mardh PA, Sparling PF, Wiesner PJ, eds. Sexually transmitted diseases. New York: McGraw-Hill Inc. 1984;496–507.
20. Gissmann L, Diehl V, Schultz-Coulon HJ, et al: Molecular cloning and characterisation of human papillomavirus DNA derived from a laryngeal papilloma. J Virol 1982;44:393.
21. Gissmann L, Wolnik L, Ikenberg H, et al: Human papillomaviruses types 6 and 11 DNA sequences in genital and laryngeal papillomas and in some cervical cancers. Proc Natl Acad Sci USA 1983;80:560.
22. Rosemberg SK: The subclinical papillomavirus infection of the male genitalia. Urology 1985;26:554.
23. Sedlacek TV, Cunnane M, Carpiniello V: Colposcopy in the diagnosis of penile condyloma. AM J Obstet Gynecol 1986;154:494.
24. Wade TR, Kopf AW, Ackerman AB: Bowenoid papulosis of the penis. Cancer 1978;42:1890.
25. Obalek S, Jablonska S, Beaudenon S, et al: Bowenoid papulosis of the male and female genitalia: risk of cervical neoplasia. J Am Acad Dermatol 1986;14:433.
26. Gross G, Ikenberg H, de Villiers EM, et al: Bowenoid papulosis: a venereally transmitted disease as reservoir for HPV 16. Banbury Rep 1986;21:149.
27. Obalek S, Jablonska S, Orth G: HPV-associated intraepithelial neoplasia of external genitalia. Clin Dermatol 1985;3:104.
28. Beaudenon S, Kremsdorf D, Croissant O, et al: A novel type of human papillomavirus associated with genital neoplasias. Nature 1986;321:246.

29. Beaudenon S, Kremsdorf D, Obalek S, et al: Plurality of genital human papillomaviruses: characterisation of two new types with distinct biological properties. Virology 1987;161:374.
30. Syrjänen SM, von Krogh G, Syrjänen KJ: Detection of human papillomavirus DNA in anogenital condylomata in men using in situ DNA Hybridization applied to paraffine sections. Genitourin Med 1987;63:32.
31. Campion MJ, McCance DJ, Mitchell HS, et al: Subclinical penile human papillomavirus infection and dysplasia in consorts of women with cervical neoplasia. Genitour Med 1988;64:90.
32. Cobleigh MA, Braun DP, Harris JE: Age-dependent changes in human peripheral blood B cells and T cells subsets: correlation with mitogen responsiveness. Clin Immunol Immunopathol 1980;15:162.
33. Jablonska S, Majewski S, Obalek S, et al: Age-related variability of ano-genital lesions induced by potentially oncogenic human papillomaviruses. Giorn Ital Chir Derm Oncol 1987;2:347.
34. Graham JH, Helwig EB: Erythroplasia of Queyrat: A clinicopathological and histochemical study. Cancer 1973;32:1396.
35. Crum CP, Liskow A, Petras P, et al: Vulvar intraepithelial neoplasia (severe atypia and carcinoma in situ): a clinicopathologic analysis of 41 cases. Cancer 1984;54:1429.
36. Buschke E, Loewenstein L: Über carcinomähnliche Condylomata acuminata des Penis. Arch Dermatol Syph (Berlin) 1931;163:30.
37. Davies SW: Giant condylomata acuminata: incidence among cases diagnosed as carcinoma of the penis. J Clin Pathol 1965;18:142.
38. Dawson DF, Duckworth JK, Bernhardt H, et al: Giant condyloma and verrucous carcinoma of the genital area. Arch Pathol 1965;79:225.
39. Youngberg GA, Thonnthwaite JT, Inoshita T, et al: Cytologically malignant squamous cell carcinoma, verrucous carcinoma of the penis. J Dermatol Surg Oncol 1983;9:474.
40. Johnson DE, Lo RK, Srigley J, et al: Verrucous carcinoma of the penis. J Urol 1985;133:216.
41. Kraus FT, Perez-Mesa C: Verrucous carcinoma: clinical and pathologic study of 105 cases involving oral cavity, larynx and genitalia. Cancer 1986;19:26.
42. Okagaki T: Female genital tumors associated with human papillomavirus infection, and the concept of genital neoplasm papilloma syndrome (GENPS). Pathol Annu 1984;19:31.
43. Boshart M, zur Hausen H: Human papillomaviruses in Buschke-Löwenstein tumors: Physical state of the DNA and identification of a tandem duplication in the non coding region of a human papillomavirus 6 subtype. J Virol 1986;58:363.
44. Rando RF, Groff DE, Chirikjian JG, et al: Isolation and characterisation of a novel human papillomavirus type 6 DNA from an invasive vulvar carcinoma. J Virol 1983;57:353.
45. Abramson AL, Brandsma J, Steinberg B, et al: Verrucous carcinoma of the larynx. Acta Otolaryngol 1985;111:709.
46. Beljaards RC, van Dijk E, Hausman R: Is pseudoepitheliomatous micaceous and keratotic balanitis synonymous with verrucous carcinoma? Br J Dermatol 1987;117:641.
47. Teokharov BA: Non-gonococcal infections of the female genitalia. Br J Vener Dis 1969;45:334.
48. Meisels A, Fortin R, Roy M: Condylomatous lesions of the cervix. II. Cytologic, colposcopic and histopathologic study. Acta Cytol 1977;21:379.
49. Campion MJ, Singer A, Clarkson PK, et al: Increased risk of cervical neoplasia in consorts of men with penile condylomata acuminata. Lancet 1985;i:943.
50. Sand PK, Bowen LW, Blischke SO, et al: Evaluation of male consorts of women with genital human papillomavirus infection. Obstet Gynecol 1986;68:679.
51. Schneider A, Sawada E, Gissmann L, et al: Human papillomaviruses in women with a history of abnormal papanicolau smears and in their male partners. Obstet Gynecol 1987;69:554–62.
52. Wickenden C, Taylor-Robinson D, Harris JRW, et al: Sexual transmission of human papillomaviruses in heterosexual and male homosexual couples, studied by DNA hybridization. Genitourin Med 1988;64:34.

53. Nahhas WA, Marshall ML, Ponziani J, et al: Evaluation of urinary cytology of male sexual partners of women with cervical intraepithelial neoplasia and human papilloma virus infection. Gynecol Oncol 1986;24:279.

54. Grussendorf-Conen El, de Villiers EM, Gissmann L: Human papillomavirus genomes in penile smears of healthy men. Lancet 1986_:1092.

55. Rosemberg SK, Reid R, Greenberg M, et al: Sexually transmitted papillomaviral infection in the male: II. The urethral reservoir. Urology 1988;32:47.

CHAPTER 7

Clinical Spectrum of HPV Infection in the Neonate and Child

Larry S. Hirschfield, MD and Bettie M. Steinberg, PhD

With the dramatic increase in incidence of human papillomavirus (HPV) infections in adults, one would logically expect a parallel increase in the incidence of childhood infections. Indeed, there is some indication that although it is rare in the pediatric age group, the incidence of anogenital condyloma acuminata may be increasing. It is difficult to determine whether cases of juvenile onset respiratory papillomatosis are increasing. They have not been reported with increased frequency, but this is not a legally mandated, reportable disease. A future increase in incidence of this serious condition may also be on the horizon. The practicing obstetrician and gynecologist should be aware of the clinical features of HPV-induced diseases in children and recognize the possible routes of acquisition of these childhood infections. Only with this knowledge can intelligent recommendations regarding management of pregnancy and delivery be made.

CLINICAL SPECTRUM OF HPV-INDUCED DISEASE IN CHILDREN

Juvenile Onset Respiratory Papillomatosis

Laryngeal papillomas are rapidly growing benign epithelial tumors caused by HPV. They are usually located on the true vocal cords and epiglottis but can involve the entire larynx as well as the tracheobronchial tree and even the lungs. Figure 7–1 shows the appearance of papillomas on the vocal folds, in contrast to a normal larynx. Although the actual incidence of the disease in the United States is unknown, estimates place the figure at approximately 1/100,000 people. In spite of its relatively low incidence, laryngeal papillomatosis is of major concern because of the significant morbidity and mortality with which it is associated. Laryngeal papillomas have a bimodal

Clinical Practice of Gynecology: **2,** 102–116, 1989

ISSN 1043-3198/89/$3.50

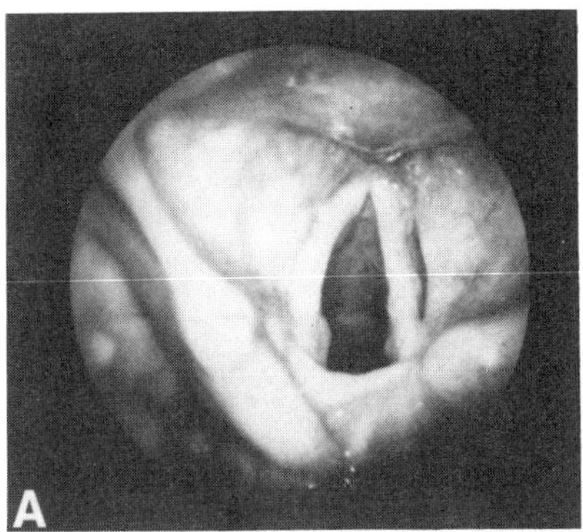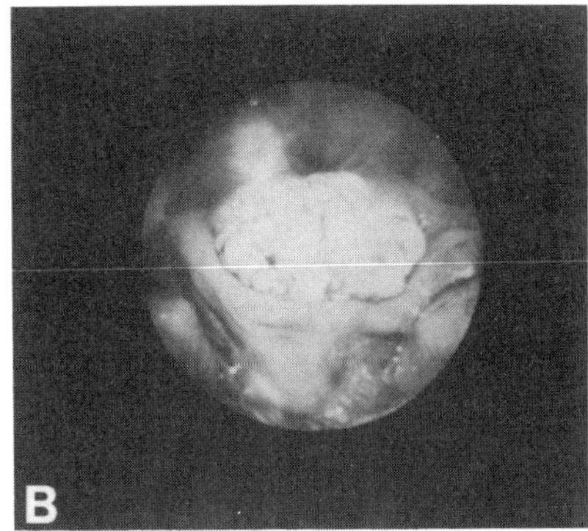

FIGURE 7–1 (A) Normal vocal cords; (B) laryngeal opening completely obstructed by papilloma.

age distribution with the first major peak occurring in children between 2 and 5 years of age and the second peak occurring in the second decade.[1] In a series of 90 children with laryngeal papillomatosis, 61 (68%) of the children developed symptoms prior to 4 years of age.[2] The male to female ratio is about equal in the juvenile onset group, but a 2 to 1 male predominance is noted in the adult onset group.[3] Clinical symptoms usually start as hoarseness or abnormal cry with subsequent respiratory distress, stridor, and aphonia. In rare instances, a child may present with severe airway obstruction requiring tracheostomy. Further morbidity results from extension of laryngeal papillomas into the tracheobronchial tree and lung parenchyma. Extension of disease from the larynx to the trachea has been reported to occur between 2% and 36% of cases.[4,5] All studies agree that the incidence of tracheal disease is greater than 50% in patients who have undergone a tracheotomy to establish and maintain an airway. For this reason, tracheotomy is avoided as far as is possible in the management of these patients. Pulmonary extension, while rare, is extremely difficult to manage and frequently fatal.

Laryngeal papillomas appear as white or pink/red, glistening wartlike masses composed of vascular connective tissue cords covered by a hyperplastic stratified squamous epithelium (Figure 7–2). On the basis of the histologic appearance and the absence of submucosal invasion, papillomas are classified as benign tumors. A mild degree of cellular atypia is not unusual, particularly in juvenile onset papillomas and is not felt to indicate a malignant potential. Several well-documented cases of malignant transformation of laryngeal papillomas, however, have been reported in the literature. The incidence of spontaneous transformation is very low, although radiation markedly increases the risk of malignant conversion. In a large study of patients at the Mayo Clinic from 1914 to 1960, 14% of 43 treated with radiation therapy developed squamous cell carcinoma, while a control

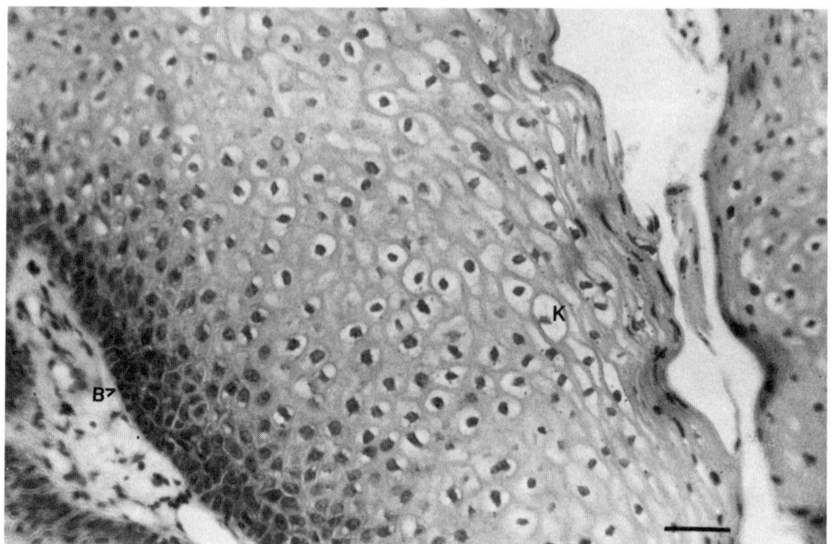

FIGURE 7–2 Histological section of hyperplastic stratified squamous epithelium of laryngeal papilloma. K, cells with cytoplasmic halos resembling koilocytes; B, Basal cell layer.

group of 58 papilloma patients treated with surgery alone showed no malignant conversion.[6] The low rate of spontaneous malignant change of respiratory papillomas is in contrast to that of cervical condylomas, which have a significant risk of conversion.

The most notable characteristic of laryngeal papillomas is their tendency to recur following surgical removal. Table 7–1A,B summarizes some of the clinical data for 57 patients at Long Island Jewish Medical Center.[7] The pattern is typical for this disease. The need for repeated surgery is seen in both the adult onset and childhood onset group. The majority of patients in both groups required surgery at least once or twice per year. Juvenile onset disease tends to recur with greater frequency, but some adult onset patients also have rapid recurrences.

Another characteristic of recurrent laryngeal papillomas is their tendency to regress spontaneously in the majority of patients. Remission can be temporary, or it can last for the lifetime of the patient. Since there is always the possibility of recurrence, we talk only about remission, not cure. It is possible that hormonal status plays some role in the course of laryngeal papillomatosis. It is generally believed that juvenile onset disease regresses around the time of puberty, although this is by no means the rule. Hormonal changes during pregnancy may also affect the clinical course of laryngeal papillomas. The patients described in Table 7–1A,B include 10 who became pregnant. Of the six who were already in remission, only one had a reac-

TABLE 7–1A. Clinical History of Juvenile Onset Papilloma

Age at Onset (Years)	Sex	No. of Operative Procedures	Years with Active Disease	NED* (Years)
4 Mo	M	4	2	3
5 Mo	F	7	2	5
11 Mo	M	10	2	2
1½	F	2	2	1
1½	F	7	3	6
2	F	15	8	6
2	F	19	4	5
2½	F	38	11	**
2½	F	62	26	**
2½	M	23	3	5
2½	F	5	3	**
2½	F	54	27	**
3	M	5	5	6
3	M	7	4	4
3	M	118	23	**
3	M	21	5	**
3	F	7	3	6
3	M	46	5	5
3	F	35	20	5
4	F	11	45	5
4	F	11	8	3
4	M	85	12	**
5	F	12	4	7
6	F	2	2	2
7	M	2	2	**
9	M	5	5	3
9	M	41	27	**
9	M	1	1	1
10	F	2	6	8
13	M	1	1	2
13	M	3	2	*

*NED, no evidence of disease.
**Active disease.

tivation of disease. Three of the four with active disease required increased frequency of surgery during pregnancy, and one was unchanged. In all cases where pregnancy aggravated the disease, frequency of surgery returned to previous levels as soon as the babies were born.

Although a viral etiology has long been suspected in laryngeal papillomas, only recently has clearcut evidence of the presence of virus in these lesions been provided. Lack et al[8] found HPV antigens in laryngeal papillomas from 26 of 35 patients (74%). Further evidence that laryngeal papillomas are caused by HPV is the homology between DNA probes prepared from known HPVs and the DNA isolated from laryngeal papillomas. In 1980 Quick et al, using Southern blot hybridization, reported that HPV 2 hybridized to

TABLE 7–1B. Clinical History of Adult Onset Papilloma

Age at Onset (Years)	Sex	No. of Operative Procedures	Years with Active Disease	NED* (Years)
20	M	7	3	**
20	F	19	5	1
21	M	5	5	6
23	F	10	5	**
24	F	6	3	6
26	F	4	3	3
26	M	3	3	4
27	M	4	3	3
27	F	3	1	10
27	M	2	2	**
27	F	2	2	7
29	M	2	7	2
30	F	5	5	2
30	F	2	6	10
31	M	2	2	**
32	M	5	7	**
32	M	7	9	**
33	M	8	5	1
35	M	14	3	**
37	M	7	26	**
38	F	2	3	5
39	M	2	2	5
46	F	55	31	1
49	F	12	2	**
56	M	5	2	**
60	M	6	3	2
67	M	7	6	3

*NED, no evidence of disease.
**Active disease.

two of nine laryngeal papillomas under stringent conditions.[9] In 1982 Mounts et al[10] analyzed 20 laryngeal papillomas for the presence of HPV DNA using Southern blot hybridization. Using a HPV 6 probe that had been isolated from a genital condyloma and cloned into the plasmid pBR322, they detected HPV-6-related DNA in all 20 samples under stringent conditions (Tm, 28°C). Gissman et al[11] isolated and cloned viral DNA from a laryngeal papilloma and classified it as HPV 11. They found this HPV 11 DNA in seven of 14 laryngeal papillomas and in the same study detected similar HPV sequences in tissue taken from genital lesions, including condyloma acuminata and cervical condyloma (cervical flat warts). Human papillomavirus 11 shares a great deal of homology with HPV 6, and it is possible that some of the HPV 6 subtypes described by Mounts et al in actuality represent HPV 11. Definite proof of the HPV etiology of laryngeal papillomas is provided by the recent report of Kreider et al.[12] They showed that infection of either laryngeal or foreskin fragments by purified HPV 11 results in condylomatous growths after implantation into nude mice.

It is currently accepted that HPV 11 is predominant in laryngeal papillomas, an inverse of the ratio in genital HPV infection where HPV 6 is more often found. Because laryngeal papillomas are presumed to be transmitted from genital condyloma, this difference in ratio of HPV 6/11 suggests that laryngeal tissues are more susceptible to infection by HPV 11.

The frequent regrowth of papillomas following surgical removal is probably not due to any seeding of virus during surgery, but rather it may reflect the transforming activity of HPV, which has been present in the laryngeal tissues since the initial viral infection. Steinberg et al[13] examined biopsy samples from 20 patients with a history of laryngeal papillomas by Southern blot hybridization. Human papillomavirus DNA sequences were found not only in the papillomas but also in biopsies from clinically uninvolved sites. Eight samples from patients in remission, and four samples from uninvolved sites in two patients, contained viral DNA. These findings explain the frequent recurrences observed even after long-term remission in laryngeal papillomatosis. Thus, it is obvious that surgery can only help control the symptoms of laryngeal papillomas, not cure the disease. The clinical pattern of laryngeal papillomatosis can be summarized as follows: a serious disease with a high degree of morbidity and a great deal of unpredictability.

Anogenital Papillomavirus-associated Diseases

Although condyloma acuminata is rare in prepubertal children, cases of childhood venereal warts have been reported with increased frequency in recent years.[14] In 1982 De Jong[15] reported four new cases of childhood condyloma acuminata and reviewed 30 cases previously reported in the literature. Since De Jong's review, 23 additional cases of childhood genital papillomavirus infections have been reported, to bring the current total to 57 cases.[16–22] Of the 57 cases, 33 were female, 20 were male, and in four the sex was not stated.

All but one of the reported cases have described the lesions as resembling condyloma acuminata, ie, warty exophytic lesions involving various genital sites. A single report[16] describes a 2-year-old male child with bowenoid papulosis of the genitalia. Human papillomavirus 16 DNA, the type most frequently seen in cervical carcinomas, was identified in the lesion, using high-stringency-hybridization techniques. The child's mother gave a history of having genital warts prior to delivery of the patient. In addition, the child had atopic dermatitis, and it was postulated that he may have acquired the infection at the time of birth. His susceptibility to HPV was thought to be related to his severe atopic tendency.

Table 7–2 lists the cases of childhood anogenital HPV infections in which viral typing was performed. It is evident that the same viral types

TABLE 7–2. HPV Types Isolated from Anogenital Condylomas of Children

Author/Case No.	Age at Onset or Diagnosis (Yr)	Sex	Location	Sexual Abuse	Viral Type
Rock et al[18]/1	8	M	Anus	+	6
Rock et al[18]/2	3	F	Labia and anus	+	6
Rock et al[18]/3	8 mo	F	Labia majora, inner thigh	−	6a
Rock et al[18]/4	2	F	Hymenal ring, urethal meatus	+	6/11
Rock et al[18]/5	3	F	Perianal skin, buttock	−	16
Breneman et al[16]/6	1	M	Penis, scrotum, perineum, and suprapubic/ Bowenoid papulosis	U	16
Vallejos et al[19]/7	7	F	Labia minora	−	6
Vallejos et al[19]/8	6	F	Labia minora	−	6/11
Vallejos et al[19]/9	2.5	F	Vulvar, vaginal	U	6/11
Vallejos et al[19]/10	1.5	F	Labial, anal, inguinal	U	6
Vallejos et al[19]/11	2.5	F	Perianal	+	6
Vallejos et al[19]/12	9	M	Perianal	+	6/11/16/18
Vallejos et al[19]/13	3	F	Perianal	−	6/11
Fleming et al[22]/14	5	M	Anal margin	−	2

present in adult genital HPV infections can be identified in the childhood cases. This suggests a common etiology for condyloma acuminata in children and adults through contact with the same viral pool. Conversely, these tissues might be more susceptible to infection by HPV 6, 11, and 16 than by other HPVs. As in condyloma acuminata of adults, HPV 6 appears to be more common than HPV 11. This is in contradistinction to laryngeal papillomatosis, in which HPV 11 is more frequently identified.

Other Diseases Caused by HPV

In addition to their well-defined role in anogenital and upper-respiratory-tract infections, HPVs are associated with other childhood lesions. Skin warts are common and for the most part caused by HPV 2. There are many other HPV types also associated with cutaneous lesions. In addition to its presence in laryngeal papillomas and anogenital condylomas, HPV 11 has been identified in a conjunctival papilloma of a 33-month-old child.[23] The presence of HPV 11 in conjunctival papillomas is of interest, as it is a further indicator that specific viral types may be associated with different lesions in different sites. Although squamous cell papillomas of the esophagus have been described in children,[24] there is no data suggesting that these lesions are induced by HPVs.

TABLE 7–3. Likely Modes of Acquisition of Childhood Genital HPV Infections (57 Cases)

Mode of Acquisition	No. of Cases (%)	Age Group
Sexual abuse	17 (30)	11 mo–12 yr
Transmission at birth	6 (10)	<2½ yr
Contact with relative with warts "innocent transmission"	9 (16)	All age groups
Self-inoculation	1 (<2)	5 yr
Unknown	24 (42)	All age groups

POSSIBLE MODES OF TRANSMISSION

There are both epidemiologic and molecular data that suggest that transmission of HPVs from mother to child occurs. Transmission during birth was first suggested in 1956 by Hajec,[25] who reported a case of laryngeal papilloma that became evident in a child during the first year after birth to a mother with extensive genital condylomas in late pregnancy. The almost invariable onset of laryngeal papillomas and genital condylomas in children older than 3–4 months of age is not inconsistent with neonatal HPV infections. This "later than expected" onset is readily explicable in terms of the incubation period and well-known latency period of these infections.[13,26] It is also possible that papilloma growth is usually slow, and symptoms only occur when a tumor of sufficient size is reached. Although the exact manner of acquisition of respiratory and genital papillomavirus infection in the neonate and child is unknown, it is conceivable that this transmission could occur in a number of different ways:

1. Direct contact with an infected maternal genital tract (intrapartum transmission).
2. Transplacental transmission of maternal infection (in utero transmission).
3. Postnatal contact with an infected individual.

The likely modes of acquisition of the reported cases of childhood genital HPV infections is shown in Table 7–3. Sexual abuse was suspected in 30% of the cases, no age group being exempt. A definite age pattern is noted in the cases in which transmission at birth is suspected. This subgroup comprised 10% of the total group, and all children were less than 2.5 years of age at the time of diagnosis. In these six children, a maternal history of condyloma during pregnancy was forthcoming, and acquisition during pregnancy or delivery was suspected. In nine cases there was a history of warts at some or other time in a close relative, although sexual abuse was not suspected. A single case report describes a 5-year-old child with anogenital warts in which autoinoculation from a hand wart was the likely route of

TABLE 7–4. Series Relating Juvenile Onset Respiratory Papillomatosis Cases to History of Associated Maternal Genital HPV Infection

Author	No. with History of Documented Maternal HPV Infection	No. of Juvenile Onset Respiratory Papillomatosis Cases	% of Cases With Maternal History of HPV Infections
Cook et al[27]	5	9	56
Quick et al[9]	20	31	65
Strong et al[1]	18	36	50
Hallden and Majmudar[28]	15	28	54
Abramson et al[7]	9	31	29

transmission. In this case, HPV 2 was identified using biotinylated probes at moderate stringency (Tm, 25°C) in both the hand wart and anogenital wart. In the vast majority of cases (42%), the route of transmission was unknown. This is not surprising in view of the long incubation period of the virus (1–20 months), difficulty in obtaining accurate history, and high incidence of unrecognized maternal genital HPV infection. Data supporting each of the three proposed modes of transmission will be presented.

Intrapartum Transmission

Table 7–4 relates the number of cases of juvenile onset laryngeal papillomatosis to the number of cases with an associated history of maternal genital HPV infection. In general, it seems that at least one-half of the cases have a history of documented prior maternal genital HPV infection. It must be emphasized that these are indeed conservative estimates, as asymptomatic maternal genital HPV infections are common. Fife et al[29] examined an unselected population of 234 pregnant women during the first trimester of pregnancy. They screened cervical scrape specimens for the presence of HPV DNA 6, 11, 16, 18, and 31 by using three different blot hybridization methods, and found 26 specimens (11.1%) to contain HPV DNA sequences. Only two of the 26 positive specimens were obtained from patients with genital warts.

Thus, it appears that intrapartum infection during fetal passage through an infected birth canal is the most common manner of transmission of juvenile onset laryngeal papillomatosis. Indeed, the vast majority of neonatal infections with herpes simplex virus are acquired in a similar fashion.[30] The virus could be transported to the fetal larynx as the neonate takes its first breath or during routine suctioning of mucous from the nasopharynx. The hypothesis that intrapartum transmission is the most frequent route of acquisition of juvenile onset respiratory papillomatosis is supported by Shah's study[31] on the incidence of cesarean section delivery in such patients. Only one of 109 cases of juvenile onset respiratory papillomatosis gave a history of birth by cesarean section, whereas ten cesarean deliveries would have been expected for this group on the basis of national rates.

In contrast to respiratory papillomatosis, genital condyloma appears to have a much lower incidence of intrapartum transmission. As mentioned previously, only 10% of cases are transmitted in this fashion, most cases being acquired postpartum.

In Utero Transmission

The single cesarean section among the 109 cases reviewed by Shah indicate that although rare, in utero transmission of HPV is indeed possible. Although transplacental hematogenous infection could conceivably occur, the HPV is known to proliferate locally at the site of entry and not known to be blood-borne. Thus, ascending infection through an unperceived tear in the membranes is a more likely manner of infection than transplacental hematogenous dissemination. Abramson et al[7] mention one further case of juvenile onset laryngeal papillomatosis who was born by cesarean section. A single case of congenital condyloma acuminata is reported in the literature.[32] In this case, which was reported by Tang et al,[32] the mother was noted to have a single labial condyloma during pregnancy, which was untreated at the time of delivery. Although the vaginal delivery occurred 24 hours after the membranes had ruptured, it is obvious that infection occurred in utero, as the condyloma in the child clearly could not have developed within 24 hours. Although these authors suggested hematogenous transmission, ascending infection seems more likely for reasons mentioned above. Roman and Fife[33] reported that 4% of the foreskins they analyzed from 70 unselected male infants undergoing routine circumcision contained HPV DNA. No correlation could be identified between abnormal Pap smears of the mothers and the HPV positive foreskins. This data support the concept of transmission of virus from mother to child in the absence of overt signs of disease. It cannot, however, distinguish between acquisition of infection in utero or during passage down the birth canal.

Postnatal Infection

Analysis of the data presented in Table 7–3 indicates that postnatal childhood infection by genital HPV can be acquired by sexual or "innocent" means. Sexual abuse accounts for the majority of cases when the mode of transmission is known. Oral–genital sexual contact may also play a role in recurrent respiratory papillomatosis. Strong et al[1] obtained a history of oral–genital contact with an infected partner in four patients with adult onset laryngeal papillomatosis. The literature does not refer to this as a possible means of transmission in juvenile onset respiratory papillomatosis. It is evident, however, from Table 7–3 that a significant number of childhood genital HPV infections are acquired through innocent nonsexual contact. They have been recorded in children who have been bathed by women relatives with genital warts,[18] and a case of autoinoculation from a hand wart has been reported.[22]

In summary, the available evidence indicates that most cases of juvenile onset laryngeal papillomatosis are acquired during contact with an infected birth canal, but intrauterine infection is also possible. While most cases of childhood anogenital papillomavirus infections are acquired by sexual abuse, intrapartum infection and nonveneral contact account for a significant number of cases.

ANOGENITAL WARTS AND THE ASSESSMENT OF CHILD ABUSE

Over 1,000,000 children are victims of child abuse each year in the United States. Sexual abuse constitutes 12% of these cases with underreporting the rule.[34] While a review of the literature indicates that sexual encounters are responsible for no more than 30% of childhood anogenital condylomas, it must be emphasized that many of the remaining 70% of cases in these reviews did not have documentation of thorough investigation for possible sexual child abuse. Indeed, experts have estimated that 40–80% of cases of childhood condyloma acuminatum result from noninnocent sexual encounters.[35]

As opposed to the situation with gonorrhea, in which each childhood case is almost certainly an indication of sexual abuse, an association between anogenitial warts and child abuse cannot be documented with this degree of certainty. However, the association is significant, and at least 50% of cases can be documented by knowledgeable investigators. Thus, although anogenital warts in children are not a certain indicator of abuse, the possibility of sexual abuse must be borne in mind. A work-up should be performed to exclude associated sexually transmitted diseases, such as gonorrhea, chlamydial infections, trichomonas, and syphilis. The coexistence of one of these infections in a child makes sexual abuse a near certainty. When child abuse is recognized or suspected, the law in all states requires that such cases be reported to the authorities. The "authorities" vary in each state, but usually they are in a separate section of the Department of Public Welfare known as the Child Protection Service. To help the clinician decide whether child abuse is likely or not in a given case, Schachner et al[35] have drawn up a set of subjective and objective criteria. A discussion of these criteria is beyond the scope of this review, and interested readers are referred to that communication.

THERAPEUTIC AND PREVENTATIVE CONSIDERATIONS

The frequent existence of a history of maternal condyloma and the rarity of cesarean section delivery in cases of juvenile onset respiratory papillomatosis has been well documented[31] (Table 7–4). The immediate impression on evaluation of this data is that juvenile onset respiratory papillomatosis is acquired at the time of delivery and that cesarean section would prevent the disease. When one considers the incidence of the two diseases (maternal condyloma and childhood papilloma), however, it immediately becomes evident that the problem is not that simple. Juvenile onset laryngeal papillomatosis is a rare disease, and the incidence is many orders of magnitude less than that of genital-tract infections. Shah et al[31] calculated that the risk of juvenile onset respiratory papillomatosis is one in several hundred to even more than one in 1000 in children born to infected mothers. In other words, because genital papillomavirus infection is common and respiratory papillomatosis is rare, the risk of intrapartum transmission is undoubtedly low. Thus, the benefit of cesarean section is extremely low when one considers the entire group of mothers with documented infection, and it does not outweigh the risks of a cesarean section. The other major problem is the high incidence of asymptomatic and unrecognized genital HPV infection during pregnancy.[29] This makes it possible for pregnant women to transmit the virus to their newborns without knowing they are infected. Clearly, the question of cesarean section would not even be entertained in this group of patients in whom no infection is suspected.

The treatment of genital condyloma during pregnancy is advisable, not only because of its precancerous potential, but also because during pregnancy, condylomas may rapidly enlarge, obliterate the birth canal, and thereby preclude vaginal delivery. Ferenczy[36] evaluated the therapeutic effectiveness of laser therapy in 43 pregnant women with extensive urogenital and anal condylomas. He noted a recurrence rate of 33, 17, and 0% for patients treated during the first, second, and third trimesters of pregnancy, respectively. Thus, carbon dioxide laser vaporization seems to be an attractive method of treating genital condylomas during pregnancy, if cesarean section delivery is to be avoided. This form of therapy is associated with a very low rate of complications, and best results are obtained when treatment is carried out near term. However, it is uncertain whether successful laser treatment will decrease the risk of HPV transmission at delivery and, thus, the subsequent development of respiratory papillomatosis. One cannot help but question the effectiveness of laser therapy in preventing transmission of HPV infection, given the evidence that laser treatment fails to eliminate papillomavirus from the margins of clinically evident lesions.[26] Clearly, it would be desirable to be able to distinguish between infectious lesions and latent infections with a low probability of transmission.

In summary, the most effective management of condyloma during pregnancy, and the most efficient means of preventing transmission to the newborn, are uncertain. While elective cesarean section would undoubtedly reduce the incidence of neonatal HPV infection, this therapeutic option should be considered in the light of the low risk of intrapartum transmission, the possible effectiveness of laser therapy, and the risks associated with cesarean delivery.

MAJOR UNANSWERED QUESTIONS

There are many unanswered questions regarding genital HPV transmission to the fetus or neonate. These relate directly to management of the patient's disease during pregnancy as well as optimum protection of the infant during and immediately after birth. These questions include the following:

Is there equal infectivity of overt and subclinical infection? If not, and it probably is not equal, what are the best methods available to detect infectious patients? Is detection of HPV structural protein, using antibodies to capsid antigen on a biopsy specimen or Pap smear, a reasonably sensitive measure of infectivity? If so, perhaps we could identify those patients who should be treated aggressively during pregnancy. If we did have a good marker for infectivity, when should it be used? Early in the pregnancy? Just before delivery? Several times during the pregnancy? Answers to these questions could alter the management of expectant mothers with HPV infections.

The high incidence of subclinical and overt maternal HPV infection, and the very low incidence of laryngeal and genital lesions in the infant, suggest a low rate of transmission. Is the rate of transmission to the newborn actually so low, or are most infections subclinical? If the transmission is truly rare, why? What factors influence or determine infection of the neonate? Could overambitious aspiration of mucous, or the stress and trauma associated with a difficult labor, enhance infection? If the transmission rate is not low, and most infections remain subclinical, what factors determine expression of disease in a small subset of infected neonates? Clearly, if we had answers to these and similar questions, we might be able to prevent the serious disease sequelae seen in some infants.

REFERENCES

1. Strong SM, Vaughan CW, Cooperband SR, et al: Recurrent respiratory papillomatosis. Ann Otol 1976;85:508–516.
2. Cohen SR, Seltzer S, Geller KA, et al: Papilloma of the larynx and tracheobronchial tree in children. Ann Otol 1980;89:497–503.
3. Holinger PH, Schild JA, Maurizi DG: Laryngeal papilloma: Review of etiology and therapy. Laryngoscope 1968a;78:1462–1467.
4. Lynn BR, Takita H: Tracheal papilloma: A case report and review of the literature. Can Med Ass J 1967;97:1354–1357.

5. Singer DB, Greenberg SD, Harrison GM: Papillomatosis of the lung. Am Rev Resp Dis 1966;94:777–783.

6. Majoros M, Parkhill EM, Devine KD: Malignant transformation of benign laryngeal papillomas in children after radiation therapy. Surg Clin North Am 1963;43:1019–1061.

7. Abramson AL, Steinberg BM, Winkler B: Laryngeal papillomatosis: Clinical, histopathologic and molecular studies. Laryngoscope 1987;97:678–685.

8. Lack EE, Jenson AB, Smith HG, et al: Immunoperoxidase localization of human papillomavirus in laryngeal papillomas. Intervirology 1980;14:148–154.

9. Quick CA, Krzyzek RA, Watts SL, et al: Relationship between condylomata and laryngeal papillomata. Ann Otol 1980;89:467–471.

10. Mounts P, Kashima H: Association of Human papillomavirus subtype and clinical course in respiratory papillomatosis. Laryngoscope 1984;94:28–32.

11. Gissmann L, Wolnik L, Ikenberg H, et al: Human papillomavirus types 6 and 11 DNA sequences in genital and laryngeal papillomas and in some cervical cancers. Proc Natl Acad Sci USA 1983;80:560–563.

12. Kreider JW, Howett MK, Stoler MH, et al: Susceptibility of various human tissues to transformation in vivo with human papillomavirus type 11. Int J Cancer 1987;39:459–465.

13. Steinberg BM, Toff WC, Schneider PS, et al: Laryngeal papillomavirus infection during clinical remission. N Engl J Med 1983;308:1261–1264.

14. Stumpf PG: Increasing occurrence of condylomata acuminata in premenarchal children. Obstet Gynecol 1980;56:262–264.

15. DeJong AR, Weiss JC, Brent RL: Condyloma acuminata in children. Am J Dis Child 1982;136:704–706.

16. Breneman DL, Lucky AW, Ostrow RS, et al: Bowenoid papulosis of the genitalia associated with human papillomavirus DNA type 16 in an infant with atopic dermatitis. Pediatr Dermatol 1985;2:297–301.

17. Baruah MC, Sardari L, Selvaraju M, et al: Perianal condylomata acuminata in a male child. Br J Vener Dis 1984;60:60–61.

18. Rock B, Naghashfar Z, Barnett N, et al: Genital tract papillomavirus infection in children. Arch Dermatol 1986;122:1129–1132.

19. Vallejos H, Del Mistro A, Kleinhaus S, et al: Characterization of human papillomavirus type in condyloma acuminata in children by in situ hybridization. Lab Invest 1987;56:611–615.

20. Zamora S, Baumgartner G, Shaw M, et al: Condyloma acuminatum in a 2½ year old girl. J Urol 1983;129:145–146.

21. McCoy CR, Applebaum H, Besser AS: Condyloma acuminata: An unusual presentation of child abuse. J Pediatr Surg 1982;17:505–507.

22. Fleming KA, Venning V, Evans M: DNA typing of genital warts and diagnosis of sexual abuse of children. Lancet 1987;ii:454.

23. Lass, JH, Grove AS, Papale JJ, et al: Detection of human papillomavirus DNA sequences in conjunctival papilloma. Am J Ophthalmol 1983;96:670–674.

24. Arima T, Ikeda K, Satoh T, et al: Squamous cell papilloma of the esophagus in a child. Int Surg 1985;70:177–178.

25. Hajek E: Contribution to the etiology of laryngeal papilloma in children. J Laryngol 1956;70:166–168.

26. Ferenczy A, Mitao M, Nagai N, et al: Latent papillomavirus and recurring genital warts. N Engl J Med 1985;313:784–788.

27. Cook TA, Cohn AM, Brunschwig JP, et al: Laryngeal papilloma: Etiologic and therapeutic considerations. Ann Otol Rhinol Lar 1973;82:649–655.

28. Hallden C, Majmudar B: The relationship between juvenile laryngeal papillomatosis and maternal condylomata acuminata. J Reprod Med 1986;31:804–807.

29. Fife KH, Rogers RE, Zwickl BW: Symptomatic and asymptomatic cervical infections with human papillomavirus during pregnancy. J Infect Dis 1987;156:904–911.

30. Nahmias AJ, Alford CA, Korones SB: Infection of the newborn with Herpes hominis. Adv Pediatr 1970;17:185–220.

31. Shah K, Kashima H, Polk BF, et al: Rarity of cesarean delivery in cases of juvenile onset respiratory papillomatosis. Obstet Gynecol 1986;68:795–799.

32. Tang CK, Shermeta DW, Wood C: Congenital condyloma acuminata. Am J Obstet Gynecol 1978;131:912–913.

33. Roman A, Fife K: Human papillomavirus DNA associated with the foreskins of normal newborns. J Infect Dis 1986;153:855–861.

34. Greenberg NH: The epidemiology of childhood sexual abuse. Pediatr Ann 1979;8:17–28.

35. Schachner L, Hankin DE: Assessing child abuse in childhood condyloma acuminatum. J Am Acad Dermatol 1985;12:157–160.

36. Ferenczy A: Treating genital condyloma during pregnancy with the carbon dioxide laser. Am J Obstet Gynecol 1984;148:9–12.

CHAPTER 8

Cytology of Genital HPV Infections

Alexander Meisels, MD, FRCPC, FIAC

TECHNICAL NOTES

Routine smears submitted to the Cytopathology Laboratory at St. Sacrement Hospital, Quebec, Canada, for screening of cancer of the cervix are usually adequate to detect symptomatic human papillomavirus (HPV) infections. The smears must however be prepared, fixed, and stained in such a way that the subtle cellular changes are well preserved. For this purpose, it is best to use the V-C-E technique:[1]

Excess secretions should be gently removed. With the use of wooden or plastic spatulas, the posterior fornix and the whole circumference of the exocervix at the transformation zone are consecutively scraped; the two samples are kept separately on the spatulas. The endocervical canal is then sampled with a cotton applicator or an endocervical brush. This last sample is the first one to be smeared on the glass slide, at the opposite end from the frosted part. The exocervical sample is then extended on the midportion of the same glass slide, and the sample from the posterior fornix is finally placed on the side nearest to the frosted end. The glass slide is then *immediately* placed in 96% alcohol or fixed with an appropriate spray fixative. Speed is of the essence, to avoid drying artifacts that make it difficult, if not impossible, to recognize the finer shadings of cytoplasmic staining. The V-C-E smear gives the best results for cancer detection, identification of the vaginal flora, hormonal assessment, and diagnosis of HPV infections.[2]

In the laboratory, care must be taken to use a good quality Papanicolaou staining procedure. A smear that is properly taken, fixed, and stained is essential for an accurate diagnosis.

Clinical Practice of Gynecology: **2,** 117–125, 1989
© 1989 Elsevier Science Publishing Co., Inc.
655 Avenue of the Americas, New York, NY 10010

ISSN 1043-3198/89/$3.50

HOW COMMON IS HPV INFECTION?

In the *asymptomatic* HPV infection, in which colposcopy and biopsy fail to reveal any epithelial lesion, the cell spread is usually normal. In population screening with DNA hybridization techniques, 10% of the population was found to carry HPV DNA.[3] However when screening is done by cytology, only about 4% of women show cellular evidence of HPV infection.

It can be argued that the asymptomatic patients carry bare DNA, which may be either integrated into the host genome or found as an episome within the nucleus, but which lacks the protein envelope necessary for its survival outside of the cells. When cellular manifestations of the disease are present, complete virions can be demonstrated in about 50% of the patients by the immunoperoxidase reaction using a common capsid antigen[4] or by electron microscopy.[5]

Complete virions are produced exclusively in mature squamous cells, on or near the epithelial surface. When these cells are shed, the virions can be transmitted to the sexual partner. It would appear that although the asymptomatic patients carry the virus DNA, they cannot transmit it, and it does not have any visible effect on their own epithelium. It is not clear at this time whether the asymptomatic patient will eventually develop morphologic signs of HPV infection and whether this might depend on the state of her immunological defenses.

CYTOMORPHOLOGY

A definitive diagnosis of HPV infection can be made on the strength of the cellular pattern. Smears in pure HPV infection have a "clean" background: There is no necrosis, no signs of inflammation, no exudate. The characteristic cell types are described below.

1. The *koilocyte* (Figure 8–1) was first described in 1949 by Ayre[6] under the name *of nearo-carcinoma.* This designation did not survive and was replaced 7 years later by the term *koilocytotic atypia.*[7] It is a mature squamous cell that presents a large, irregular, sharply demarcated perinuclear cavity, which appears almost empty. The cytoplasm in the periphery of the cell is usually very dense and amphophilic, taking both the pink and the green color of the Papanicolaou cytoplasmic stains. Sometimes the hue is a mixture of both colors. There are often two nuclei per cell. The nuclear chromatin looses its sharp detail and becomes smudged and maybe darkly stained. The nuclear membrane is not apparent. There is often some degree of anisonucleosis but no marked nuclear atypias. These nuclear changes are the result of degenerative phenomena. Koilocytes do not contain nucleoli, nor does the HPV produce any visible inclusions. These cells may be found isolated or in small groupings. They are pathognomonic for HPV infection; they are never seen in other conditions.

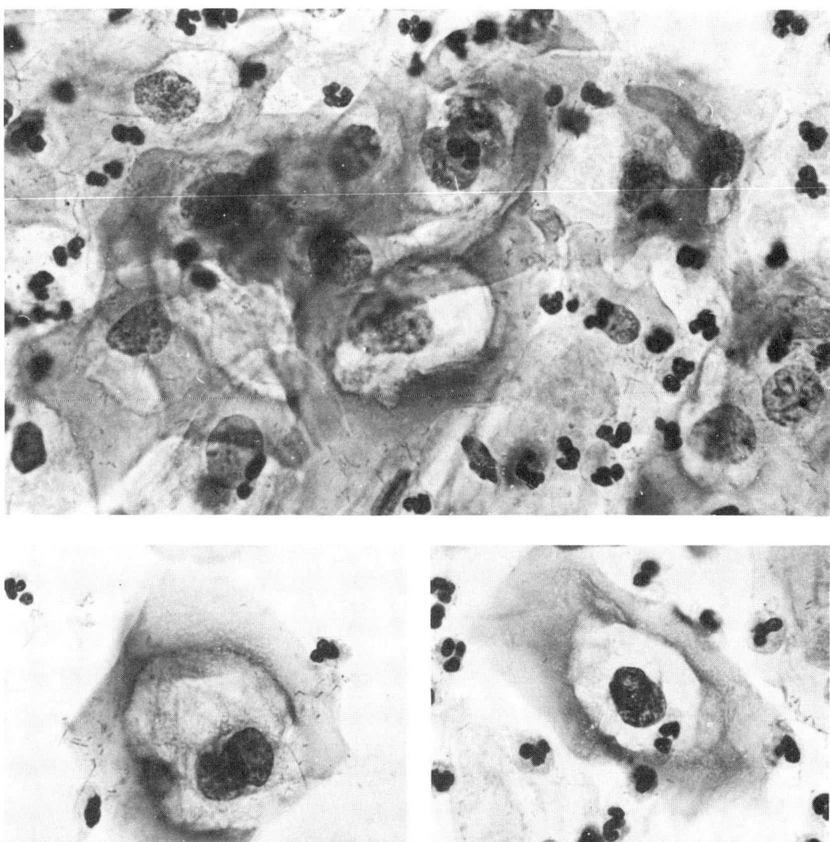

FIGURE 8–1 Koilocytes. Note frequent binucleation, indistinct chromatin pattern, inapparent nuclear membrane, sharply demarcated perinuclear cavity, and dense peripheral cytoplasm.

2. The *dyskeratocyte* (Figure 8–2) was first described as a sign of HPV infection in 1976.[8] It is also a mature squamous cell with dense orange-ophilic or eosinophilic cytoplasm. There is no perinuclear cavity. The nuclear changes are very similar to those described for the koilocytes. The dyskeratocytes are most often seen in dense, multilayered groupings. They are also diagnostic for HPV infection but should not be confused with the nonspecific dyskeratosis, which is not significant, and consists of a few cells either forming tiny pearllike arrangements or small sheets in which the cells lay parallel to each other. This is a surface phenomenon and has no diagnostic significance.

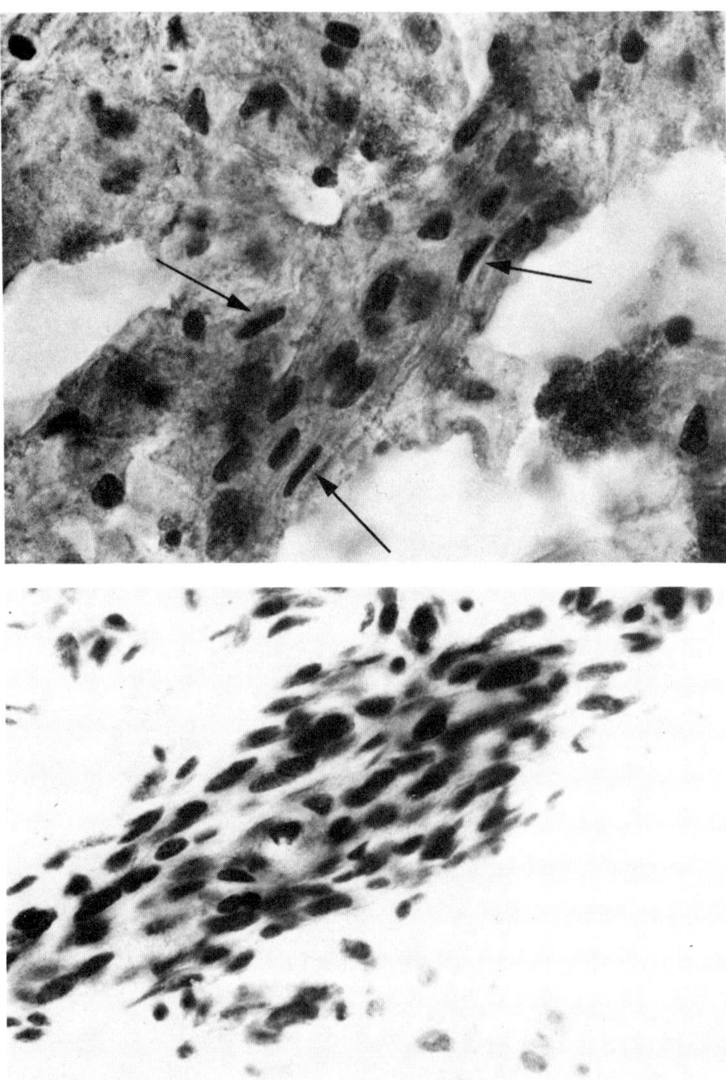

FIGURE 8–2 Dyskeratocytes. They usually present in sheets or three-dimensional clusters of keratinized cells, containing darkly stained, homogenous, often cigar-shaped nuclei (arrows).

3. *Parabasal condylomatous cells*[8] are immature squamous cells with nuclear characteristics similar to those described for the two previous cell-types. The cytoplasm is often amphophilic, but there is no perinuclear cavity (Figure 8–3). When the nuclear changes are marked, these cells may be confused with cells derived from an intraepithelial neoplasia. However, the

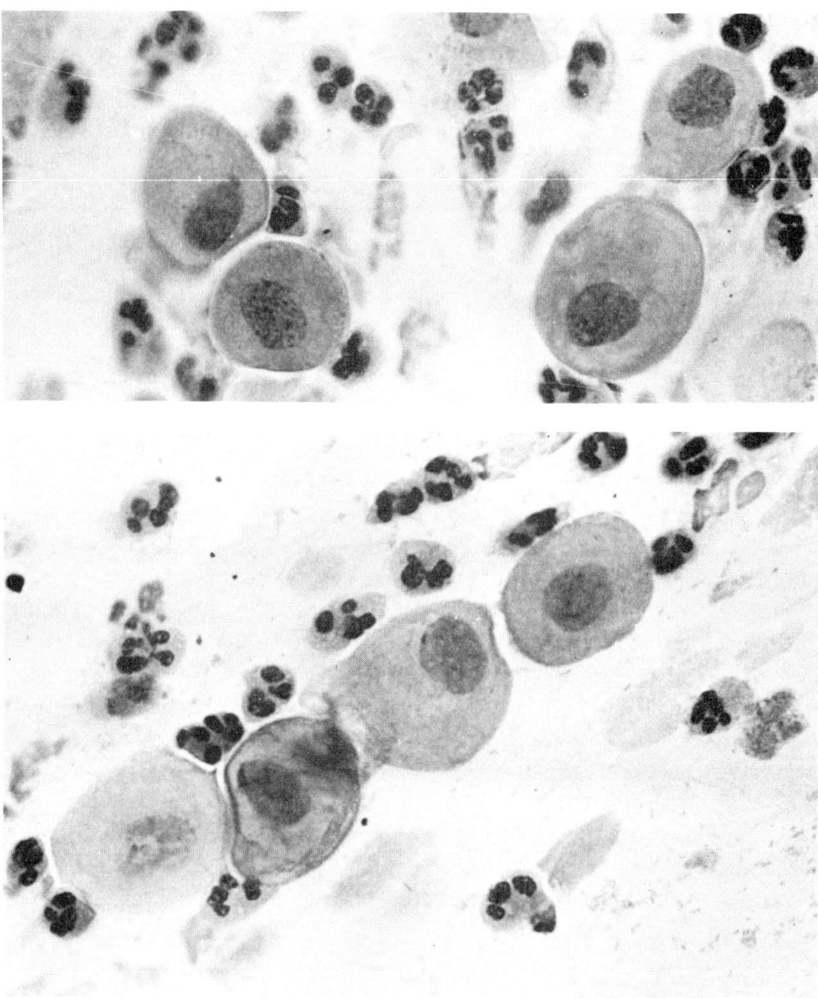

FIGURE 8–3 Parabasal condylomatous cells. The cytoplasm is eosinophilic or even orangeophilic. Nuclear structure is indistinct. Mono- and binucleated forms may be seen.

latter have a well defined, somewhat irregular nuclear membrane, and the chromatin detail is sharp and clearly visible.

4. *Nonspecific changes* help to identify HPV infection. When cell spreads from patients with positive HPV DNA hybridization are carefully scrutinized, and none of the above cell-types can be found, more subtle changes become visible.[9] They consist of mild nuclear enlargement and binucleation of intermediate cells with sometimes a few isolated dyskeratotic cells. These changes are not sufficient to identify clearly an HPV in-

fection, but they may represent the earliest morphologic manifestation of viral activity.

CYTO-HISTOLOGIC CONFRONTATION

There is not a perfect correlation between the cytologic pattern and the results of colposcopically directed biopsies. Even when the cytology is conclusive for HPV infection, there may not be a visible lesion on the cervix, and biopsies fail to reveal the characteristic viral manifestations. This may be due to a diffuse type of infection, a condylomatous cervicitis or colpitis, without a single well-defined lesion. DNA hybridization will usually demonstrate HPV in those cases.

Another more serious situation exists when the smear displays only the characteristic patterns of HPV infection, but the histologic findings are consistent with an intraepithelial neoplasia (CIN). These cases can be explained by the vertical association of CIN and HPV infection: The condylomatous epithelium is being replaced from the basal layers upward by a neoplastic epithelium, in a way similar to the reserve cells, differentiating towards a squamous epithelium, which eventually replace the columnar cells of the transformation zone, to produce squamous metaplasia. CIN may occupy most of the thickness of the epithelium, but the most superficial layers—those that will be scraped by the spatula—still retain the morphologic pattern of HPV infection. This can be demonstrated by the immunoperoxidase reaction, which will be positive in the upper layers, even when the section has all the appearance of a typical CIN.

Because of the possibility of such a vertical association, patients with cytological evidence of HPV infection need to be examined under the colposcope, and colposcopically directed biopsies must be taken in order to rule out a coexistent CIN.

In other cases, the two lesions—CIN and HPV infection—exist at different sites on the cervix. This is the horizontal association. Smears will usually contain cells typical of HPV infection and cells with the characteristics of CIN. Each of the cell types is discrete. No cell can simultaneously display both changes.

THE ATYPICAL CONDYLOMA[10]

In about 10–15% of all cases of HPV infection, the cell spreads display highly atypical mature keratinized cells. They contain one or several very hyperchromatic, irregular, enlarged nuclei, with indistinct chromatin. Bizarre forms may be seen (Figure 8–4). Most often these cells are shed in dense, tridimensional clusters, but isolated cells can also be found. There are no koilocytes in atypical condyloma, only markedly altered dyskeratocytes. Sometimes the smear contains cells that at first look seem to point

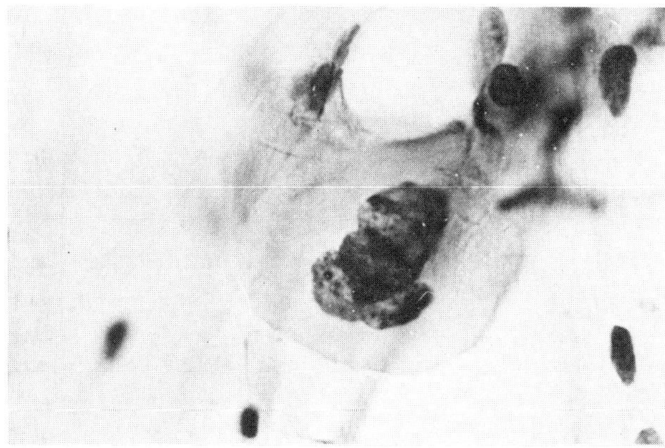

FIGURE 8–4 Atypical condyloma. The cytoplasm is vividly orangeophilic. The nuclei are irregular, darkly stained, and several times larger than nuclei from normal intermediate cells.

towards an intraepithelial neoplasia, but the groups contain a few binucleated cells with clearing of the cytoplasm in the perinuclear area (Figure 8–5). These cases represent a coexistence between atypical condyloma and CIN, or a transitional stage from the former to the latter.

The differential diagnosis is with an invasive keratinizing squamous carcinoma. It may be extremely difficult for the cytopathologist to come to

FIGURE 8–5 Atypical condyloma. Binucleated cells with perinuclear clearing can be seen next to denser parabasal cells, suggestive of associated CIN.

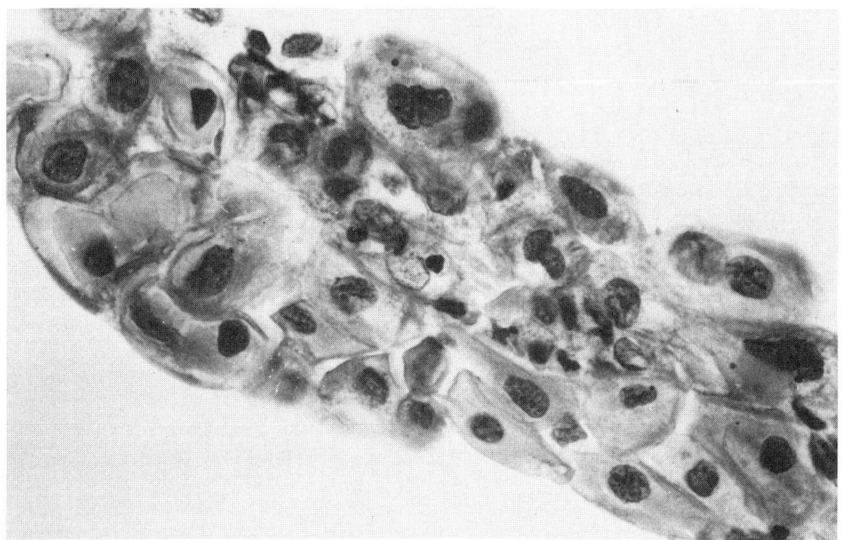

a correct conclusion. These cases mostly contain HPV type 16 DNA, the same that is also found in cervical cancers. However, biopsies will not demonstrate any stromal invasion. The epithelium contains many koilocytes, sometimes with very atypical nuclei, which may reach deep into the lower layers. The nucleo/cytoplasmic ratio remains low. The upper layers are keratinized and may contain very atypical nuclei. Even on sections, the chromatin is usually smudged and indistinct. This is very different from CIN, in which the cell population is immature and uniform from the basal layers up to the surface. In CIN the chromatin detail is sharp, and there are often small nucleoli. Mitotic figures, even atypical ones, can be found in CIN, in atypical condyloma, and even in the other types of HPV infection.

CONCLUSION

Most symptomatic cases of HPV infection can be accurately diagnosed with the routine V-C-E smear, if all the characteristic signs are taken into consideration. Although koilocytes are pathognomonic, they may be absent, and only the presence of dyskeratocytes will then permit a correct diagnosis. It must be understood that cytology underestimates the real incidence of HPV infection in the population, but the fate of the asymptomatic women is not known at the present time. When cytology detects an HPV infection, the patient must be referred to colposcopy, and biopsies must be obtained to rule out the presence of CIN, which may not be revealed on the smear. Atypical condyloma can represent a cause of error. The cytopathologist sometimes will overcall this lesion and diagnose an invasive squamous carcinoma. The reverse also happens: The early keratinizing carcinoma may be undercalled and reported as condyloma. This situation again emphasizes the need of colposcopy and biopsies in all patients with HPV infection.

REFERENCES

1. Wied GL, Bahr GF: Vaginal, cervical and endocervical cytologic smears on a single slide. Obstet Gynecol 1959;14:361–367.
2. Meisels A, Desbiens V: Superiority of the V-C-E smear. Acta Cytol 1969;13:1–2.
3. de Villiers EM, Wagner D, Schneider A, et al: Human papillomavirus infections in women with and without abnormal cervical cytology. Lancet 1987;ii:703–705.
4. Sato S, Okagaki T, Clark BA, et al: Sensitivity of koilocytosis, immunocytochemistry and electron microscopy, as compared to DNA hybridization in detecting human papillomavirus in cervical and vaginal condyloma and intraepithelial neoplasia. Intern J Gynecol Pathol 1986;5:297–307.
5. Hills E, Laverty CR: Electron microscopic detection of papilloma virus particles in selected koilocytotic cells in a routine cervical smear. Acta Cytol 1979;23:53–56.
6. Ayre JE: The vaginal smear. "Precancer" cell studies using a modified technique. Amer J Obstet Gynecol 1949;58:1205–1219.
7. Koss LG, Durfee GR: Unusual patterns of squamous epithelium of the uterine cervix: cytologic and pathologic study of koilocytotic atypia. Ann NY Acad Sci 1956;63:1245–1261.

8. Meisels A, Fortin R: Condylomatous lesions of the cervix and vagina. I. Cytologic patterns. Acta Cytol 1976;20:505–509.

9. de Villiers EM, Wagner D, Schneider A, et al: Human papillomavirus infections in women with and without abnormal cervical cytology. Lancet 1987;ii:703–705.

10. Meisels A, Roy M, Fortier M, et al: Human papillomavirus infection of the cervix: The atypical condyloma. Acta Cytol 1981;25:7–16.

CHAPTER 9

Molecular/Morphologic Correlation of HPV Infection of the Genital Tract

Gerard J. Nuovo, MD

The rapid expansion of knowledge on the molecular biology of human papillomavirus (HPV)-related lesions of the genital tract has given us insights into the dynamics of the disease. However, relatively speaking, we are still in the early stages of an understanding of the molecular biologic aspects of genital tract HPV infection and of being able to apply such knowledge to the diagnosis and management of patients with this disease. As a result, we have a great deal of information that was not available until recently, but we are not always quite sure how to use it. This chapter will discuss the correlation of the clinical and pathologic aspects of HPV infection with the relevant molecular biologic information about this disease. The following points will be stressed: 1) There is a relationship between certain histologic features and certain HPV types. 2) This relationship is dependent on the site as well as histologic findings. 3) This information has clinical relevance, as certain types, such as HPV 6/11, are very rarely associated with cancer, whereas others, such as HPV 16, are. 4) Certain molecular/histologic correlates of infection by HPV, such as viral copy number and capsid antigen production, are important to consider when experiments are planned or interpreted.

BASIC PRINCIPLES

In order to elaborate on the molecular/histologic correlation of HPV infection, some basic principles need to be discussed. First, we will discuss the histologic features that are used to distinguish the different categories of HPV-related lesions. This will be followed by a discussion of the salient basic concepts in molecular biology centered around the two common methods of detecting the virus: *filter hybridization* analysis,

Clinical Practice of Gynecology: **2,** 126–151, 1989

ISSN 1043-3198/89/$3.50

655 Avenue of the Americas, New York, NY 10010

which includes *Southern blot* and *slot blot* hybridization, and in situ hybridization.

Pathologic Diagnosis of HPV-related Lesions

The diagnostic cytologic and histologic feature of early HPV infection of the genital tract is *koilocytotic atypia,* in which perinuclear halos in conjunction with nuclear atypia are found in the infected cells.[1,2] Nuclear atypia refers to variation in nuclear size, shape, and chromaticity. Bi- and multinucleate forms are also commonly seen. On histologic examination, these features are most prominent in the superficial and middle zones of the epithelium.

HPV-related lesions of the genital tract may be divided into two groups based on the histologic features. One group—the *condylomata*—are characterized by koilocytotic atypia, as just described. The basal epithelium will appear similar to that observed in normal genital tract epithelium. When such histologic features are seen on the vulva, penis, vagina, and perianal area, the term *condyloma* is used. As tradition would have it, when similar histologic changes are seen in the cervix, the term *cervical intraepithelial neoplasia* (CIN) grade 1 is used. The distinction of condylomata from the other group—the *intraepithelial neoplasms* (INs)—is based on histologic changes seen toward the basal zone. Whereas INs often show the koilocytotic atypia typical of condylomata, they have, in addition, an increased mitotic activity, atypical mitotic forms, increased cellular crowding, and nuclear atypia toward the basal zone of the epithelium. INs are typically subdivided into grades 2 and 3 based on the degree of surface maturation; in grade 3, often called carcinoma in situ, cell maturation is minimal or absent.[1-4] The histologic distinction between condylomata and INs is illustrated in Figure 9–1.

Molecular Hybridization

Several reviews have been published recently about the basics of molecular hybridization.[5,6] At its core, molecular hybridization involves attaching denatured (for DNA), single-stranded nucleic acid from a sample (called the *target*) to a labeled *probe. Homology* is a reflection of the degree of base pair matching between the target and probe. If the degree of homology is high, then the target/probe complex tends to remain hybridized under conditions that destabilize the main force keeping the complex together—hydrogen bonding. On the other hand, target/probe complexes with poor homology will disassociate. *Stringency* is the term used to reflect the relative degree of destabilization of hydrogen bonds. The high sensitivity and specificity of molecular hybridization is based on the fact that hybridized complexes with strong homology remain

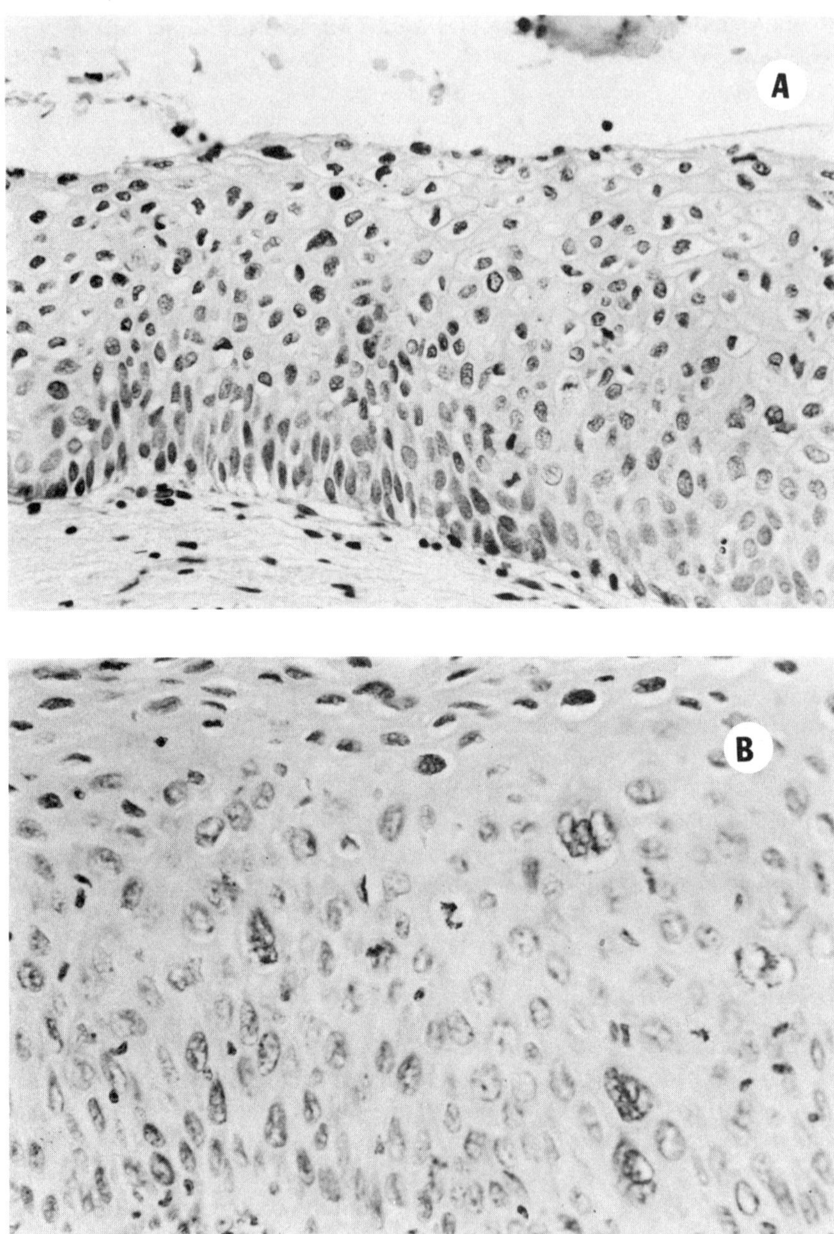

FIGURE 9–1 Histologic categories of HPV-related genital tract lesions. Panel A depicts a condyloma (CIN 1) in which nuclear atypia and perinuclear halos (koilocytotic atypia) are evident toward the surface as well as binucleate forms. The basal epithelium is unremarkable. In panel B, koilocytotic atypia is seen, but the crowding, disorganization, and increased mitotic activity at the basal area are diagnostic of CIN 2.

paired even at high stringency, whereas complexes with poor homology will separate. Stringency is often recorded in the literature as the *Tm*, which is the temperature of the hybridization (or posthybridization wash) in which one-half of a completely homologous probe/target complex will remain hybridized and the other half will dissociate. If the temperature is 40°C below this temperature, the conditions are reported as Tm-40 (*low stringency*), whereas if the temperature is 5°C below the Tm, it will be reported as Tm-5 (*high stringency*). The probe is typically labeled with nucleotides, to which radioactive isotopes or biotin have been attached. In this way, the probe/target complex can be visualized with an autoradiograph or a colorometric reaction for biotin.

Let us use an example to illustrate these points. For the purpose of this example, the probe will be radioactive (^{32}P)-labeled HPV 16 DNA, and the sample will be a vulvar condyloma that contains HPV 11 (Figure 9–2). The temperature of the hybridization is 42°C, which is about 40° less than the Tm for a probe/target complex of HPV 16/HPV 16. The HPV 16 probe will not remain bound to the human DNA target because the degree of homology is so poor. The HPV 16 probe would not even remain bound to some other HPV types (such as HPV 1) under these conditions because of insufficient homology. However, there is sufficient homology between HPV 11 and HPV 16 that enough of the probe would remain attached to the target, such that a positive signal would be obtained using autoradiography. However, if the temperature was increased to 68°C, which is 5° below the Tm, the probe would dissociate from the target because there is not sufficient base pair matching between these two HPV types to provide enough hydrogen binding to keep the molecules annealed.

There are two basic techniques that use molecular hybridization—*filter hybridization,* in which the DNA is extracted from the tissue and fixed to a filter, and in situ hybridization, in which the target DNA is not extracted from the tissue but assayed directly on a histologic section.

There are two different techniques based on filter hybridization—*slot blot* and *Southern blot* hybridization. In slot blot hybridization, the extracted DNA is transferred directly to a filter. In Southern blot hybridization, this is done after electrophoresis of the sample DNA. These tests are both highly sensitive; about 0.1 pg of HPV DNA can be detected. For a 10-μg sample of cellular DNA, this amount corresponds to about 1 viral DNA molecule (copy) for every 100 cells.[5–7]

Because there are fewer steps and less specialized equipment involved, slot blot hybridization analysis is the preferred technique for the commercially available tests for HPV based on filter hybridization (eg, Virapap). However, there are certain problems with the slot blot assay. First, there may be problems with background that would increase the false-positive rate. (Because the DNA is first separated and the specific

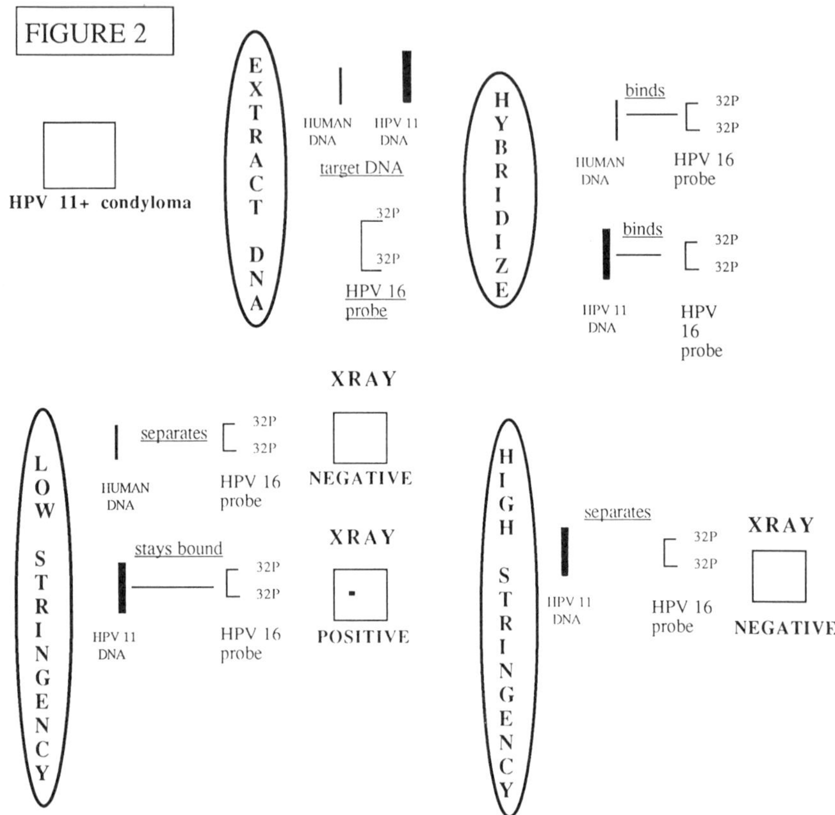

FIGURE 9–2 Graphic depiction of molecular hybridization. In this example, the DNA from a condyloma that contains HPV 11 is analyzed for HPV using a ^{32}P HPV 16 probe. The probe would bind to the HPV 11 and human DNA but would dissociate from the latter at low stringency because of poor base pair complementarity. At high stringency, the HPV 11/HPV 16 target/probe complex would likewise dissociate. Thus, one could say that the sample contained HPV DNA that was related to, but distinct from, the probe (HPV 16).

bands concentrated by size in Southern blot hybridization, there is no problem with background using this assay.) Second, there are problems if one tries to determine the specific HPV type by slot blot. It will be recalled that by using high stringency, one can determine the HPV type in that the probe and target would have to be very similar or identical for the target/probe complex to remain hybridized at high stringency. This works well in typing some HPVs, such as HPV 6/11. However, even at high stringency, there is sufficient homology between some HPV types (such as HPV 31 and 16) that if the probe was HPV 16 and the sample contained HPV 31, the sample could incorrectly be called HPV 16 positive because the hybridization signal would persist at high stringency.[6]

The way to determine unequivocally the HPV type is to do Southern blot hybridization analysis of the extracted DNA after the sample is digested with one or more restriction endonucleases. Restriction endonucleases are enzymes that cut DNA at specific sites. Thus, after endonuclease digestion, one would observe a pattern of band(s) corresponding to the number of sites in the DNA that are cut by a given endonuclease. By comparing this to the distinct patterns that have been deduced for the different HPV types[8–11] as well as doing a high-stringency wash, one can unequivocally determine the HPV type.

The main advantages of in situ hybridization are that it can be done in 1 day compared to the approximately 1 week needed for filter hybridization analysis, it does not use radioactive probes, and one can directly compare the histology to the tissue being analyzed for the virus.

In order for a hybridization signal to be evident with in situ analysis, 20–50 viral copies per cell must be present using either biotin or ^{35}S labeled probes.[12–15] This number range is based on the ability to detect the HPV 18 DNA in HeLa cells via in situ hybridization;[6] the actual threshold may be less. Although there are reports of higher sensitivity for ^{3}H-labeled probes,[6] these require 1-month exposure times and, thus, are of limited usefulness for diagnostic work.[16,17] Therefore, it would seem that in situ hybridization would be less sensitive than filter hybridization for the detection of HPV because of this 100-fold difference in the threshold detection level. However, it has recently been reported that in situ hybridization is as sensitive as filter hybridization for detecting HPVs for cases that contain HPV 6, 11, or 16.[18] It is now realized that the sensitivity of the two methodologies is equivalent for CIN 1s and condylomata—each at least 95%—if enough HPV types are included in the probe cocktails.[18–22] Thus, it is clear that in these lesions, many of the cells will contain at least 50 viral copies per cell. However, filter hybridization is still more sensitive than in situ hybridization for INs 2/3 and invasive carcinomas.[1,16,17,23,24] The explanation for this is that, for reasons that are now unclear, there are fewer viral copies per cell in these less differentiated lesions.

Before we finish this discussion of the different molecular hybridization techniques used for the detection of HPV, brief mention should be made of the polymerase chain reaction (PCR).[5] This test is based on the ability of an enzyme—Taq polymerase—to amplify a target DNA sequence if the appropriate complementary sequence (primer) is present. This enzyme can work at a temperature high enough to denature the newly synthesized target. Hence, by successive synthesis and denaturing cycles, extraordinary amplification of the target DNA can occur. Whereas filter hybridization can detect 1 viral particle per every 100 cells, PCR can theoretically detect 1 viral particle in the *entire tissue section.* Needless to say, there is the potential for a high false-positive rate caused by contamination. The utility of this test should become more evident in the near future.

HPV TYPES AND HISTOLOGICALLY DEFINED LESIONS

Condylomata

Association with HPV

CIN 1, vulvar, perianal, penile, and vaginal condyloma are strongly correlated with the presence of HPV; up to 100% of such cases having detectable HPV DNA are detected by either filter or in situ hybridization.[14,20,25–32]

Correlation of HPV Type with Condylomata

Many studies have examined the segregation of the HPV types most commonly found in the genital tract (HPV 6/11, 16, and 18) with condylomata.[14,20,25–34] As detailed in Table 9–1, most of these studies have demonstrated that HPV 6/11 are the most common types associated with condylomata of the genital tract. However, one will note that in some studies, HPV 16 and HPV 18 are also noted frequently in these lesions. Although Sutton et al[35] noted HPV 16 in 60% of cervical condylomata, most studies have noted this HPV type in a maximum of 20% of such lesions.

It is clear from Table 9–1 that there is much variability in the data comparing the HPV type with condylomata from different laboratories. What are the reasons for this? When one is analyzing molecular/morphological correlations in HPV infection of the genital tract, it is important to know the technique used to detect the virus. Most of the information listed in Table 9–1 comes from Southern blot hybridization analysis where the tissue used for the DNA analysis cannot be examined histologically. Thus, it is very possible that the tissue used for the Southern blot analysis may not be the same histologically as the adjacent piece that was used for histologic analysis. One reason this may happen is that HPV-related lesions can be very focal. They can also be very variable, with regions of condyloma seen in some areas and INs seen in adjacent areas. The latter is quite common; 60% of CIN 2/3 lesions will have areas that, if examined separately, would be diagnosed as CIN 1.[23,28,36] These problems inherent with Southern blot hybridization no doubt explain some of the variability in the segregation pattern reported by different groups for the various HPV types found in the genital tract.

The way around these problems is to do in situ hybridization, where the section used for histological analysis is only 4 μm from the section analyzed for HPV. However, there are still problems with this technique when one group's HPV type segregation patterns is compared to that of

TABLE 9–1. Association of HPVs 6/11, 16, and 18 with Genital Tract Condylomata and Intraepithelial Neoplasms

Study	Histology	HPV (%)		
		6/11	16	18
DelMistro[20]	Condyloma	100	0	0
Buscema[27]	Condyloma	77	12	9
	VIN	0	81	6
Barasso[25]	Condyloma	38	0	—
	P(penile)IN	0	77	—
Crum[28]	CIN 1	45	0	—
	CIN	0	61	—
Fuchs[33]	CIN 1	21	3	6
	CIN	4	45	18
Lorincz[24]	CIN 1	9	20	0
	CIN	13	43	0
	Cervix SCC*	0	47	17
	adenocarcinoma	0	44	22
Syrjanen[22]	CIN 1	41	0	—
	CIN	51	40	—
Pater[39]	CIN 1	—	0	23
	CIN 2	—	23	20
	CIN 3	—	50	26
DiLuca[41]	Cervix SCC	—	46	—
	VIN	—	100	—
	Condyloma	—	0	—
	Vulvar cancer	—	20	—
Tase[44]	Cervix SCC	—	54	0
	adenocarcinoma	—	3	40
Wilczynski[45]	Cervix SCC	0	50	7
	adenocarcinoma	0	13	50
Sutton[35]	CIN 1	00	60	30
	CIN	75	50	0
	Cervix SCC	33	58	4
	SCC vulva	78	33	22
Twiggs[90]	VIN	12	40	—
Nuovo[91]	CIN 1	27	36	0
	CIN	0	23	0
	Condyloma	95	0	0
	VIN	0	100	0

*SCC, squamous cell carcinoma.

another. There is some (more than we may care to admit) subjectivity in histologically defining the different categories of HPV-related lesions; one person's CIN 1 may be another's CIN 2. Still, because in situ hybridization affords the opportunity to compare the morphology and HPV type in serial sections, it is the best way to analyze this area.

In situ hybridization analysis of condylomata has shown that in general, HPV 6 and 11 are the most common types. However, the HPV

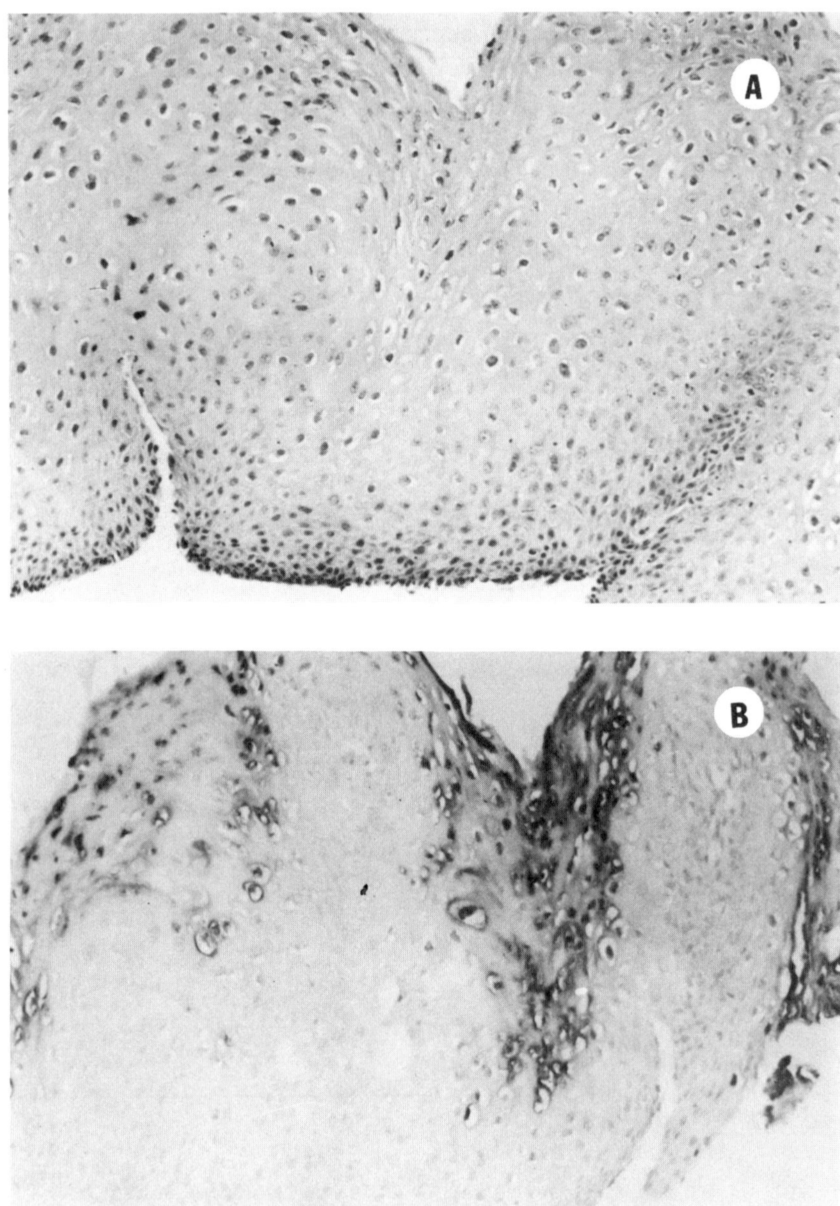

FIGURE 9–3 Correlation of histology and HPV type in "low-grade" lesions. Panel A is a CIN 1 lesion that contained HPV 11 as demonstrated by in situ hybridization (panel B).

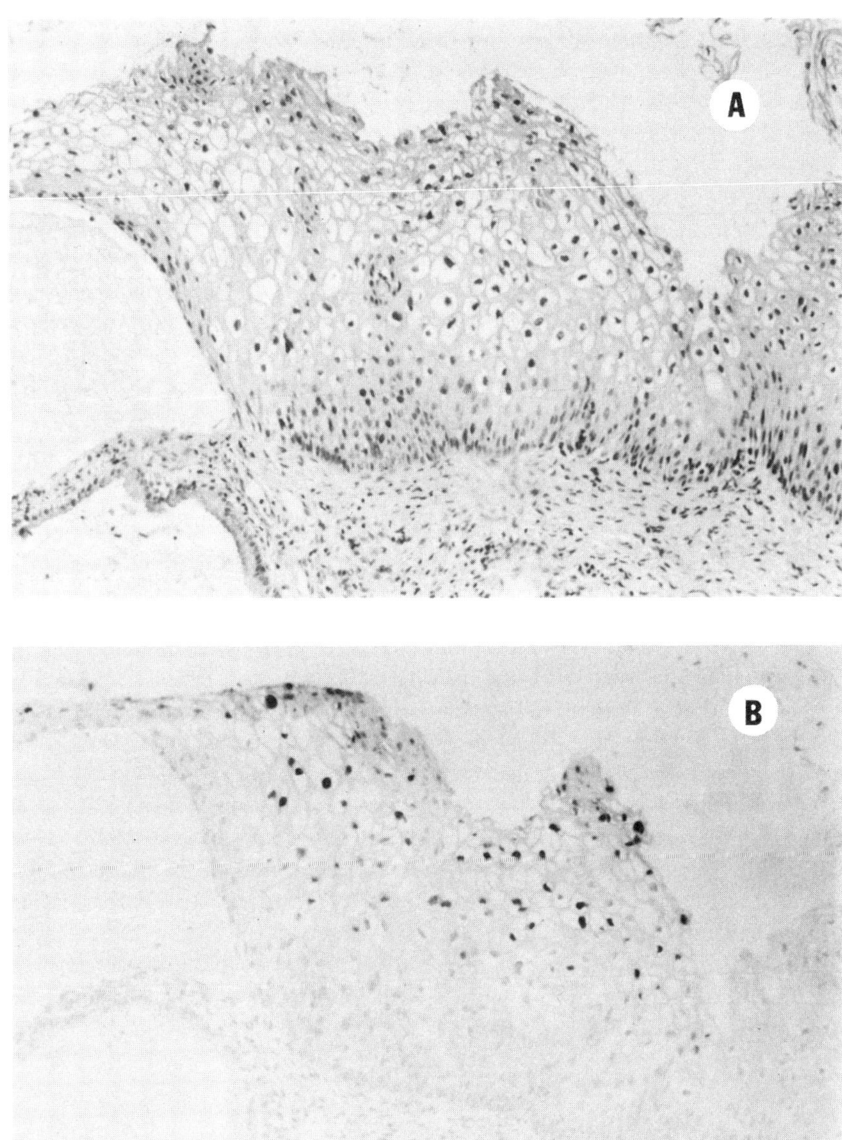

FIGURE 9–4 Correlation of histology and HPV type in "low-grade" lesions. Panel A is a CIN 1 lesion that contained HPV 16 as demonstrated by in situ hybridization (panel B). Compare with Figure 9–3, in which similar histologic features were seen.

types found vary markedly according to the site of the lesion. In cutaneous genital tract condyloma (vulva, perianal, penis), HPV 6 or 11 are found in the vast majority of cases.[14,20,29,32] In our experience, 96% of these lesions have HPV 6 or 11, with type 6 predominating.[29] The "oncogenic" HPV types, such as HPV 16, 31, 33, and 35, are rarely found in cutaneous genital tract condyloma. On the other hand, in CIN 1 lesions, the "oncogenic" HPVs predominate, with HPV 16 often being the most common type identified. In our experience, HPV 6 and 11 is found in 19% of such lesions, which compares to 35% for HPV 16 and 31% for HPV 31, 33, and 35.[29] Because these lesions are very similar histologically, one cannot differentiate the HPV 6/11 lesions from the HPV 16 lesions by histology. This is illustrated in Figures 9–3 and 9–4, in which CIN 1 lesions that contain HPV 11 and HPV 16, respectively, are illustrated. Another difference in the pattern of the HPV types found in CIN 1 versus cutaneous condyloma is that the less common HPV types, such as HPV 42, 43, 44, 45, 51, 52, and 56, are very rarely found on the vulva or perianal area but, relatively speaking, are more commonly found on the cervix.

At this time it is unclear why lesions with equivalent histologic features—cutaneous condyloma and CIN 1 lesions—should be so different in the distribution of HPV types found in such lesions. Part of the explanation may relate to the larger histologic variability seen in CIN lesions as compared to cutaneous HPV-related lesions. As noted previously, it is not unusual to see in a given case CIN 1 in some areas, and CIN 2 or 3 in other areas of the biopsy. Thus, a lesion diagnosed as CIN 1 may have other areas of CIN 2/3 that are not seen. It is presumed that such cases would rarely have types 6 or 11, which, as will be discussed, are very rarely found in such cases. On the other hand, in our experience vulvar condyloma rarely have other areas in the tissue that have the histologic features of vulvar intraepithelial neoplasia (VIN). Whatever the reasons, these observations do illustrate the point that the correlation of histology and molecular biology (HPV DNA segregation patterns) is by no means absolute but dependant on site.

INTRAEPITHEIAL NEOPLASMS

Association with HPV

Intraepithelial neoplasms are distinguished from condylomata by their increased mitotic rate, parabasal nuclear atypia, and abnormal mitotic figures. As in condylomata, such changes are strongly correlated with the presence of HPV with up to 100% of such cases having detectable HPV DNA sequences.[23,24,28,33,37–40]

Correlation of HPV Type with Intraepithelial Neoplasms

As is clear from Table 9–1, HPV 16 is the most common HPV type detected in genital tract INs. Much of this information was obtained from Southern blot hybridization analysis. The data with in situ hybridization analysis shows similar tendencies, ie, that HPV 16 predominates in such lesions, whereas the types commonly found in condylomata, HPVs 6 and 11, are very rarely found in these higher-grade lesions.[23,24,28,33,37–40] Using in situ hybridization analysis, we did not detect HPV 6 or 11 DNA in any of 132 cases of CIN or VIN[29] (Nuovo, unpublished observations).

As for the condylomata, the site of the lesion is important when one is analyzing the pattern of the HPV types in INs. CINs have a more heterogeneous pattern of HPV types with HPV 31, 33, 35, and others found relatively commonly.[8,10,24,27,28,33,41] However, in VIN lesions, HPV 16 is found in the vast majority, with the other types less commonly found.[27,38,42] Interestingly, the predominance of HPV 16 over the other "oncogenic" types in INs appears to be the case at other cutaneous sites including the penis and, interestingly, the periungual region of the finger.[25,43]

In summary, the following observations have been made regarding the histologic/molecular correlation of HPV type in genital tract lesions: 1) whereas HPV 16 can be associated with the histologic features of a condyloma (CIN 1), INs or, as will soon be discussed, cancer, the histologic range of HPV 6 or 11 appears to be more limited, being restricted to condylomata; 2) cervical lesions have a more heterogeneous group of HPV types, whereas cutaneous lesions will contain either HPV 6/11 (cutaneous condyloma) or HPV 16 (cutaneous INs). These findings may have important clinical significance in that HPV 6/11 associated lesions rarely, if ever, progress to cancer, whereas HPV 16-associated lesions are at an increased risk for the development of an invasive tumor[2] (see discussion below on HPV and cancer). Because most cutaneous condylomata have HPV 6/11, and very few INs have HPV 6/11, this distinction of "oncogenic" versus "nononcogenic" types can be made in these instances by histology quite reliably. It is with CIN 1 lesions that histology *cannot* reliably distinguish HPV 6/11 from the other HPV types. Thus, it is in these cases that HPV typing may help predict the clinical course.

CARCINOMA OF THE GENITAL TRACT

Association with HPV

The association of HPV with invasive squamous cell carcinoma of the genital tract is as strong as condylomata and intraepithelial neoplasms.

Lorincz et al[24] noted that 89% of such lesions had detectable HPV DNA sequences. Two recent reports have documented that a less common histologic variant of invasive carcinoma of the cervix—adenocarcinoma—is also strongly associated with HPV.[44,45] Stoler et al (personal communication) have made an interesting observation about an even rarer histologic variant of cervical cancer—small cell carcinoma. This tumor, which is commonly rapidly fatal,[46–49] was demonstrated usually to contain HPV DNA.

Correlation of HPV Type with Genital Tract Carcinoma

An association between CIN and invasive squamous cell carcinoma of the cervix has been suggested by epidemiologic data.[50–53] Obviously, there are many histologic similarities between CIN and invasive squamous cell cancer.[1,2] Given these observations, it is not surprising that the segregation of HPV types in invasive genital squamous malignancies parallels that found in INs. Specifically, HPV 16 predominates in these lesions, whereas HPV 18 is detected in 0 to 17% of these cancers (Table 9–1).[24,44] As noted with INs, invasive cervical cancers have a more heterogeneous grouping of HPV types with certain types, such as HPV 31, 33, 35, and 51 routinely being isolated from such cancers. On the other hand, genital cutaneous invasive squamous cell carcinomas are much more likely to be associated with HPV 16; the other types are typically present in lower percentages when compared to cervical squamous cell cancers.[8,9,24,54–56] To our knowledge, there are no unequivocally documented cases (including endonuclease restriction enzyme digestion analysis) of HPV 6/11 in genital squamous cell carcinomas, although there is a case report of such an occurrence in the trachea.[57] However, HPV 6/11 has been reported in a rare histologic variant of squamous cell cancer of the genital tract—verrucous carcinoma.[27] This lesion, although locally aggressive, rarely metastasizes and, thus, has a biologic behavior quite different from the typical invasive squamous cell cancer from this site.[58,59]

The most common HPV type identified in adenocarcinomas is HPV 18, with HPV 16 being the second most common.[24,44,45] Figure 9–5 depicts an adenocarcinoma of the cervix that contained HPV 18. Interestingly, HPV 18 is also the most common type in the highly lethal small-cell carcinoma of the cervix (Stoler, personal communication). Thus, HPV 18 appears to be associated with cancers that have glandular, as opposed to squamous, differentiation and that have a poorer prognosis. Indeed, it has been shown that squamous cell cancers that contain HPV 18 have a poorer prognosis than the corresponding tumor that contains HPV 16.[60] Because of this observation, plus the fact that HPV 18 is rarely associated with precancerous lesions (intraepithelial neoplasms), HPV 18

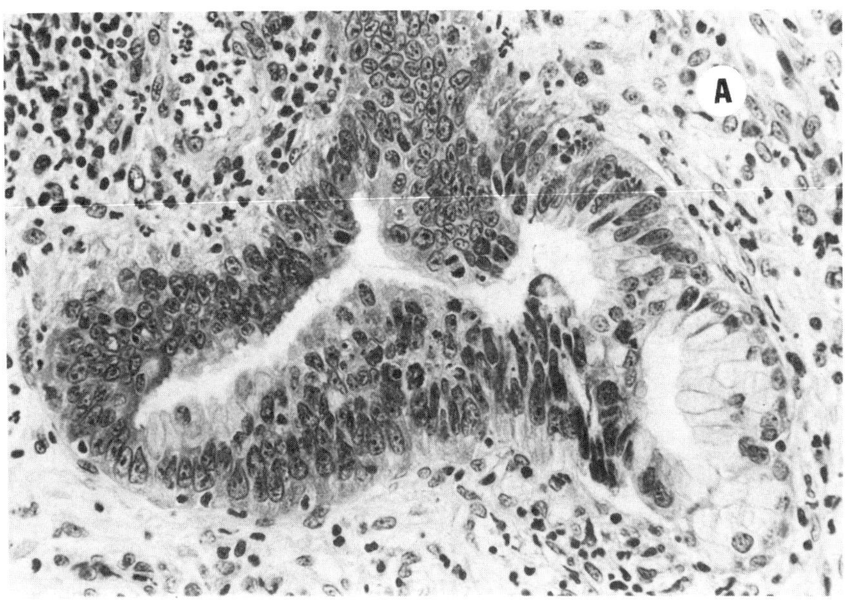

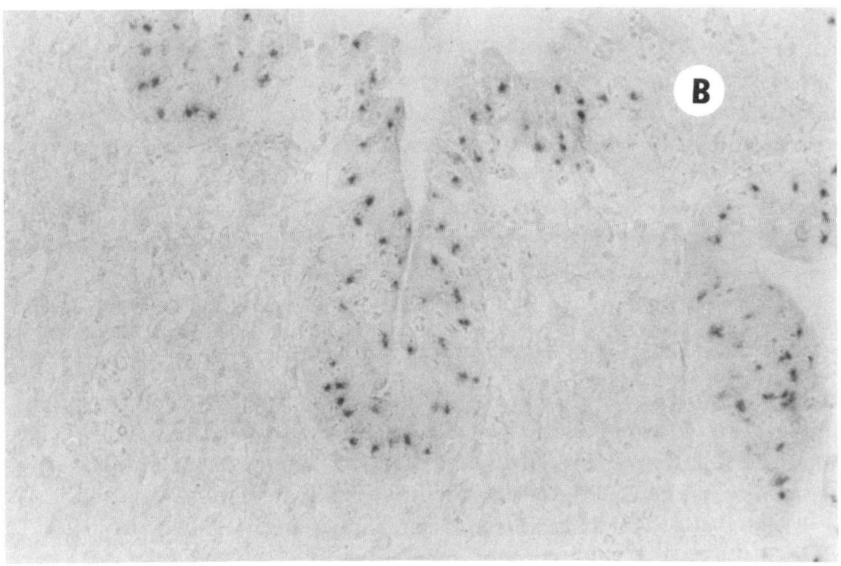

FIGURE 9–5 HPV analysis of a cervical adenocarcinoma. Panel A depicts the nuclear stratification, nuclear atypia, and mitotic activity of a cervical adenocarcinoma. The lesion contained HPV 18 as demonstrated by in situ hybridization (panel B).

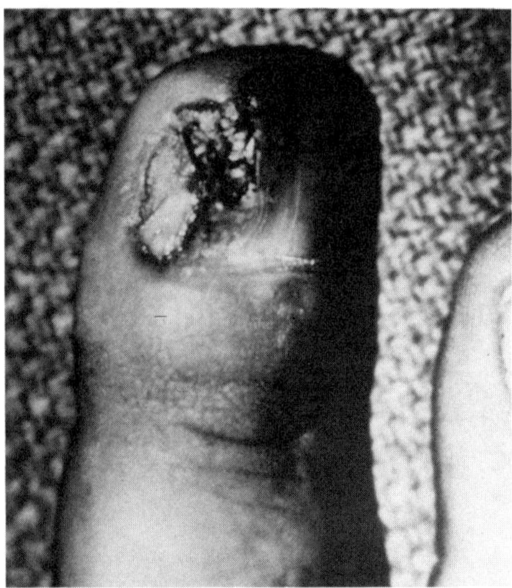

FIGURE 9–6 Clinical appearance of a squamous cell carcinoma of the periungual region of the finger. This lesion, as is the case for most of the squamous cell neoplasms from this site, contained HPV 16.

has been referred to as an HPV type with a "high oncogenic risk," as compared to HPV 16, which has been described as a type with an "intermediate oncogenic risk." The molecular basis for this paucity of HPV 18 is in histologically defined precursors, but its preponderance in certain types of cervical cancer remains an enigma. Tase et al[61] searched for precursors to cervical adenocarcinomas by analyzing microglandular hyperplasia and glandular dysplasia for HPV 18. However, most of the tissues with these histologic findings were HPV negative.

Squamous Cell Carcinoma at Other Sites

The few published studies analyzing nongenital tract squamous cell carcinomas for HPV have failed to demonstrate an association with a few notable exceptions. One is the rare clinical syndrome of epidermodysplasia verruciformis, marked by impaired cellular immunity and multiple verrucae plana, which bear some semblance histologically to INs.[62–68] Many HPV types, although not ones found in the genital tract, have been detected in such lesions. Such patients are at a high risk of developing squamous malignancies; HPV 5 is most commonly detected in these malignancies. The other exception is squamous cell carcinoma of the finger. As noted previously, the majority of such cases (either in situ or invasive) contain HPV 16 (Figure 9–6). Because HPV was associated with squamous cell cancers of the genital tract and the periungual region of the finger, but not with such tumors from other skin sites, the authors concluded that the finger lesions may be acquired by sexual transmission.[43] Two other recent reports have also documented the presence of genital tract HPVs (HPV 16 and 35) in periungual cancers.[69,70] In one such report, the same HPV type was found in a vulvar carcinoma in situ, lending further credence to a link between squamous cell neoplasms from the genital tract and finger.

OTHER MOLECULAR/HISTOLOGIC CORRELATIONS IN HPV-RELATED LESIONS

Copy Number

As mentioned earlier, the number of viral DNA molecules per cell decrease from the "low-grade" condylomata to the "higher-grade" INs to the "least differentiated" carcinomas (Figure 9–7). The reason for this is unclear. It may be related to the observation that the HPV DNA in condylomata is episomal, whereas it often is integrated in INs and carcinomas.[38,71–75] Perhaps integration "turns off" some factor required for the continued synthesis of the viral DNA.

Whatever the explanation, the variation in viral copy number with the different histologic categories of HPV-related lesions explains why in situ hybridization is equally effective to filter hybridization for detecting HPV DNA in condylomata, where the copy number is high. However, in situ hybridization is less effective compared to filter hybridization in analyzing INs and much less effective in analyzing carcinomas where the viral copy number tends to be below the threshold of in situ hybridization (about 20–50 copies per cell) but above that for filter hybridization (about 1 copy per every 100 cells).[24,28,29,36,44,45]

Transcription and Translation

Because there are differences in viral copy number among the condylomata, INs, and carcinomas, one might expect similar differences in viral RNA and protein patterns. The protein that has been studied most extensively is the capsid antigen, since it has been used to detect HPV in tissues. The capsid antigen is detected in much higher rates in condylomata as compared to INs.[26,40,76,77] Gupta[28,51] noted an 83% detection rate of the capsid antigen for HPV 11 lesions and 62% for HPV 16 lesions. It is very unusual to detect the capsid antigen in invasive carcinomas. Thus, use of anticapsid antigen antibodies for research has limited value, as there will be many false-negative cases with the CIN lesions.

Much attention has recently been focused on the viral translation patterns in condyloma as compared to INs. The reasoning is that since the

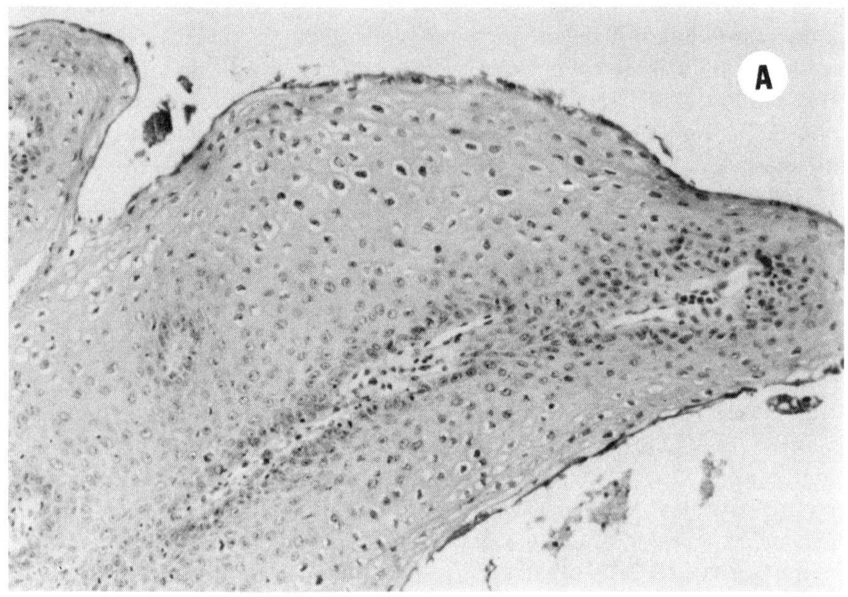

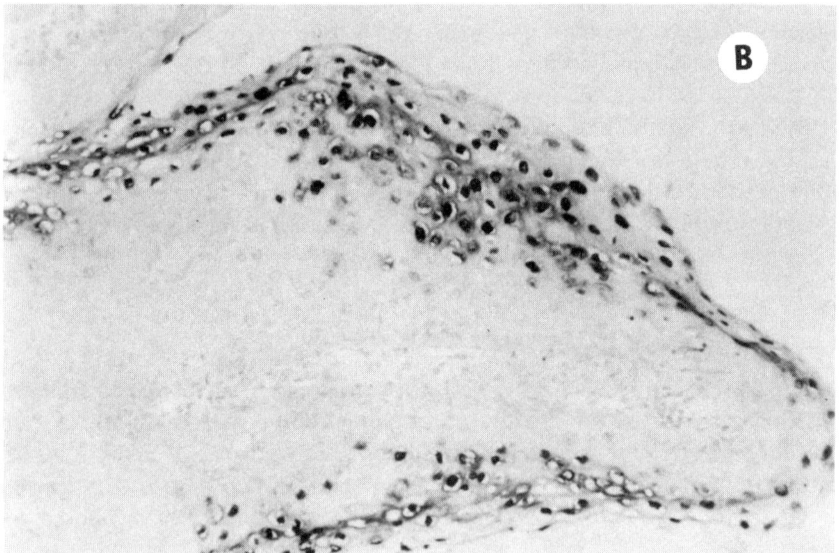

FIGURE 9–7 Copy number of HPV as it relates to histology. Panel A shows a vulvar condyloma in which many of the cells contain detectable HPV DNA in relatively large amounts based on the intensity of the hybridization signal (panel B). Compare this to panels C and D, which demonstrate a VIN 2 lesion that contained HPV 16 as detected by in situ hybridization analysis.

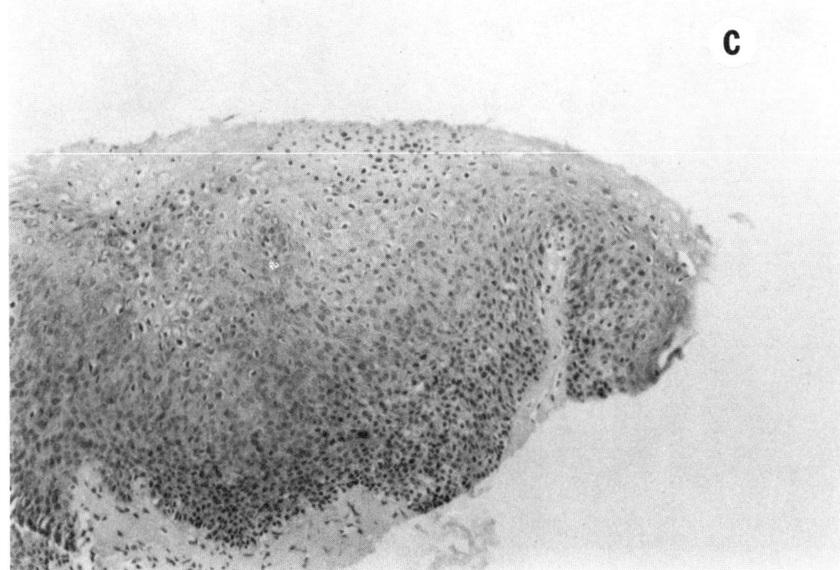

former is often benign and the latter has a high risk of progression, one might be able to identify differences in the translation patterns that would explain the different clinical courses. It has been noted that all the viral transcripts (referred to as open reading frames—ORFs) are detectable in condylomata.[78–80] However, the E4, E5, E6, and E7 transcripts are typically

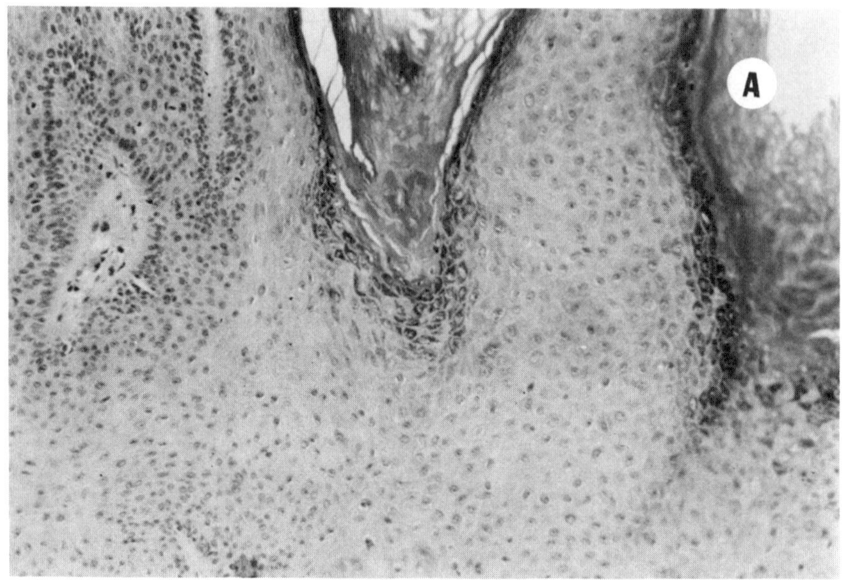

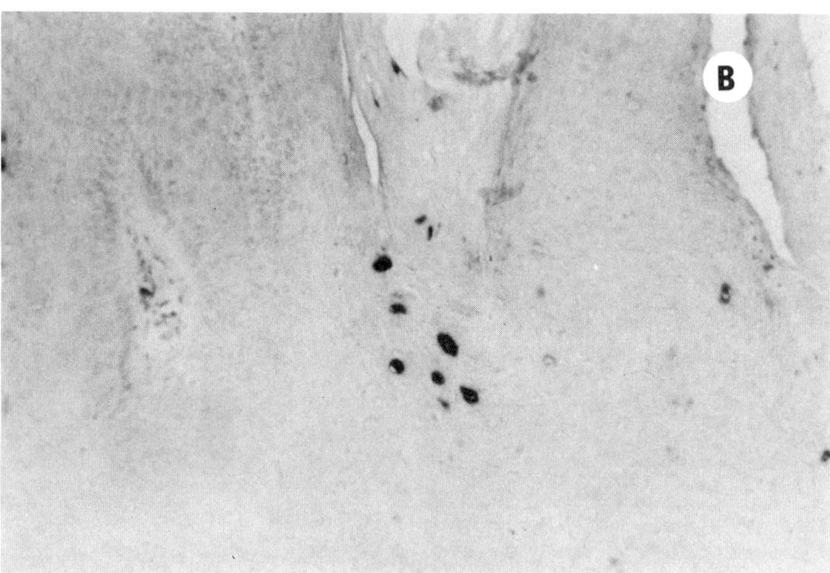

FIGURE 9–8 HPV DNA in tissues lacking clear-cut koilocytotic atypia. In this vulvar lesion, HPV DNA is noted by in situ hybridization cells that lacked unequivocal koilocytotic atypia.

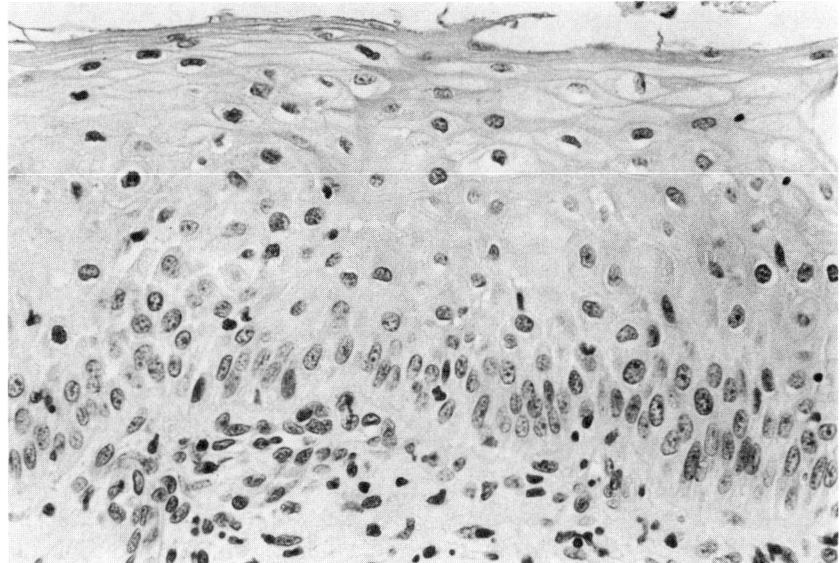

FIGURE 9–9 Mimics of koilocytotic atypia. This cervical lesion, in which there are perinuclear halos, is suggestive of CIN 1, but the degree of nuclear atypia is not sufficient for this diagnosis. HPV DNA was not detected by in situ hybrization, which is true for the vast majority of such cases.

the most prevalent in the INs; E2 is often absent.[14,72,79–81] Because the virus integrates at the site of its' E2 ORF, it is theorized that integration is responsible for the decreased translation of the E2 ORF. This in turn may permit the expression of other viral transcripts, such as E7, which has recently been shown to bind to and likely inactivate the retinoblastoma gene product.[79] This may be an important event in the evolution to a malignant state. Needless to say, extensive research is now ongoing in this area.

Given the observation that HPV 6- or 11- related lesions rarely progress to cancer but HPV 16, 18, 31, and other types may, much attention has been focused on deducing the reason for this at the molecular level. One important difference may be at E7, in which certain DNA binding motifs as well as an E6 splice site have been identified in "oncogenic" HPV types such as HPV 16 but not in HPV 6 or 11.[89]

In situ hybridization analysis has allowed us to correlate the amount of viral DNA, RNA, and protein production with cellular morphology. Such analysis has made it clear that viral DNA, RNA, and protein production is more prominent in cells that demonstrate the perinuclear halos and nuclear atypia characteristic of the disease. The less differentiated cells toward the base typically do not contain detectable viral DNA, RNA, or protein.[36,82] The reasons again are enigmatic, but it likely reflects a cooperation of these viral processes with cellular processes resulting in cell maturation.

HPV and Occult Infection

Occult infection by HPV is defined as detecting the virus in the absence of the diagnostic pathologic features of such infection—ie, perinuclear halos and nuclear atypia. HPV has been detected by many investigators in tissues that histologically are normal or, at least, lack clear-cut koilocytotic atypia. With the use of filter hybridization analysis, about 10% of men and women with no clinical or pathologic evidence of HPV infection can be shown to harbor the virus on the cervix or penis.[5,24,33,83–87] It is important to realize that this 10% value comes from filter hybridization. If one uses in situ[18,29] hybridization, it is *very* unusual to detect the virus if the histologic features of an HPV infection are lacking. We have never detected the virus in tissues using in situ in "truly" latent infection-negative history of an abnormal pap smear and genital wart—even if the virus has been demonstrated in the case by filter hybridization.[86,87] Even in cervical lesions from patients with abnormal Pap smears, in whom HPV DNA can be detected by filter hybridization in about 40% of cases that lack the histologic features of CIN, the viral DNA is very rarely detected (about 4%) by in situ hybridization.[29,88] In our experience, HPV DNA can be detected by in situ hybridization somewhat more commonly in vulvar lesions in areas that lack clearcut koilocytotic atypia (Figure 9–8). Most likely, the viral copy number in the "nondiagnostic" infected tissue is below the 20–50-copy threshold; again, this likely relates to the absence of the clearcut koilocytotic atypia that is associated with an apparent increase in synthesis of viral DNA, RNA, and proteins. As a practical rule, one should be *suspicious* of claims that HPV DNA, RNA, or its proteins are being routinely identified in tissues that lack the histologic features of the infection (Figure 9–9).

REFERENCES

1. Nuovo GJ, Crum CP, Silverstein SJ: Papillomavirus infection of the uterine cervix. Microbial Pathogenesis 1987;3:71–78.
2. Richart RM: Causes and management of cervical intraepithelial neoplasia. Cancer 1987;60:1951–1959.
3. Fu YS, Huang I, Beaudenon S, et al: Correlative study of human papillomavirus DNA, histopathology, and morphometry in cervical condyloma and intraepithelial neoplasia. Int J Gynecol Pathol 1988;7:297–307.
4. Winkler B, Crum CP, Fujii T, et al: Koilocytotic lesions of the cervix: The relationship of mitotic abnormalities to the presence of papillomavirus antigens and nuclear DNA content. Cancer 1984;53:1081–1087.
5. Lorincz AT: Detection of human papillomavirus infection by nucleic acid hybridization. Obstet Gynecol Clin N Am 1987;14:451–469.

6. Nuovo GJ, Richart RM: Human papillomavirus: A review. Yearbook of Obstetrics and Gynecology 1989. In: Mishell DR, Kirschbaum TH, Morrow CP, eds. Chicago: Year Book Medical Publishers Inc., 1989.

7. Ostrow RS, Zachow KR, Niimura M, et al: Detection of papillomavirus DNA in human semen. Science 1986;231:731–733.

8. Beaudenon S, Kremsdorf D, Croissant O, et al: A novel type of human papillomavirus associated with genital neoplasias. Nature 1986;321:246–249.

9. Lorincz AT, Quinn AP, Lancaster WD, et al: A new type of papillomavirus associated with cancer of the uterine cervix. Virology 1987; 159:187–190.

10. Nuovo GJ, Crum CP, deVilliers EM, et al: The isolation of a novel human papillomavirus (HPV 51) from a cervical condyloma. J Virol 1988;62:1452–1455.

11. Dartmann K, Schwartz E, Gissmann L, et al: The nucleotide sequence and genomic organization of human papilloma virus type 11. Virology 1986;151:124–130.

12. Crum CP, Nagai N, Levine RU, et al: In situ hybridization analysis of human papillomavirus 16 DNA sequences in early cervical neoplasia. Am J Pathol 1986;123:174–182.

13. Crum CP, Nuovo GJ, Friedman D, et al: A comparison of biotin and isotope labeled ribonucleic acid probes for in situ detection of HPV 16 ribonucleic acid in genital precancers. Lab Invest 1988;58:354–359.

14. Stoler MH, Broker TR: In situ hybridization detection on human papillomavirus DNAs and messenger RNAs in genital condylomata and a cervical carcinoma. Human Pathol 1986;17:250–258.

15. Walboomers JMM, Melchers WJG, Mullink H, et al: Sensitivity of in situ detection with biotinylated probes of human papillomavirus type 16 DNA in frozen tissue sections of squamous cell carcinoma of the cervix. Am J Pathol 1988;131:587–594.

16. Ostrow RS, Manias DA, Clark BA, et al: The analysis of carcinomas of the vagina for human papillomavirus DNA. Int J Gynecol Pathol 1988;7:308–314.

17. Ostrow RS, Manias DA, Clark BA, et al: Detection of human papillomavirus DNA in invasive carcinomas of the cervix by in situ hybridization. Cancer Res 1987;47:649–653.

18. Nuovo GJ, Richart RM: A comparison of slot blot, Southern blot and in situ hybridization analyses for human papillomavirus DNA in genital tract lesions. Obstet Gynecol 1989;74:673–678.

19. Burns J, Graham AK, Frank C, et al: Detection of low copy human papillomavirus DNA and mRNA in routine paraffin sections of the cervix by non-isotopic in situ hybridization. J Clin Pathol 1987;40:865–869.

20. DelMistro A, Braunstein JD, Halwer M, et al: Identification of human papillomavirus types in male urethral condylomata acuminata by in situ hybridization. Hum Pathol 1987;18:936–940.

21. Gupta JW, Gupta PK, Rosenshein N, et al: Detection of human papillomavirus in cervical smears. A comparison of in situ hybridization, immunocytochemistry and cytopathology. Acta Cytol (Baltimore) 1987;31:387–395.

22. Syrjanen S, Syrjanen K: An improved in situ DNA hybridization protocol for detection of human papillomavirus (HPV) DNA sequences in paraffin-embedded biopsies. J Virol Methods 1986;14:293–304.

23. Crum CP, Ikenberg H, Richart RM, et al: Human papillomavirus type 16 and early cervical neoplasia. N Engl J Med 1984;310:880–883.

24. Lorincz AT, Temple GF, Kurman RJ, et al: Oncogenic association of specific human papillomavirus types with cervical neoplasia. JNCI 1987;79:671–677.

25. Barrasso R, DeBrux J, Croissant O, et al: High prevalence of papillomavirus associated penile intraepithelial neoplasia in sexual partners of women with cervical intraepithelial neoplasia. N Engl J Med 1987;317:916–923.

26. Beckmann A, Myerson B, Daling J, et al: Detection and localization of human papillomavirus

DNA in human genital condylomas by in situ hybridization with biotinylated probes. J Med Virol 1983;16:265–273.

27. Buscema J, Naghashfar Z, Sowada E, et al: The predominance of human papillomavirus type 16 in vulvar neoplasia. Obstet Gynecol 1988;71:601–605.

28. Crum CP, Mitao M, Levine RU, et al: Cervical papillomaviruses segregate within morphologically distinct precancerous lesions. J Virol 1985;54:675–681.

29. Nuovo GJ, O'Connell M, Blanco JB, et al: Correlation of histology and human papillomavirus DNA detection in condyloma acuminatum and condyloma-like vulvar lesions. Am J Surg Pathol 1989;13:700–706.

30. Sato S, Okagaki T, Clark BA, et al: Sensitivity of koilocytosis, immunocytochemistry, and electron microscopy as compared to DNA hybridization in detecting human papillomavirus in cervical and vaginal condyloma and intraepithelial neoplasia. Int J Gynecol Pathol 1987;5:297–307.

31. Sfameni S, Ostor A, Chanen-Fortune D: The association between vulvar condylomata acuminata, cervical wart virus infection and cervical intraepithelial neoplasia. Aust NZ J Obstet Gynaecol 1986;26:149–150.

32. Vallejos H, DelMistro A, Kleinhaus S, et al: Characterization of human papilloma virus types in condylomata acuminata in children by in situ hybridization. Lab Invest 1987;56:611–615.

33. Fuchs PG, Girardi F, Pfister H: Human papillomavirus DNA in normal, metaplastic, preneoplastic and neoplastic epithelia of the cervix uteri. Int J Cancer 1988;41:41–45.

34. Syrjanen S, Syryjanen K, Lamberg M: Detection of human papillomavirus DNA in oral mucosal lesions using in situ DNA hybridization applied on paraffin sections. Oral Surg Oral Med Oral Pathol 1986;62:660–667.

35. Sutton G, Stehman F, Ehrlich C, et al: Human papillomavirus deoxyribonucleic acid in lesions of the female genital tract: Evidence for type 6/11 in squamous carcinoma of the vulva. Obstet Gynecol 1987;70:564–568.

36. Crum CP, Friedman D, Nuovo GJ, et al: Morphological correlates of genital human papillomavirus infection: Viral replication, transcription, and gene expression. In: Gallo R, Hazeltine W, Klein G, et al, eds. Viruses and human cancer. New York: Alan R Liss, 1986.

37. Seedorf K, Krammer G, Durst M, et al: Human papillomavirus type 16 DNA sequence. Virology 1985;145:181–185.

38. Bergeron C, Naghashfar Z, Canaan C, et al: Human papillomavirus type 16 in intraepithelial neoplasia (bowenoid papulosis) and coexistent invasive carcinoma of the vulva. Int J Gynecol Pathol 1987;6:1–11.

39. Pater MM, Dunne J, Hogan G, et al: Human papillomavirus types 16 and 18 sequences in early cervical neoplasia. Virology 1986;155:13–18.

40. Mitao N, Nagai N, Levine RU, et al: Human papillomavirus type 16 infection: A morphological spectrum with evidence for late gene expression. Int J Gynecol Pathol 1987;5:287–296.

41. DiLuca DR, Pilotti L, Stafanon B, et al: Human papillomavirus type 16 DNA in genital tumors: A pathological and molecular analysis. J Gen Virol 1986;67:583–589.

42. Beckmann AM, Kiviat NB, Daling JR, et al: Human papillomavirus type 16 in multifocal neoplasia of the genital tract. Int J Gynecol Pathol 1988;7:39–47.

43. Moy RL, Eliezri YD, Nuovo GJ, et al: Squamous cell carcinoma of the finger is associated with human papillomavirus type 16 DNA. JAMA 1989;261:2669–2673.

44. Tase TT, Okagaki T, Clark BA, et al: Human papillomavirus types and localization in adenocarcinoma and adenosquamous carcinoma of the uterine cervix: A study by in situ DNA hybridization. Cancer Res 1988;48:993–998.

45. Wilczynski SP, Bergen S, Walker J, et al: Human papillomaviruses and cervical cancer: Analysis of histopathologic features associated with different viral types. Hum Pathol 1988;19:697–704.

46. Groben P, Reddick R, Askin F: The pathologic spectrum of small cell carcinoma of the cervix. Int J Gynecol Pathol 1985;4:42–57.

47. Gersell DJ, Mazoujian G, Mutch DG, et al: Small cell undifferentiated carcinoma of the cervix. A clinicopathologic, ultrastructural, and immunocytochemical study of 15 cases. Am J Surg Pathol 1988;12:684–698.

48. Sheets E, Berman M, Hrountas C, et al: Surgically treated, early-stage neuroendocrine small-cell cervical carcinoma. Obstet Gynecol 1988;71:10–14.

49. Ulich T, Liao S, Layfield L, et al: Endocrine and tumor differentiation markers in poorly differentiated small cell carcinoids of the cervix and vagina. Arch Pathol Lab Med 1986;110:1054–1057.

50. Oriel JD: Condylomata acuminata as a sexually transmitted disease. Dermatol Clin 1983;1:93–102.

51. Skegg D, Corwin P, Paul-Doll A: Importance of the male factor in cancer of the cervix. Lancet 1982;ii:581–583.

52. LaVecchia C, Franceschi S, DeCarli A, et al: Sexual factors, venereal diseases, and the risk of intraepithelial and invasive cervical neoplasia. Cancer 1986;58:935–941.

53. Kessler I: Venereal factors in human cervical cancer. Cancer 1977;39:1912–1919.

54. Boshart M, Gissmann L, Ikenberg H, et al: A new type of papillomavirus DNA, its presence in genital cancer biopsies and in cell lines derived from cervical cancer. EMBO J 1984;3:1151–1157.

55. deVilliers EM, Weidauer S, Otto N, et al: Papillomavirus DNA in human tongue carcinomas. Int J Cancer 1985;36:575–577.

56. Ikenberg H, Gissmann L, Gross M, et al: Human papillomavirus type 16 related DNA in genital Bowen's disease and in bowenoid papulosis. Int J Cancer 1983;32:563–565.

57. Byrne J, Tsao M, Fraser R, et al: Human papillomavirus 11 DNA in a patient with chronic laryngotracheobronchial papillomatosis and metastatic squamous cell carcinoma of the lung. N Engl J Med 1987;317:873–878.

58. Gupta J, Pilotti S, Shah KV, et al: Human papillomavirus-associated early vulvar neoplasia investigated by in situ hybridization. Am J Surg Pathol 1987;11:430–434.

59. Brisigotti M, Moreno A, Murcia C, et al: Verrucous carcinoma of the vulva: A clinico-pathologic and immunohistochemical study of five cases. Int J Gynecol Pathol 1989; 8:1–7.

60. Barnes W, Delgado G, Kurman RJ, et al: Possible prognostic significance of human papillomavirus type in cervical cancer. Gynecol Oncol 1988;29:267–273.

61. Tase T, Okagaki T, Clark BA, et al: Human papillomavirus DNA in glandular dysplasia and microglandular hyperplasia: Presumed precursors of adenocarcinoma of the uterine cervix. Obstet Gynecol 1989;73:1005–1008.

62. Jablonska S, Orth G, Obalek S: Cutaneous warts: Clinical, histologic and virologic correlations. Clin Dermatol 1985;3:71–82.

63. Orth G: Epidermodysplasia verruciformis: A model for understanding the oncogenicity of human papillomavirus. Ciba Found Symp 1986;120:157–174.

64. Ostrow RS, Bender M, Niimura M, et al: Human papillomavirus DNA in cutaneous primary and metastasized squamous cell carcinomas from patients with epidermodysplasia verruciformis. Proc Natl Acad Sci USA 1982;79:1634–1638.

65. Ostrow RS, Manias D, Mitchell AJ, et al: Epidermodysplasia verruciformis: A case study associated with primary lymphatic dysplasia, depressed cell-mediated immunity, and Bowen's disease containing human papillomavirus 16 DNA. Arch Dermatol 1987;123:1511–1516.

66. Pfister H, Gassenmaier A, Nurnberger F, et al: Human papillomavirus 5 DNA in a carcinoma of an epidermodysplasia verruciformis infected with various human papilloma virus types. Cancer Res 1983;43:1436–1441.

67. Pfister H, Iftner T, Fuchs PG: Papillomavirus from epidermodysplasia verruciformis patients and renal allograft recipients. In: Howley P, Broker TR, eds. Papillomaviruses: Molecular and clinical aspects. New York: Alan R Liss, Inc, 1985.

68. Ruiter M: On malignant degeneration of skin lesions on epidermodysplasia verruciformis. Dermatol Venerol 1986;49:309–314.

69. Ostrow RS, Shaver K, Turnquist S, et al: Human papillomavirus-16 DNA in a cutaneous invasive carcinoma. Arch Dermatol 1989;125:666–669.

70. Rudlinger R, Grob R, Yu YX, et al: Human papillomavirus-35-positive bowenoid papulosis of the anogenital area and concurrent human papillomavirus-35-positive verruca with bowenoid dysplasia of the periungual area. Arch Dermatol 1989;125:655–659.

71. Durst M, Croce CM, Gissmann L, et al: Papillomavirus sequences integrate near cellular oncogenes in some cervical carcinomas. Proc Natl Acad Sci USA 1987;84:1070–1074.

72. ElAwady MK, Kaplan JB, O'Brien SJ, et al: Molecular analysis of integrated human papillomavirus 16 sequences in the cervical cancer line SiHa. Virology 1987;159:389–398.

73. Lehn H, Villa LL, Marziona F, et al: Physical state and biological activity of human papillomavirus genomes in precancerous lesions of the female genital tract. J Gen Virol 1988;69:187–196.

74. McCance D, Kopan A, Fuchs R, et al: Human papillomavirus type 16 alters human epithelial cell differentiation in vitro. Proc Natl Acad Sci USA 1988;85:7169–7173.

75. Meanwell C, Cox M, Blackledge R, et al: HPV 16 DNA in normal and malignant cervical epithelium: implications for the aetiology and behaviour of cervical neoplasia. Lancet 1987;i:703–707.

76. Firzlaff JM, Kiviat NB, Beckmann AM, et al: Detection of human papillomavirus capsid antigens in various squamous epithelial lesions using antibodies directed against the L1 and L2 open reading frames. Virology 1988;164:467–477.

77. Kadish AS, Burk RD, Kress Y, et al: Human papillomavirus of different types in precancerous lesions of the uterine cervix: Histologic, immunocytochemical and ultrastructural studies. Human Pathol 1986;17:384–392.

78. Giri I, Danos O: Papillomavirus genomes: From sequence data to biological properties. Trend Gene 1986;2:227–232.

79. Dyson N, Howley PM, Munger K, et al: The human papilloma virus-16 E7 oncoprotein is able to bind to the retinoblastoma gene product. Science 1989;243:934–936.

80. Crum CP, Nuovo GJ, Friedman D, et al: Accumulation of RNA homologous to human papillomavirus type 16 open reading frames in genital precancers. J Virol 1988;62:84–90.

81. Nuovo GJ, Friedman D, Silverstein SJ, et al: Transcription of human papillomavirus type 16 in genital precancers. Cancer Cells (Cold Spring Harbor) 1987;5:337–343.

82. Nagai N, Nuovo GJ, Friedman D, et al: Detection of papillomavirus nucleic acids in genital precancers with the in situ hybridization technique: A review. Int J Gynecol Pathol 1987;6:366–379.

83. deVilliers EM, Schneider A, Miklaw H, et al: Human papillomavirus infections in women with and without abnormal cervical cytology. Lancet 1987;i:703–706.

84. Grussendorf-Conen EI, deVilliers EM, Gissmann L: Human papillomavirus genomes in penile smears of healthy men. Lancet 1986;i:1092.

85. Lorincz AT, Temple GF, Patterson JA, et al: Correlation of cellular atypia and human papillomavirus deoxyribonucleic acid sequences in exfoliated cells of the uterine cervix. Obstet Gynecol 1986;68:508–512.

86. Nuovo GJ, Cottral S, Richart RM: Occult infection of the uterine cervix by human papillomavirus in postmenopausal women. Am J Obstet Gynecol 1989;160:340–344.

87. Nuovo GJ, Nuovo MA, Cottral S, et al: Histological correlates of clinically occult human papillomavirus infection of the uterine cervix. Am J Surg Pathol 1988;12:198–204.

88. Nuovo GJ: Correlation of histology with human papillomavirus DNA detection in the female genital tract. Gynecol Oncol 1988;31:176–181.

89. Goldsborough MD, DiSilvestre D, Temple GF, et al: Nucleotide sequence of human papillomavirus type 31: A cervical neoplasia-associated virus. Virology 1989;171:306–311.

90. Twiggs LB, Okagaki T, Clark B, et al: A clinical, histopathological, and molecular biological investigation of vulvar intraepithelial neoplasia. Int J Gynecol Pathol 1988;7:48–55.
91. Nuovo GJ, Richart RM: In situ hybridization analysis of HPV DNA segregation patterns in lesions of the female genital tract. Gynecol Oncol (in press).

CHAPTER 10

Natural History and Clinicopathologic Correlations of HPV-Related Changes

Yao-Shi Fu, MD and Lee H. Hilborne, MD, MPH

Papillomaviruses are a family of DNA viruses that naturally infect a variety of animal hosts, including humans. Human papillomavirus (HPV) is responsible for a broad range of epithelial manifestations, including the verruca vulgaris and the genital condyloma. We are most concerned in this chapter with the role HPV plays in genital infections and subsequent neoplasia.

Human papillomavirus usually comes to the attention of the patient and physician either by the presence of visible genital warts or a suggestive abnormality (eg, koilocytosis or dyskeratotic cells) on routine Papanicolaou cytology. The natural history of HPV may follow five possible scenarios, once the infection is established and detected. There may be persistent active infection, evidenced by persistent genital warts or abnormal clinical signs, including colposcopy, cytology and histology; some genital HPV infections, like their counterparts in other locations, persist for years without evidence of neoplastic transformation. Following active infection, one may also observe regression of detectable disease with molecular or ultrastructural evidence of viral persistence, suggesting a latent viral persistence. There may be active infection for some period of time, followed by regression and complete resolution of the infection. It is difficult, if not impossible, to distinguish between complete absence of the virus following infection and its persistence in a latent stage.

Some sexual partners of individuals with definitive HPV infection demonstrate only molecular or ultrastructural evidence of disease; thus, one possible situation is a latent infection without an observed period of cytologic or visible disease. The last possible scenario, and the most clinically important, is infection of the external genital tract followed by progression to epithelial neoplasia. Epidemiologic evidence strongly suggests that HPV, either latent or expressed, plays a major role in the development of these neoplasms. It is the nature of this association that is the basis of the following discussion.

ISSN 1043-3198/89/$3.50

Clinical Practice of Gynecology: **2,** 152–173, 1989
© 1989 Elsevier Science Publishing Co., Inc.
655 Avenue of the Americas, New York, NY 10010

EPIDEMIOLOGY OF HPV INFECTION

Human papillomavirus is highly contagious in the genital tract. In a follow-up study of 97 patients who had intercourse with known infected partners, 62 (64%) developed subsequent evidence of HPV infection.[1] The incubation period ranged from 3 to 33 weeks with an average period of 2.8 months. Not all patients were followed for the duration of the study; thus, the risk of infection may in fact be higher than 64%. In a study of 15 virgin women exposed to men with penile HPV, all subsequently developed vulvar warts.[1]

Human papillomavirus infectivity appears to decrease with duration of infection. Among women who developed HPV infections following exposure to infected men, the male genital lesions had been present for an average of 3.5 months. The HPV infection was present for an average of 12 months in men whose partners, when exposed, failed to develop clinical evidence of infection.[1] In common skin warts, the number of HPV particles reaches a peak at about 12 months and decreases thereafter; therefore, it is reasonable to postulate that the same process occurs in the genital tract.[2]

Molecular pathology confirmation of infection was not available when these early studies were performed. Although population-dependent, a more recent study demonstrated the presence of detectable HPV DNA from genital washings or cervical scrapings in 9% of women with negative cytologic smears.[3] This suggests that latent infection may be more prevalent than had previously been suspected.

A number of prospective studies have been performed to evaluate the potential risk of associated future neoplasia once HPV infection is established. Vayrynen and colleagues[4] colposcopically followed 271 women who, on routine Papanicolaou smears, had cytologic changes consistent with HPV infection. The HPV incidence peaked in women between 22 and 24 years of age; 60% were under 30 years old. During the initial study evaluation, following referral based on cytology suggesting HPV infection, 35% (197/556) of the repeat smears were determined to be class I (normal). Of these, 63% (124/197) showed no colposcopic evidence of atypia (ie, warty, punctate, mosaic, leukoplakial, or a combination of these changes). When viewed from the standpoint of colposcopic appearance, when colposcopy was negative, 46% of follow-up smears were class I (normal); 46%, class II (inflammatory atypia); 7%, class III (dysplasia); and 0.4%, class IV (carcinoma in situ). When colposcopy showed an abnormality, 25% of follow-up smears were class I; 60%, class II; 15%, class III; and 0.3%, class IV. When the authors studied 271 biopsy specimens (from an unspecified number of patients, although they biopsied only patients with cervical intraepithelial neoplasia [CIN] and HPV), only 190 (70%) contained histologic evidence of HPV infection. The remaining 81 biopsies from patients with cytologic evidence of CIN were histologically negative for HPV, and only 38% (31/

81) of these showed any colposcopic suggestion of atypia. Although the authors suggest that biopsy may have removed small lesions (ie, nonspontaneous regression), colposcopic evidence of regression was also observed in situations where biopsy was not taken.

Schneider and colleagues[5] suggest that colposcopy may be superior to cytology when one is evaluating patients for HPV infection. Of 2232 women with no evidence of CIN by conventional cytology, 11% demonstrated the presence of HPV DNA by nucleic acid hybridization. Of these, 150 patients had an adequate colposcopic examination. Abnormal findings were observed in 70%.

A number of studies have discussed the biologic behavior of HPV infection. The study duration, variables examined, and criteria for inclusion vary considerably between studies. A few significant studies will be presented, followed by a discussion of the implications of the findings.

Syrjanen et al[6] prospectively followed 513 consecutive women with cytologic changes suggestive of HPV for an average of 25.6 ± 17.9 (1 SD) months. When HPV was the only initial finding, regression was observed in 30% of patients, persistence in 62% and progression to CIN in 8%. When CIN accompanied the HPV infection on the initial evaluation, regression was observed in 13% of patients, persistence in 59%, progression to more advanced CIN in 24%, and recurrence in 3%. Since biopsy was included in the initial evaluation of some patients, the reported regression rate may not fairly represent the spontaneous regression rate because the viral infection site may have been surgically excised. The authors also published another report, using the same patients, describing the natural history of HPV infection based on the Papanicolaou smear at the time of entry into the study.[7]

Nash and colleagues[8] studied 45 patients who, on initial cytology, had findings compatible with HPV infection. Patients were excluded when there was cytologic evidence of any additional pathology. Histologic confirmation was required for entry into the study. There were 412 new patients who sought care from the Bethesda Naval Hospital during the study, 87 (21%) of whom had cytologic evidence of HPV as the only abnormality. Of these, 52 patients had histologic confirmation of the infection, and follow-up was available for 45. Of the 45 patients at the time of entry into the study, CIN was already present in 5. Of the remaining 40 patients, resolution occurred in 18 (45%) over an average period of 13.7 months, persistence in 7 (18%) over an average period of 21 months, and progression to CIN in 15 (38%) over an average period of 10.9 months.

The exact natural history of HPV infections remains unclear from the studies presented. It is clear that some HPV lesions regress, while others persist or progress. Cervical intraepithelial neoplasia, when present, is associated with a decreased likelihood of regression and an increased chance of progression to more advanced disease. When CIN is present, severity of dysplasia inversely correlates with regression and directly correlates with progression to higher grades of CIN.[6] The above findings clearly suggest that CIN alone, determined by conventional cytology and histology, is inadequate to accurately predict the behavior of HPV infections. The infection pattern, the type of HPV present, and DNA ploidy pattern are likely candidates for influencing neoplastic behavior in these lesions. Establishment of neoplasia requires a favorable interaction between the host and the neoplasm. The host's ability to mount an immune response to destroy HPV and associated neoplasia must be of significance in predicting tumor behavior. The remaining portion of this chapter discusses other factors related to the pathogenesis of HPV-induced changes and their clinicopathologic correlations.

HPV TYPES AND OUTCOME OF CERVICAL CONDYLOMA AND CIN

With the growth of modern molecular pathology, it is now possible to study HPV infections at the molecular level. Such investigations have identified well over 50 HPV types.[9] The prevalence of HPV types varies from study to study and is influenced by geographic location, the population, detection techniques, and morphologic criteria; nevertheless, a general trend exists. HPV types 6 and 11 are most frequently associated with exophytic warts and low-grade dysplasia, whereas HPV subtypes 16, 18, 31, 33, 35, 39, and those in the 40s more frequently result in higher-grade dysplasias. Genital HPV infection is a venereal disease, and the manner of acquisition does not vary between different types. Since the risk factors for all genital HPV types are similar, the frequency of mixed HPV infection, using the Southern blot technique for detection, is between 15–20%.[6,7]

When the natural history of HPV infection is compared with HPV type, an increased likelihood of progression or persistence is observed with HPV types 16 and 18. The results of Syrjanen's study comparing HPV type to neoplastic progression are presented (Table 10–1). Campion and colleagues[10] examined HPV type and the natural history of CIN I (Table 10–1). This study followed 100 women for a minimum of 19 months and included hybridization for only HPV 6 and 16. At least one of these viruses was detected in 58% of women with persistent disease and 88% of women with progressive disease. Of 26 women with evidence of progression to CIN III, 85% of patients were infected with HPV 16. Of the nine HPV-6-positive patients who progressed to CIN III, eight were also infected with HPV 16. Since other HPV types (eg, 18, 31, 33) were not studied, this latter patient may also have been infected with a second, undetected virus. In this study, 15% of women who subsequently developed CIN III had two consecutive false-negative cervical smears. This suggests that women with CIN I should be aggressively evaluated; complacency is inappropriate in

TABLE 10–1. Natural History of Different HPV Types

Author/Disease	HPV Type	Regress (%)	Persist (%)	Progress (%)	Recur (%)
Syrjanen et al[6]	6/11	26	26	48	—
(HPV & HPV + CIN)	16	6	56	33	6
	18	11	67	22	—
	31	—	100	—	—
	Dbl Infect	27	55	18	—
Campion et al[10]	6,N = 46	7	74	20	—
(CIN I)	16,N = 39	0	36	54	10
	6 + 16,N = 20	0	60	40	—
Schneider et al[11]					
HPV only	6/11,N = 7	43	57	0	—
	16/18,N = 3	66	0	33	—
	6/11 + 16/18,N = 7	14	71	14	—
CIN I/II	6/11,N = 5	60	40	0	—
	16/18,N = 17	53	24	24	—
	6/11 + 16/18,N = 4	25	25	50	—
CIN III	16/18,N = 4	0	100	0	—
	6/11 + 16/18,N = 1	0	100	0	—

the study of any patient with CIN. Although the numbers are small, Schneider et al[11] similarly found that progressive cases were more likely to contain HPV 16 or 18 than HPV 6 or 11.

While the details of all the studies presented are somewhat variable, they all support the existence of two general categories of HPV infection. Human papillomaviruses 6 and 11 are associated with a more benign process, and HPV 16 and 18 appear to possess more oncogenic potential. While HPV type cannot entirely predict the future behavior of all infections, it is clear that knowledge of the HPV type may be useful in guiding therapeutic decisions. The HPV type, especially in CIN I lesions, can be of value in deciding between a more conservative intensive follow-up program and a more aggressive treatment regimen.

IMMUNE RESPONSE AND HPV INFECTION

The biologic behavior of neoplastic growths involves a variety of host interactions in addition to the presence or absence of an inciting or promoting agent. We know, from multiple other studies, that patients who are immunosuppressed for any reason (eg, transplant patients, patients with acquired or inherited immunodeficiencies) are at increased risk for the development of malignancy. Some of the variability seen in neoplastic behavior of lesions in HPV-infected patients, therefore, may well represent an inability of the woman's immune system to effectively eliminate or suppress the viral expression. Several findings suggest that host immune responses do occur and play a major role in the natural history of HPV infection. Immunosuppressed women are 10–15 times more likely to develop cervical condyloma and neoplasia than are their nonimmunosuppressed counterparts. Spontaneous regression of skin and genital warts frequently occurs, confirming the host's ability to deal effectively with the viral assault. Pregnant women are relatively immunosuppressed; increased growth of genital warts during pregnancy frequently occurs with subsequent regression following childbirth. Evidence of a cell-mediated dermal immune response in regressed skin warts attests to the ability of the immune system to recognize the foreign virus and destroy the infection. Patients with epidermodysplasia verruciformis, a particular group of skin warts, develop in situ and invasive squamous cell carcinoma in sun-exposed areas; these patients also have a recessive genetic T-cell deficiency. These patients are infected with a number of HPV types (mostly 5 and 8) that are not seen in immunologically competent individuals.[12] Following radiation, HPV-infected laryngeal and genital tissues frequently undergo malignant transformation.[13,14] Unfortunately, there is only limited information available on the specific immune factors that play a role neoplastic growth in the presence of HPV.

Lancaster and Jenson[15] review the natural history of HPV infection. Within their review, they consider the host immune response. Viral-coded polypeptides have been identified in vitro on the cytoplasmic membranes of HPV-infected cells.[16] One would expect recognition of foreign viral proteins to induce a vigorous immune response, yet many CIN lesions persist for some time. Latency may represent an abnormal immune response to the viral infection. Human papillomavirus antigens were detected in nearly one-half of laryngeal papilloma patients on single biopsy; however, with repeated biopsy over time in the same patients, all demonstrated viral antigens on at least one biopsy.[17] Possible explanations for this finding include sampling and sporadic viral antigen expression, perhaps cyclical and related to the immunotolerance of the local environment.

Syrjanen and colleagues[7] studied subepithelial stromal inflammatory infiltrates surrounding HPV infections. Stromal immunocompetent cell infiltrates were studied using fresh frozen biopsy specimens. Infiltrates in the subepithelium consist of helper (OKT-4) and cytotoxic/suppressor T-lymphocytes, B lymphocytes (Leu-10), NK and K (HNK-1) cells, and monocyte/macrophages (MPS cells), including Langerhans cells (OKT-6). The relative proportions of OKT-4 and OKT-8 cells (helper/suppressor ratio) bear some relationship to the degree of cellular atypia, with a decreasing ratio associated with increasing cellular atypia. When CIN was present in the initial biopsy, there was a trend toward smaller T-helper/suppressor ratios. While an association appears to exist between the lymphocyte population and the presence and degree of dysplasia, further studies are needed to determine the exact nature of this observed correlation.

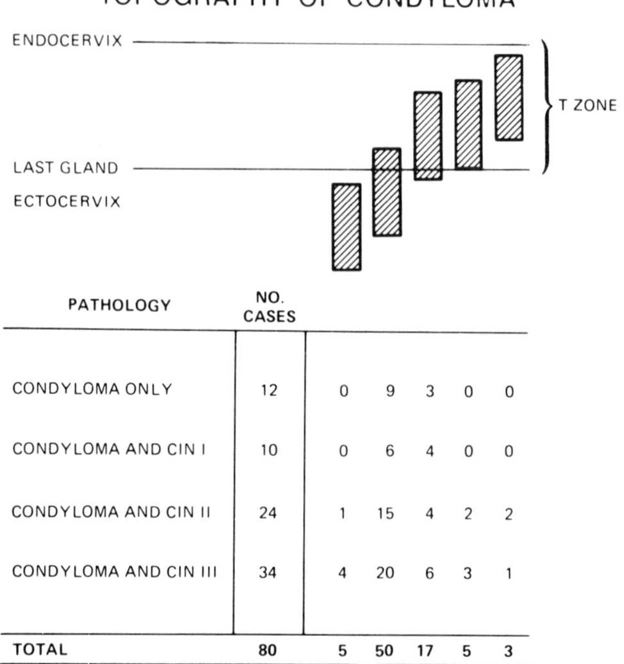

PATHOLOGY	NO. CASES					
CONDYLOMA ONLY	12	0	9	3	0	0
CONDYLOMA AND CIN I	10	0	6	4	0	0
CONDYLOMA AND CIN II	24	1	15	4	2	2
CONDYLOMA AND CIN III	34	4	20	6	3	1
TOTAL	80	5	50	17	5	3

FIGURE 10–1 Topography of condyloma in relation to the transformation zone. The majority occur in the vicinity of the last endocervical gland, which earmarks the original squamocolmnar junction. The ectocervical mucosa is usually involved. (Reprinted with permission from the American Cancer Society, Saito et al: Cancer 1987; 59:2064.)

TOPOGRAPHIC RELATIONSHIP BETWEEN CERVICAL CONDYLOMA AND INTRAEPITHELIAL NEOPLASIA

Studies performed in the 1950s and 1960s based on careful mapping and reconstruction of cervical biopsies and colposcopic examination demonstrated that a great majority of cervical intraepithelial neoplasias occur within the transformation zone. The topographic relationship between cervical condyloma and CIN is not entirely clear because flat condylomas were an unrecognized entity in these earlier studies. Recently, 101 consecutive conization specimens with CIN were mapped to determine where HPV infects cervical epithelium, the sites where CIN develop, and the topographic relationship between condyloma and CIN.[18] In this study, the last endocervical gland marked the original squamocolumnar junction. Condylomatous changes were present in 85% of cervices with CIN. In 75 of 80 (94%) specimens, the condylomatous changes involved the transformation zone (Figure 10–1). The majority (63%) of condylomas extend distally to involve the original squamocolumnar junction. Condylomatous

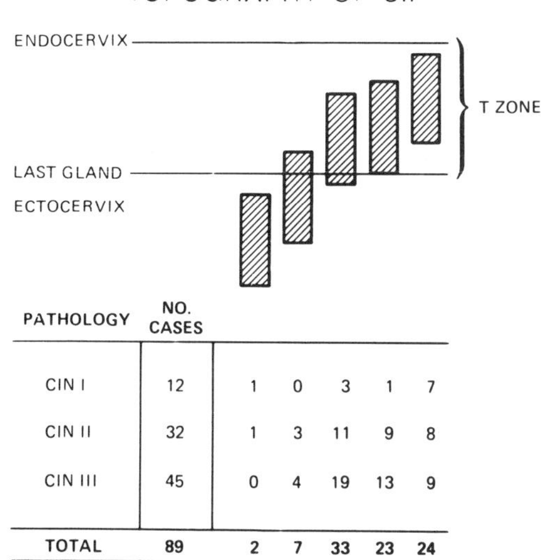

PATHOLOGY	NO. CASES					
CIN I	12	1	0	3	1	7
CIN II	32	1	3	11	9	8
CIN III	45	0	4	19	13	9
TOTAL	89	2	7	33	23	24

FIGURE 10–2 Topography of CIN, on the other hand, is predominantly proximal to the last endocervical gland. (Reprinted with permission from the American Cancer Society, Saito et al: Cancer 1987; 59:2064.)

lesions were completely isolated on the ectocervix in only five (5%) of cases (Figure 10–1).

Condylomatous change can be distinguished from the adjacent normal ectocervical mucosa by slight thickening, increased cellular proliferation in the parabasal layers, and koilocytosis. The histologic extent of condylomatous change is more extensive than colposcopically observed changes; the outer borders are clearly delineated microscopically. The inner borders of condyloma merge with squamous metaplasia, CIN, and the endocervical mucosa.

When CIN was evaluated topographically, in contrast with condyloma, 80 of 89 (89%) were proximal to the original squamocolumnar junction (Figure 10–2).[18] Seven (8%) of the remaining CINs involved predominantly the mucosa overlying the last endocervical gland and ectocervix. Only two (2%) CINs were located in the ectocervix without any involvement of the transformation zone (Figure 10–2). When condyloma coexists with CIN, the former is always distal (ectocervical side) to the latter. The most common topographic relationship between the two is a gradual transition from condyloma to atypical condyloma to CIN (37 specimens, 42%). A sharp transition between condyloma and CIN was observed in 23 (26%) specimens studied. Therefore, nearly 70% of all CINs in this study were in direct contact with condyloma. Less commonly (15 specimens, 17%), CIN was separated from the condyloma by a squamous metaplasia zone. Only 14 (15%) CINs were not associated with condyloma or atypical condyloma.

Most of these cases were either grade II or grade III CIN. Over 90% of CIN I and CIN II biopsies also contained koilocytes, compared with 78% of those with CIN III.[18] Parenthetically, earlier topographic studies performed when koilocytosis was unrecognized as the hallmark of HPV infection, reported clear cells with perinuclear vacuoles in 50% of dysplasias.[19]

Topographic studies demonstrate that the severity and degree of CIN differentiation is influenced by the affected epithelium location. Lesions at or adjacent to the squamocolumnar junction tend to show more koilocytotic change and less severe dysplasia when compared with those CINs higher in the endocervical canal.

The well-defined proximal condyloma borders observed in these topographic studies do not support the concept that HPV infection induces a diffuse field change involving the entire cervical mucosa. In situ hybridization studies would be helpful to further confirm this observation and other unanswered questions.

IN SITU AUTORADIOGRAPHIC EVALUATION OF CERVICAL INTRAEPITHELIAL NEOPLASIA

Representative sections of 70 cervical conization specimens with sufficient intraepithelial neoplasia were studied by in situ hybridization using an ^{35}S-labeled nucleic acid probe and an autoradiographic technique. The findings of these cases, and in vulvar intraepithelial neoplasia (VIN), demonstrate that HPV DNA is detected only in condyloma and intraepithelial neoplasia and not in normal cervical or vulvar epithelium (Figure 10–3).[20,21] When detected, HPV DNA was greatest toward the surface and weakest toward the basal layers (Figure 10–4). The DNA amount expressed was directly related to the degree of differentiation and the viral antigen expression. Invasive carcinomas were essentially negative, and areas of carcinoma in situ demonstrated variable hybridization. In less differentiated lesions, the number of silver particles is fewer. The authors suggest the detection limits of their particular assay system is 100 DNA copies per cell.[21]

With the use of a similar technique and ^{35}S-labeled probes, HPV DNA was detected in 71% of cervical conization specimens removed for CIN. When it was examined by HPV type, 41% were HPV type 16, 14% HPV type 18, 7% HPV type 31, and 7% were mixed with more than one HPV type.[22] When evaluated by degree of dysplastic change, over 90% of HPV types 16, 18, 31, and mixed infections were associated with CIN II and CIN III (Figure 10–4). HPV types 6 and 11 were detected primarily in cases of mixed infections.[20] Mixed infections were observed, in this study, in only 7% of all CINs and in 16% of CINs in which HPV DNA was detected.[20] This frequency is lower than the 15–20% of mixed infections observed in cervical condyloma or CIN by Southern blot analysis. This variation may be explained by the different sensitivity of the two techniques.

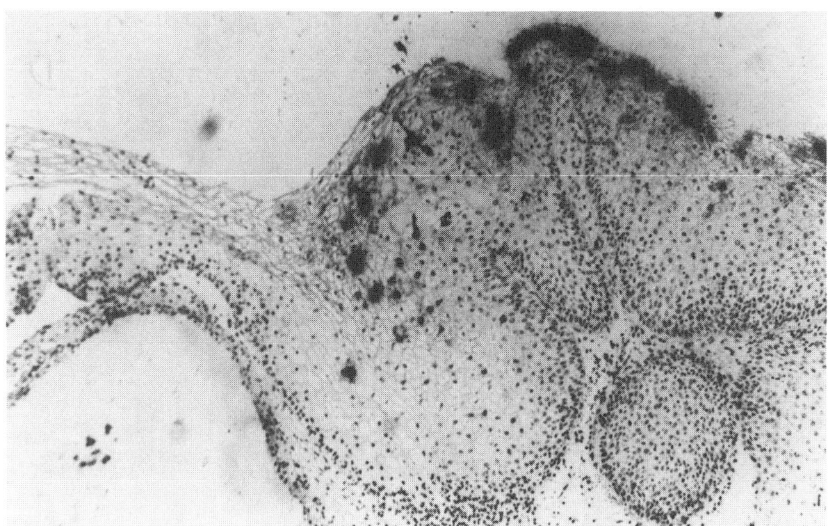

FIGURE 10–3 Autoradiographic preparation using ^{35}S-labeled HPV DNA type 6. Note heavy concentrations of silver grains in the superficial layers and a sharp border with normal mucosa. ($\times$ 80).

Most CINs histologically have benign condylomatous changes; when dysplasia is present in cervical biopsies, different degrees or grades of dysplasia are frequently seen in close proximity. The HPV type in each of these lesions is usually the same. This suggests that all HPV types initially cause mild changes. Those that subsequently progressed to CIN spread proximally to the cervical canal. Irrespective of HPV type, then, it is essential to adequately sample affected areas to determine the maximum degree of dysplastic changes present.

HPV TYPES AND DNA PLOIDY PATTERNS

In order to directly correlate DNA ploidy patterns with HPV type, paraffin blocks histologically containing CIN and autoradiographically shown to contain HPV DNA were selected for further analysis. Autoradiographic in situ hybridization was used to determine both the presence and type of HPV virus present. DNA ploidy was studied using 44 conization specimens from which 10–12 micron paraffin sections were cut, stained by the Feulgen technique, and analyzed by computerized digital imaging using a 560-nm light. Eighty-eight percent of CINs with HPV type 16 (23/26) (Figure 10–5), 88% of HPV type 18 (7/8), 86% of HPV type 31 (6/7), and all mixed HPV infections (3/3) had aneuploid DNA distributions. The remaining five (11%) specimens had either diploid (4 cases) or polyploid (1 case) DNA patterns. These findings are comparable with the study by Goppinger et

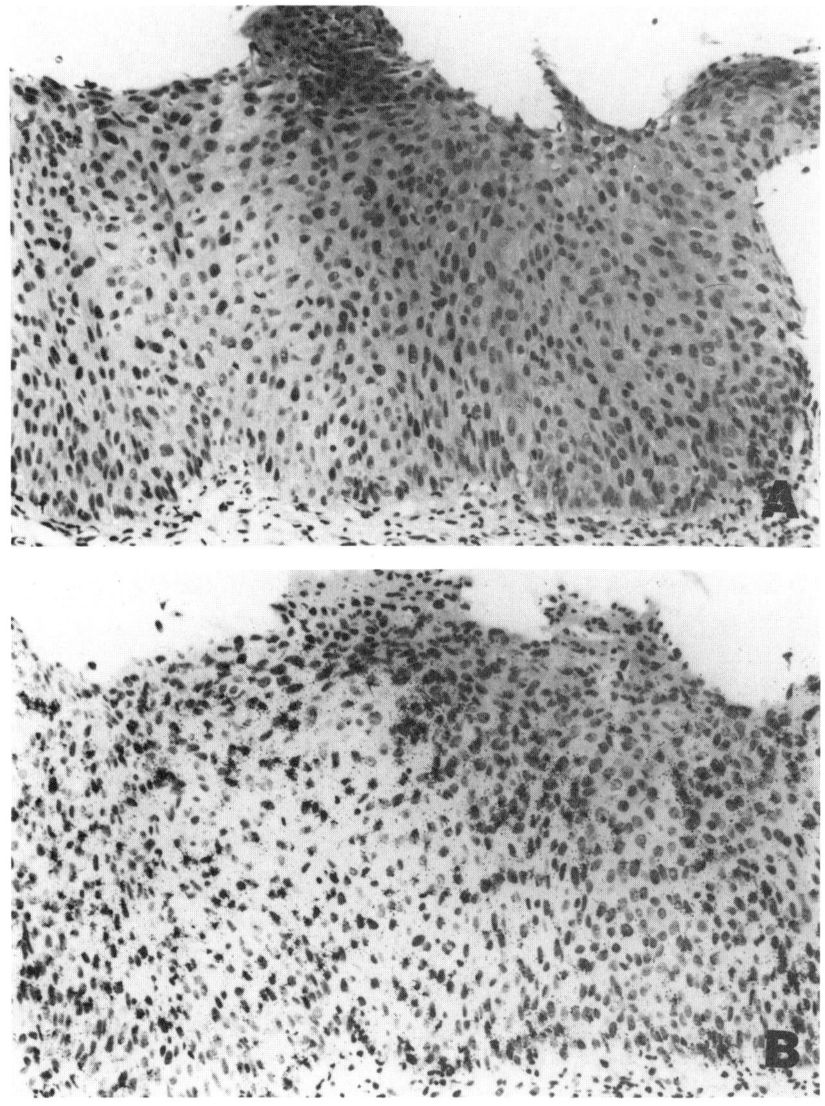

FIGURE 10–4 This CIN III prepared with autoradiographic technique using ^{35}S-labeled HPV probes is negative for HPV 6 and 11 (A), but positive for HPV 18 (B). A diffuse deposit of silver grains within the CIN is accompanied by a heavier concentration in the superficial cells. (× 250)

al,[22] who found that 88% (14/16) of CINs associated with HPV type 16 or 18 were aneuploid. In contrast, 85% (11/13) of CINs having HPV type 6/11 were diploid or polyploid (Figure 10–6), and the remaining 15% aneuploid.

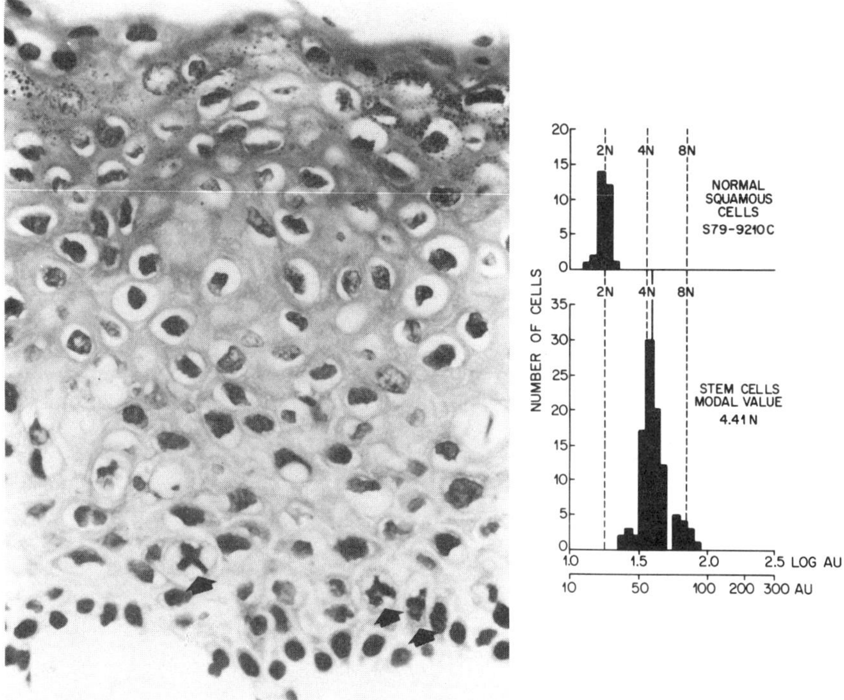

FIGURE 10–5 A CIN II associated with HPV 16 and an aneuploid DNA pattern. Abnormal cells demonstrate moderate nuclear atypia with enlargement, irregularity, and hyperchromasia. Abnormal mitotic figures (arrows) occur in the parabasal layers. The modal value of the major peak (4.41N) exceeds the expected polyploid range. (× 510)

When an aneuploid pattern is present, the stem cell modal values (the mean of a predominant peak) were significantly different from the diploid or polyploid ranges. Differences were considered significant when they exceeded the control cell coefficient of variation (standard deviation/mean). With the use of similar criteria for the interpretation of DNA histograms and DNA ploidy patterns, the latter were found to be most reliable for CIN outcome prediction.[23]

In a retrospective study of 120 women with histologically confirmed CIN and without therapy for at least 1 year, the initial cervical biopsies were studied by Feulgen microspectrophotometry for determining ploidy patterns. Among 47 CINs that returned to normal, 40 (85%) were diploid or polyploid, and seven (15%) were aneuploid. Of the 65 CINs that persisted for at least 1 year, 60 (92%) were aneuploid, and five (8%) were diploid or polyploid. All eight CINs that progressed to invasive carcinoma had an aneuploid DNA distribution.[24] Although the study by Nasiell and colleagues[25]

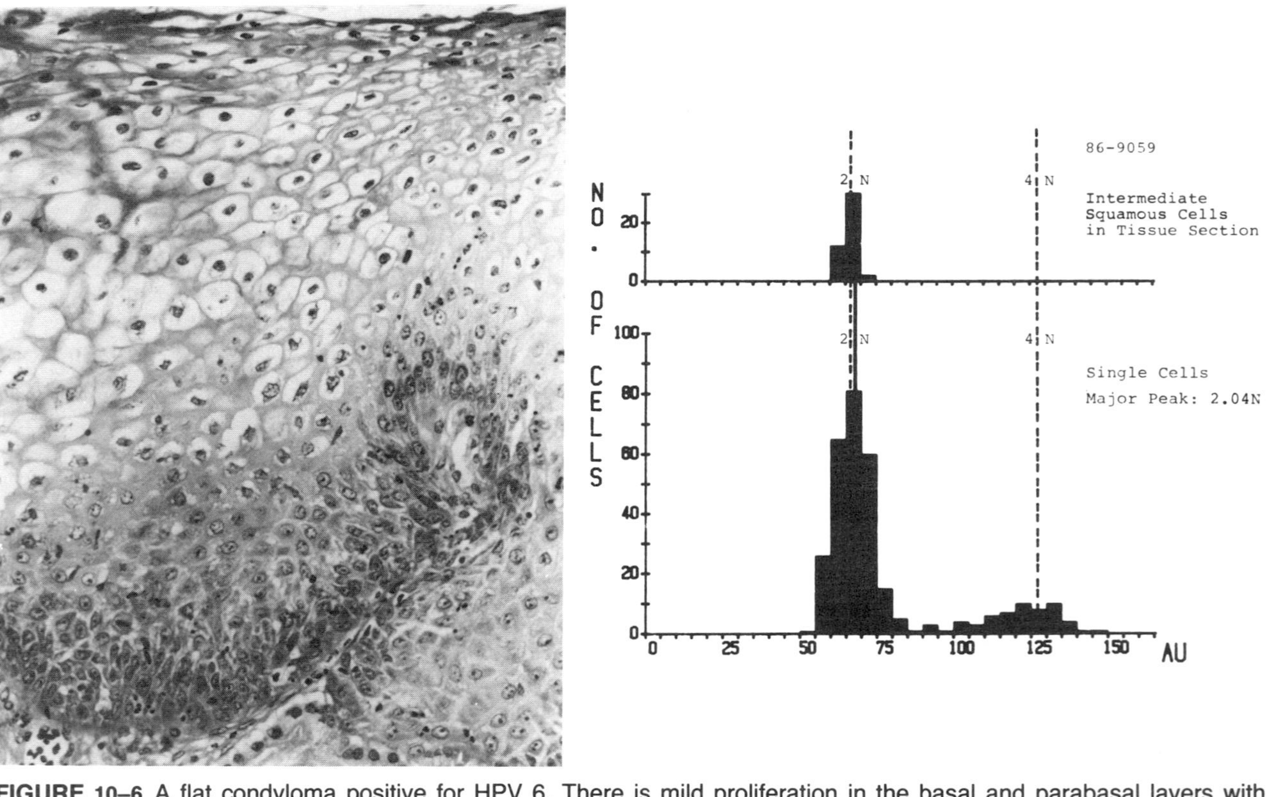

FIGURE 10–6 A flat condyloma positive for HPV 6. There is mild proliferation in the basal and parabasal layers with preservation of normal polarity. Koilocytosis is prominent in the intermediate and superficial layers. Nuclear atypia is minimal. DNA histogram reveals a diploid pattern with a predominant peak in the diploid region. Scattered values up to the tetraploid (4N) range represent S and G2 cells, corresponding to koilocytes with nuclear atypia. (× 200)

failed to demonstrate a correlation between DNA ploidy and CIN behavior, their study was based on a relatively small number of cells present on cervical smears, precluding accurate determination of the ploidy pattern in most specimens. Furthermore, abnormal cells in cervical smears tend to degenerate and are less representative of the lesion studied because of their superficial layer origin.

In a prospective study of 51 untreated women with warty atypia who were cytologically and colposcopically monitored, 53% (18/34) of lesions with a polyploid pattern regressed, whereas all five with aneuploid changes persisted at least 1 year.[26] Therefore, aneuploidy again appears indicative of malignant potential with a strong likelihood of persistence and possible progression to invasive carcinoma.

Most ordinary cervical condylomas are diploid or polyploid.[27–30] When atypia (ie, dysplasia, CIN) is present, 45% of condylomatous lesions are aneuploid.[27] These findings explain the increased frequency of persistence and progression in condylomas with atypia.

Further correlative studies of DNA ploidy with histologic features identified abnormal mitotic figures and marked nuclear atypia as the histologic counterpart of aneuploidy.[31] In cervical biopsies, abnormal mitotic figures were observed in 85% of cervical condylomas and CIN when an aneuploid pattern was present and in only 14% of specimens that were diploid or polyploid.[30] In a separate study, when abnormal mitotic figures were seen in the cervical biopsies with CIN, 18% were polyploid and 82% aneuploid.[32] The abnormal mitotic figures in polyploid lesions were usually those of dispersed or tripolar types. Other forms of abnormal mitoses, especially those in group two and three metaphase, are more common in aneuploid CIN.

MORPHOMETRY AND HPV TYPE

A strong correlation between morphology and HPV type supports the concept of low- and high-risk groups among HPV patients. Furthermore, abnormal mitotic figures are most frequently found in association with HPV type 16. Among CINs with and without abnormal mitotic figures, the frequency of HPV type 16 is 70% and 10%, respectively.[33] Other investigators, however, have found no correlation between CIN morphology and HPV type.[34] To determine the key morphologic differences between those CINs with HPV 6 and 11 and those with HPV 16, 18 and 33, cervical lesions of known HPV type were quantitated on the basis of their morphometric and mitotic parameters.[35] The mean parameter values for these two groups are summarized in Table 10–2. Useful discriminators, determined mathematically with the use of F statistics in the order of descending importance, are total mitotic index, abnormal mitotic index, cellularity index of the super-

TABLE 10–2. Mean Values of Each Parameter

Parameters	HPV 6/11	HPV 16/18/33	F-Statistics
Parabasal layer			
nu* perimeter mean (μm)	22.5	22.8	0.05
nu perimeter SD (μm)	3.8	4.0	0.35
nu area mean (μm^2)	40.5	40.5	0.00
nu area SD (μm^2)	12.6	12.8	0.01
cellularity index	68.6	80.1	0.70
Intermediate layers			
nu perimeter mean (μm)	25.5	24.7	0.15
nu perimeter SD (μm)	3.5	4.5	1.42
nu area mean (μm^2)	52.7	47.7	0.42
nu area SD (μm^2)	15.0	16.3	0.07
cellularity index	32.4	63.0	7.43
Superficial layers			
nu perimeter mean (μm)	23.9	24.0	0.00
nu perimeter SD (μm)	3.8	4.3	0.55
nu area mean (μm^2)	47.8	43.5	0.29
nu area SD (μm^2)	14.8	13.7	0.14
cellularity index	20.1	51.9	8.14
Mitotic index			
Total number	2.5	17.9	12.29
Abnormal form	0.1	7.5	8.82

Cellularity index, number of nuclei/10,000 μm^2; SD, standard deviation; nu*, nuclear; mitotic index, number of mitotic figures per 10 high power fields.

(Modified and Reprinted with permission from International Society of Gynecological Pathologists, Fu et al., Int J Gynecol Path 1988 7:297.)

ficial and intermediate layers, and standard deviation of nuclear perimeter of intermediate cells (Figures 10–4–10–6).[35]

Both the total and abnormal mitotic indices differ significantly between the HPV 6/11 and HPV 16/18/33 groups. All HPV 6 or 11 cases demonstrated a total mitotic index of less than seven per ten high-power fields (HPF, 1 HPF = 350 μm in diameter or 96,200 μm^2). Only one of seven specimens demonstrated abnormal mitotic figures with dispersed chromosomes. In HPV 16/18/33, two of 14 specimens had less than seven total mitotic figures per ten HPFs. All of these had abnormal mitotic figures (Figure 10–5). These findings support those of Bergeron and colleagues.[36] In their study of multicentric squamous intraepithelial neoplasia of the female lower-genital tract, abnormal mitotic figures were found in 16% of HPV 6/11, 87% of HPV 16, and 75% of mixed HPV types.[36]

By stepwise discriminant analysis, HPV types can be separated by six morphometric criteria. If mitotic indices are added, a total mitotic index and three other morphometric parameters suffice to distinguish the two groups. Therefore, objective, quantitative analyses of lesions associated with HPV 16/18/33 reveal higher proliferative rates and mitotic activities than those of HPV 6/11.[35]

A basic theme emerges; HPV 6/11 lesions are generally diploid or polyploid, morphologically and morphometrically less proliferative, and portend a more benign outcome. On the contrary, other HPV types are more likely to be aneuploid, more atypical with abnormal mitotic figures, and more likely to persist or progress. Among women infected by either HPV group, some patients will recover without further complication. This suggests enhancement of the neoplastic process by cocarcinogens or promotors. Recurrence or persistence of HPV-related changes following treatment is likely to result from such factors as reinfection, immunosuppression, and multifocal and multicentric disease.

MULTIFOCAL AND MULTICENTRIC INVOLVEMENT IN LOWER GENITAL TRACT

Multifocal disease in one anatomic site and multicentric involvement of more than one site (ie, cervix, vagina, vulva, and perineum) by HPV is common; failure to recognize this possibility may lead to oversights in the detection of coexistent lesions. When such infections are untreated, they serve as a site for reinfection. The possibility of progression to invasive carcinoma in these instances cannot be overlooked. Among women with squamous condyloma or neoplasia and HPV DNA detected in the lower-genital tract using autoradiography and ^{35}S probes, 13 (43%) had multicentric disease.[21] In ten (77%) of these 13 cases, the HPV type was the same in all sites within an individual patient. More than one HPV type was identified in the remaining three patients; multiple HPV types were found at the same site in 6% (3/47) of patients.

Bergerson and colleagues[36] also addressed the issue of HPV multicentricity in anogenital lesions. They studied 24 patients with 61 multicentric lesions involving the cervix, vagina, vulva, urethra, and anus. Thirteen (54%) patients had two sites involved, nine (38%) had three sites involved, and two (8%) had four sites involved. HPV DNA was found in 21 (88%) of 24 patients and 46 (75%) of 61 lesions examined. Simultaneous infection with more than one virus was found in 48% of 21 patients and in 17% of the 46 lesions. Of the ten patients with multiple infections, nine were infected by two viral types, most commonly a 6/11 type and HPV 16, and one patient was infected by four viral types. Thus, in the presence of HPV infection, the entire anogenital region is at risk of exposure to more than one type of HPV and of developing squamous and possibly glandular neoplasms.

HPV AND CERVICAL GLANDULAR NEOPLASMS

A review of six studies reported from different geographic areas demonstrates a correlation between the histologic type of cervical neoplasm and HPV type (Table 10–3).[37–42] Human papillomavirus 16 is clearly the most

TABLE 10–3. HPV Type and Cervical Invasive Carcinoma[37–42]

Histology	No. Pts.	HPV-16 (%)	HPV-18 (%)
Squamous cell carcinoma	126	57 (45)	4 (3)
Adenocarcinoma in situ	10	2 (20)	5 (50)
Micro adenocarcinoma	11	3 (27)	5 (45)
Adenocarcinoma	48	5 (10)	21 (44)
Adenosquamous carcinoma	55	10 (18)	13 (24)

common virus type among genital squamous neoplasms, being detected in 45% of invasive squamous carcinomas. Human papillomavirus 16 is followed by HPV 18 in 3%. In contrast, HPV 18 is the predominant type identified in 50% and 44% of in situ and invasive adenocarcinomas, respectively. Human papillomavirus 16 was isolated in 20% and 10% of in situ and invasive adenocarcinomas, respectively. In adenosquamous carcinomas, HPV 16 and 18 are almost equally distributed, each in the range of 20%.[40]

Because as many as 50% of cervical adenocarcinomas, in situ or invasive, have coexisting squamous neoplasia, the possibility exists that in some cases the detected HPV DNA may come from the squamous neoplasia adjacent to adenocarcinoma.[43] This event seems unlikely in those studies based on in situ hybridization, which has localized HPV DNA in the nuclei of both in situ and invasive adenocarcinoma cells.[40,41] Human papillomavirus DNA has also been found in adenocarcinoma metastases with the use of the Southern blot technique.[38,42,44,45] Women whose cervical adenocarcinoma have HPV DNA are younger than those without HPV DNA (mean age 37.3 vs 49 years, respectively).[44] Thus, HPV 18 may preferentially affect cervical glandular or subcolumnar reserve cells. The latter are believed to differentiate into glandular or squamous cells. It is of interest that the HeLa cells, which are derived from a poorly differentiated adenocarcinoma, contain integrated HPV 18.[46] Whether or not the rising incidence of cervical adenocarcinoma among women under 35 years of age is related to HPV remains to be elucidated.[47,48]

POSSIBLE SYNERGISTIC EFFECTS WITH OTHER AGENTS

The potentiating action of other infectious and chemical agents on HPV has been raised by zur Hausen.[49] Prakash and colleagues[50] examined cervical biopsies and sera from 55 women with benign or malignant disease for evidence of infection with herpes simplex virus type 2 (HSV2) or HPV 16. Additional risk factors were obtained by an interview. Sera were tested for anti-HSV1 and anti-HSV2 antibodies, and cervical biopsies were tested for HPV 16 or HSV 2 DNA by Southern blot hybridization. HSV2 titers were considered positive when the HSV2/HSV1 index was greater than or equal to 85. Hybridization for HPV 16 was performed both under stringent conditions (ie, excluding other HPV types) and under nonstringent conditions (ie, to include all HPV types, since they share many common nucleotide sequences). The study was relatively small (55 patients) but included patients with nonneoplastic conditions (ie, cervicitis, hyperplasia, or metaplasia), preinvasive neoplasia, and invasive carcinoma. Evidence of exposure to HSV2 was observed in one of six (17%) patients with condyloma, one of seven (12%) patients with nonneoplastic conditions, 4 of 12 (25%) with preinvasive neoplasia (CIN), and 8 of 19 (42%) patients with invasive carcinoma; HSV2 DNA sequences were detected less frequently. HPV DNA (ie, nonstringent hybridization) was detected in 4 of 6 (67%) condylomas, 2 of 17 (12%) nonneoplastic lesions, 6 of 12 (50%) CINs, and 13 of 20 (65%) invasive carcinomas. When the same analysis was performed using more stringent hybridization, only one of the four condylomas initially present contained HPV 16, neither of the two nonneoplastic biopsies contained HPV 16, three of the six CINs contained HPV 16, and all but one (12/13, 92%) of the invasive squamous carcinomas contained HPV 16. Although the study was small, a statistically significant relative risk of invasive cervical cancer was observed for patients with anti-HSV2 antibodies ($RR =$ 5.5, $P < .05$) and HPV-DNA sequences ($RR = 13.94$, $P < .01$). While statistical significance implies that these figures may be extrapolated to the general population, it is not clear this small Panamanian study represents a true random distribution of the population.

Kaufman and colleagues[51] examined the coexistence of HPV and HSV2 in vulvar CIS. In this study, HPV DNA was found in 38 of 46 (83%) of vulvar CIS samples; 23 of 46 specimens (50%) immunohistochemically demonstrated the presence of HSV2 antigen. Biopsies from 19 of 46 (41%) patients had evidence of both HPV and HSV2 infections. Only four of 46 (9%) biopsies demonstrated HSV2 antigen without the presence of HPV DNA. Human papillomavirus DNA in this study was most frequently type 18 (10 patients, 22%). Specific HPV types detected included 6, 11, 16, 18, and 31. Of the 38 biopsies with HPV DNA, 22 (58%) contained at least one of HPV 16, 18, and 31. Although the study suggests that HPV has a stronger association with vulvar CIS than HSV2, whether any synergistic action occurs between these two viruses remains obscure.

Kjaer and colleagues[52] performed a population based study to investigate the carcinogenic roles that HPV and HSV play in cervical cancer. They studied randomly selected women in Greenland and Denmark, since the rate of cervical carcinoma is 5.7 times greater in Greenland among women aged 20–39 years. Surprisingly, the total HPV 16/18 infection rate was higher in Denmark (13%) than it was in Greenland (8.8%); when adjusted for age, the prevalence rate in Greenland was 67% that of Denmark. Similar rates of HPV 6/11 infection and mixed infection were found between the two groups. When HSV2 was studied, 68.2% of women in Greenland were positive for antibodies to the virus, whereas only 30.9% of the Denmark population possessed anti-HSV2 antibodies. This study reconfirms that we do not completely understand the roles HPV and HSV play in genital carcinogenesis. The authors suggest that their results be interpreted with caution, and they recommend the prospective cohort be studied to fully examine the epidemiologic relationship between each virus and neoplasia.

Although speculation has existed for some time that the intracellular bacterium *Chlamydia trachomatis* may be involved in cervical carcinogenesis, the scientific basis for this theory is less clear than for HPV or HSV. Syrjanen and colleagues[53] evaluated 418 women included in their HPV study to identify a possible relationship between chlamydia and cytological atypia, determined by Papanicolaou smear. Chlamydial infection (4.1% in the cervix and 3.6% in the urethra) did not correlate positively with the degree of cytological atypia or with the degree of neoplasia associated with HPV. The authors suggest that chlamydial infection is indirectly related to dysplasia to the extent the agent is sexually transmitted in a manner similar to HPV.

Among women with CIN, there is no difference in the prevalence of condyloma acuminatum, seropositivity for cytomegalovirus, and methods of contraception between smokers and nonsmokers.[54] While 56% of women with CIN I are smokers, smokers comprise of 71% of those with CIN III ($P < 0.01$).[54] The finding of koilocytosis in the biopsies of CIN III is also more common among smokers than nonsmokers.[54] These differences are not readily explained. Although cigarette smoking coincides with rising lung cancer among females, no such trend exists for cervical cancer.

CONCLUDING REMARKS

This chapter has reviewed the features associated with HPV and genital neoplasia. Human papillomavirus appears to strongly correlate with risk of neoplastic progression. The oncogenic potential depends, although not exclusively, on the specific type of HPV present. Aneuploidy is associated with more aggressive disease, and cases with aggressive HPV types are most frequently present in aneuploid neoplasms. Host immune factors also appear to influence the risk of progression to more advanced disease. Continuing basic science and epidemiologic research will better define the specific interrelationship among host factors, HPV, and other agents associated with the pathogenesis of neoplasia.

ACKNOWLEDGMENTS

This study was supported by grants CA 34870 and 42126, awarded by the National Cancer Institute, Department of Health and Human Services (YSF) and by a grant from the Robert Wood Johnson Foundation, Princeton, New Jersey (LHH). The opinions and conclusions expressed herein are those of the authors and do not necessarily represent those of the Robert Wood Johnson Foundation.

REFERENCES

1. Oriel JD: Natural history of genital warts. Br J Vener Dis 1971;47:1.
2. Barrera-Ora JG, Smith KO, Melnick JL: Quantitation of papovavirus in human warts. J Natl Cancer Inst 1962;29:583.
3. DeVillers EM, Wagner D, Schneider A, et al: Human papillomavirus infections in women with and without abnormal cervical cytology. Lancet 1987;ii:703.
4. Vayrynen M, Syrjanen K, Castren O, et al: Colposcopy in women with papillomavirus lesions of the uterine cervix. Obstet Gynecol 1985;65:409.
5. Schneider A, Sterzik K, Buck G, et al: Colposcopy is superior to cytology for the detection of early genital human papillomavirus infection. Obstet Gynecol 1988;71:236.
6. Syjanen K. Mantyjarvi R, Vayrynen M, et al: Evolution of human papillomavirus infections in the uterine cervix during a long-term prospective follow-up. Appl Pathol 1987;5:121.
7. Syrjanen KJ, Mantyjarvi R, Vayrynen M, et al: Cervical smears in assessment of the natural history of human papillomavirus infections in prospectively followed women. Acta Cytologica 1987;31:855.
8. Nash JD, Burke TW, Hoskins WJ: Biologic course of cervical human papillomavirus infection. Obstet Gynecol 1987;69:160.
9. Koss LG: Cytologic and histologic manifestations of human papillomavirus infection of the female genital tract and their clinical significance. Cancer 1987;60:1942.
10. Campion MJ, McCance DJ, Cuzick J, et al: Progressive potential of mild cervical atypia: Prospective cytological, colposcopic, and virological study. 1986; Lancet ii:237.
11. Schneider A, Sawada E, Gissmann L, et al: Human papillomaviruses in women with a history of abnormal Papanicolaou smears and in their male partners. Obstet Gynecol 1987;69:554.
12. Orth G, Jablonska S, Jarzabek-Chorzelska M, et al: Characteristics of the lesions and risk of malignant conversion as related to the type of human papillomavirus involved in epidermodysplasia verruciformis. Cancer Res 1979;39:1074.
13. Boxer RD, Skinner DG: Condyloma acuminata and squamous carcinoma. Urology 1977;9:72.
14. Majoros M, Devine KD, Parkhill EM: Malignant transformation of benign laryngeal papillomas in children after radiation therapy. Surg Clin North Am 1963;43:1049.
15. Lancaster WD, Jenson AB: Natural history of human papillomavirus infection of the anogenital tract. Cancer Metastasis Rev 1987;6:653.
16. Smotkin D, Wettstein FO: Transcription of human papillomavirus type 16 early genes in a cervical cancer and a cancer-derived cell line and identification of the E7 protein. Proc Natl Acad Sci USA 1986;83:4680.
17. Lack EE, Jenson AB, Smith HG, et al· Immunoperoxidase localization of human papillomavirus in laryngeal papillomas. Intervirol 1980;14:148.
18. Saito K, Saito A, Fu YS, et al: Topographic study of cervical condyloma and intraepithelial neoplasia. Cancer 1987;59:2064.
19. Reagan JW, Patten SF Jr: Dysplasia: A basic reaction to injury in the uterine cervix. Ann NY Acad Sci 1962;97:662.
20. Gupta J, Saito K, Saito A, et al: Human papillomaviruses and the pathogenesis of cervical neoplasia: A study by *in situ* hybridization. Cancer, in press.
21. Gupta J, Pilotti S, Rilke F, et al: Association of human papillomavirus type 16 with neoplastic lesions of the vulva and other genital sites by in situ hybridization. Am J Pathol 1987;127:206.
22. Goppinger A, Birmelin G, Ikenberg H, et al: Human papillomavirus standardization and DNA cytophotometry in cervical intraepithelial neoplasia. J Reprod Med 1987;32:609.
23. Fu YS, Reagan JW, Richart RM: Definition of cervical pre-cursors. Gynecol Oncol 1981;12:S220.
24. Fu YS, Reagan JW, Richart RM, et al: Definition of cervical cancer precursors, In Grundmann

E, ed. Cancer campaign, Vol. 8. Cancer of the uterine cervix. Stuttgart; Gustar Fisher Verlag. 1985, 67–74.

25. Nasiell K, Auer G, Nasiell M, et al: Retrospective DNA analyses in cervical dysplasia as related to neoplastic progression or regression. Analyt Quant Cytol Histol 1979;1:103.

26. Evans AS, Monaghan JM: Spontaneous resolution of cervical warty atypia: the relevance of clinical and nuclear DNA features: a prospective study. Brit J Obstet Gynecol 1985;92:165.

27. Fu YS, Braun L, Shah KV, et al: Histologic, nuclear DNA, and human papillomavirus studies of cervical condylomas. Cancer 1983;52:1705.

28. Fujii T, Crum CP, Winkler B, et al: Human papillomavirus infection and cervical intraepithelial neoplasia: Histopathology and DNA content. Obstet Gynecol 1984;63:99.

29. Shevchuk MM, Richart RM: DNA content of condyloma acuminatum. Cancer 1982;49:489.

30. Reid R, Fu YS, Herschman BR, et al: Genital warts and cervical cancer. VI. The relationship between aneuploid and polyploid lesions. Am J Obstet Gyencol 1984;150:189.

31. Fu YS, Reagan JW, Richart RM, et al: Nuclear DNA and histopathologic studies of genital lesions in DES-exposed progeny. I. Intraepithelial squamous abnormalities. Am J Clin Pathol 1979;72:502.

32. Winkler B, Crum CP, Fujii T, et al: Koilocytotic lesions of the cervix: The relationship of mitotic abnormalities to the presence of papillomavirus antigens and nuclear DNA content. Cancer 1984;53:1081.

33. Crum CP, Ikenberg H, Richart RM, et al: Human papillomavirus type 16 and early cervical neoplasia. New Engl J Med 1984;310:880.

34. Kadish AS, Burk RD, Kress Y, et al: Human papillomaviruses of different types in precancerous lesions of the uterine cervix: Histologic, immunocytochemical and ultrastructural studies. Human Pathol 1986;17:384.

35. Fu YS, Huang I, Beaudenon S, et al: Correlative study of human papillomavirus DNA, histopathology, and morphometry in cervical condyloma and intraepithelial neoplasia. Int J Gynecol Pathol 1988;7:297.

36. Bergeron C, Ferenczy A, Shah K, et al: Multicentric human papillomavirus infections of the female genital tract: Correlation of viral types with abnormal mitotic figures, colposcopic presentation, and location. Obstet Gynecol 1987;69:736.

37. Yoshikawa H, Matsukura T, Yamamoto E, et al: Occurrence of human papillomavirus types 16 and 18 DNA in cervical carcinomas from Japan: Age of patients and histological type of carcinomas. Jpn J Cancer Res 1985;76:667.

38. Smotkin D, Berek JS, Fu YS, et al: Human papillomavirus DNA in adenocarcinoma and adenosquamous carcinoma of the uterine cervix. Obstet Gynecol 1986;68:241.

39. de Villiers EM, Schneider A, Gross G, et al: Analysis of benign and malignant urogenital tumors for human papillomavirus infection by labelling cellular DNA. Med Microbiol Immunol 1986;174:281.

40. Tase T, Okagaki T, Clark BA, et al: Human papillomavirus types and localization in adenocarcinoma and adenosquamous carcinoma of the uterine cervix: a study by in situ DNA hybridization. Cancer Res 1988;48:993.

41. Tase T, Okagaki T, Clark BA, et al: Human papillomavirus DNA in adenocarcinoma in situ, microinvaisve adenocarcinoma of the uterine cervix and coexisting cervical squamous intraepithelial neoplasia. Int J Gynecol Pathol 1989;8:8.

42. Wilczynski SP, Bergen S, Walker J, et al: Human papillomaviruses and cervical cancer: Analysis of histopathologic features associated with different viral types. Human Pathol 1988;19:697.

43. Fu YS, Reagan JW: Pathology of the Uterine Cervix, Vagina, and Vulva. Philadelphia: WB Saunders 1989.

44. Wilczynski SP, Walker J, Liao SY, et al: Adenocarcinoma of the cervix associated with human papillomavirus. Cancer 1988;62:1331.

45. Walboomers JMM, Fokke HE, Polak M, et al: In situ localization of human papilloma virus type 16 DNA in a metastasis of an endocervical adenocarcinoma. Intervirology 1987;27:81.

46. Boshart M, Gissmann L, Ikenberg H, et al: A new type of papillomavirus DNA, its presence in genital cancer biopsies, and in cell lines derived from cervical cancer. EMBO J 1984;3:1151.

47. Peters RK, Chao A, Mack TM, et al: Increased frequency of adenocarcinoma of the uterine cervix in young women in Los Angeles County. J Natl Cancer Inst 1986;76:423.

48. Schwartz SM, Weiss NS: Increased incidence of adenocarcinoma of the cervix in young women in the United States. Am J Epidemiol 1986;124:1045.

49. zur Hausen H: Human genital cancer: Synergism between two virus infections or synergism between a virus infection and initiating events. Lancet 1982;ii:1370.

50. Prakash SS, Reves WC, Sisson GR, et al: Herpes simplex virus type 2 and human papillomavirus type 16 in cervicitis, dysplasia and invasive cervical carcinoma. Int J Cancer 1985;35:51.

51. Kaufman RH, Bornstein J, Adam E, et al: Human papillomavirus and herpes simplex virus in vulvar squamous cell carcinoma in situ. Am J Obstet Gynecol 1988;158:862.

52. Kjaer SK, deVilliers EM, Haugaard BJ, et al: Human papillomavirus, herpes simplex virus and cervical cancer incidence in Greenland and Denmark. A population based cross-sectional study. Int J Cancer 1988;41:518.

53. Syrjanen K, Mantyjarvi R, Vayrynen M, et al: Coexistent chlamydial infections related to natural history of human papillomavirus lesions in uterine cervix. Genitourin Med 1986;62:345.

54. Grail A, Norval M: Significance of smoking and detection of serum antibodies to cytomegalovirus in cervical dysplasia. Brit J Obstet Gynecol 1987;95:1103.

CHAPTER 11

Cryosurgery

Duane E. Townsend, MD, FACOG

For almost three decades, profound hypothermia has been used successfully to treat a variety of human papillomavirus (HPV) infections of the visible portion of the female genital tract, including the anus. In this chapter, the principles of the technique will be reviewed, and the various methods of achieving a satisfactory therapeutic result with profound hypothermia will be discussed.

Cold as a therapeutic tool in medicine dates back to antiquity. It was used by the Egyptians in cold compresses for infected wounds and fractures and by Hippocrates to reduce hemorrhage and swelling. Richardson,[1] in 1866, introduced ether spray as a freezing agent; ethyl chloride was substituted in 1891. Openchowski[2] circulated iced saline through the vagina of a woman with a large pelvic neoplasm, noting a marked tumor reduction. Weitzner,[3] in 1940, treated chronic cervicitis placing dry ice rods on the tissues. Two years later, Hall[4] noted beneficial effects of cryosurgery with liquid freon delivered through probes in the treatment of benign cervical disease. Bobrow[5] repeated these studies several decades later with excellent healing and no abnormal cytologic findings.

From these modest beginnings, cryosurgery did not receive further attention until Cooper,[6] a neurosurgeon, developed several precise instruments that made the use of cold a therapeutic reality. Collins[7,8] was among the first to report on the success of liquid nitrogen in the treatment of benign cervical disease. Shortly thereafter, our own laboratory confirmed his studies and was the first to perform cryosurgery in an outpatient setting. Townsend[9] and Crisp[10] pointed out the value of the technique for premalignant disease of the female genital tract. These earlier studies were hampered by the size and expense of the apparatus delivering the refrigerant. Liquid nitrogen was impractical for the average physician. The burgeoning use of the technique in gynecology began with the arrival of simpler and

Clinical Practice of Gynecology: **2,** 174–186, 1989
© 1989 Elsevier Science Publishing Co., Inc.
655 Avenue of the Americas, New York, NY 10010

more economic systems in the mid-1960s. The first modern report on the use of freon was in 1968,[11] and it emphasized the simplicity, safety, and cost-saving aspects of the method. Shortly thereafter, units employing nitrous oxide or carbon dioxide gas were introduced. Since then, outpatient cryosurgery has been utilized to treat tens of thousands of women with a variety of HPV infections of the lower-female-genital tract. It is the most commonly employed method to treat premalignant disease of this organ system.

Principles of Hypothermia

Hypothermia is achieved by two methods, the basis of which are:

1. Change of the cryogen phase (evaporation of liquid or solid) achieved by circulating liquid gas with a probe.
2. Adiabatic isentropic expansion of compressed gas through a small orifice (the Julius Thompson effect).

In both systems, the heat exchange occurs at the tip of the probe (boiler) that lies at the surface of the tissue to be frozen. Heat is withdrawn by the low temperature of the cryogen, so that ice forms in the tissues. Formation of the ice occurs in the range of 0 to $-10°C$. Cell death is caused primarily by dehydration, which increases the solute concentration and destroys protein. Water crystallizes, weakening the cell membrane and making it more prone to rupture. Singularly or collectively, these changes usually result in cell death. The rate of cooling determines whether ice forms intracellularly or extracellularly. Slow cooling of tissue usually causes extracellular freezing, and rapid cooling produces intracellular icing. Cell death is more pronounced by rapid cooling. The thaw rate also plays a part in cell death; slow thawing is the most injurious; thus, a rapid freeze and slow thaw sequence is most lethal to mammalian tissue. Tissue destruction is also enhanced by repeated cycles of freezing—thawing, ie, freeze, partial thaw, refreeze.

There are several ways that profound hypothermia can be obtained. Metal probes can be dipped into liquid nitrogen and then applied to the tissues. Liquid nitrogen sprayed or directly applied to the tissue produces a satisfactory lowering of the tissue temperature.

Alternatively, the cryogen can be delivered to the tissue through instruments. Initially, the cryosurgical units were bulky and required liquid nitrogen as the cryogen and electricity to power the probes. Now, modern units use the cryogen not only to freeze and destroy the tissues but also to defrost the probe tip. The most versatile units in current use are those with a gunlike configuration (Figure 11–1) employing either carbon dioxide or nitrous oxide gas as the refrigerant. These units have the advantage that the

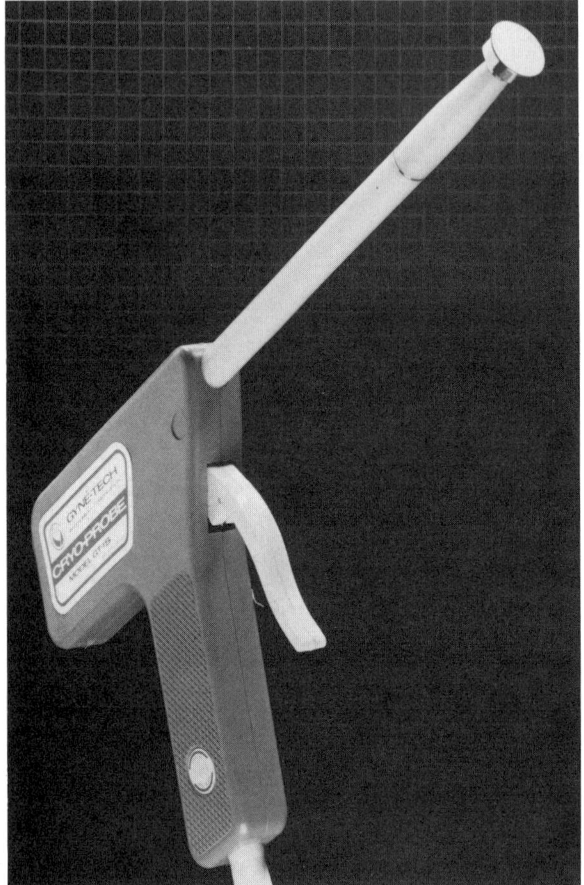

FIGURE 11–1 Gun-type cryoprobe with 18-mm flat-tip probe attached.

cryogen can be stored indefinitely. They are highly reliable, almost indestructible, and their versatility is ensured by the availability of a wide range of probe tips (Figure 11–2). In selecting a system for safe operation, it is important that all components are pressure tested to twice the cryogen pressure which varies between 700 and 900 PSI.

Clinical Application

Virtually all HPV infections can be treated by cryosurgery. Each organ system will be considered separately, and the technique for using profound hypothermia will be detailed.

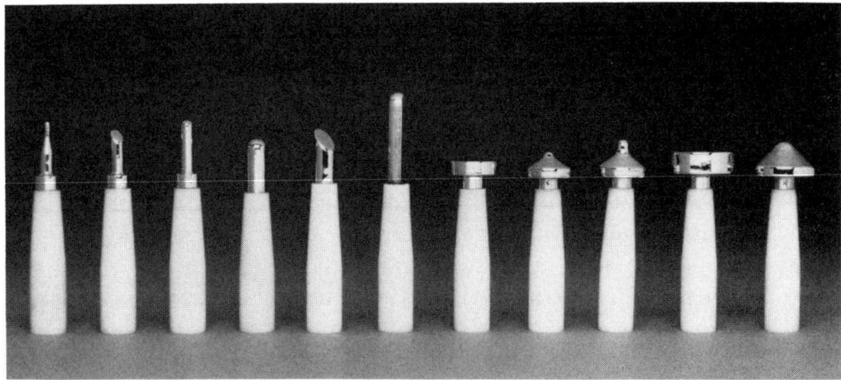

FIGURE 11–2 Probe tips available with cryoprobe from left to right: 1-mm condyloma tip, 4-mm diagonal condyloma tip, 4-mm rod tip, 8-mm rod tip, 8-mm diagonal condyloma tip, 6-mm rod tip, 18-mm flat tip, 18-mm convex tip, 18-mm extended nipple tip, 25-mm flat tip, 25-mm convex tip.

VULVA

Because of their accessibility, HPV infections of the vulva are easily treated by freezing. The first report on the successful use of cryosurgery for the acuminate wart of the vulva was in 1969. Ostergard and Townsend[12] treated a number of patients with this technique and achieved a high cure rate. They treated both patients with a few lesions and those with extensive disease. However, when the disease was extensive, severe vulvar edema often developed after treatment. Consequently, it is recommended that when cryosurgery is used, the area treated be limited to individual lesions or groups of lesions no more than 2 cm in diameter.

Methods of Cryosurgery

Prior to the employment of profound hypothermia or any technique, persistent lesions of the genital tract should be sampled to exclude the possibility of a precancerous or cancerous lesion. There have been patients who were treated for "benign" condyloma and subsequently were found to have invasive cancer. Colposcopy is strongly recommended in such patients. Once it has been determined that the patient has a benign acuminate lesion that has not been responsive to chemical therapy, cryosurgery may be undertaken.

When cryosurgery is employed, the gun-type units are preferred with nitrous oxide as the refrigerant. A 4-mm or 8-mm rod-tipped probe is recommended. The area or lesion to be treated is identified. Local analgesia is seldom used unless the lesion is broad-based. Then, a small amount of local anesthesia is injected directly in the base of the wart. The lesion is moistened with saline or lubricating jelly to insure adequate heat transfer. The probe tip is placed on the tissue, and gentle pressure is applied to ensure proper probe surface to tissue surface contact. Refrigerant is circulated. The probe will immediately adhere to the tissue. Slight traction is applied to the probe to elevate the lesion. This reduces pain associated with the treatment; freezing is continued until the ice ball extends to at least 3–4 mm onto normal tissue. During freezing, patients occasionally experience a mild burning sensation, but pain is not a problem in most cases. Once the iceball has extended the necessary 3–4 mm onto normal tissue, the probe is defrosted; additional areas are treated. In the first 24–36 hours, edema is noted around the lesion and surrounding tissue. In a rare patient, extensive vulvar swelling will occur. Within 4 days, the lesion turns dark. By the end of a week, the treated area will begin to slough, leaving a shallow ulcer. Patients are advised to keep the vulva as clean and dry as possible. Discomfort following cryosurgery is seldom a problem. Wet tea bags directly applied to the treated areas for 20–30 minutes, 3–4 times a day, is particularly soothing.

Discomfort from the raw surfaces is relieved with topical analgesic gel. Healing generally occurs within 3–4 weeks after freezing. In some cases, depigmentation of the treated area occur.

If very large areas are treated by cryosurgery, the invariable edema occurs. This lasts for several days and can be quite uncomfortable, although it usually does not interfere with normal activities. Because of the vulvar edema and the fair degree of necrosis and pain that can occur with extensive cryosurgery, these large areas are best managed by other destructive techniques. Examples of cryosurgery for the acuminate wart are depicted in Figures 11–3–11–8.

Other methods of delivering cold to these lesions include dipping a metal rod into liquid nitrogen and then applying it to the lesion. Liquid nitrogen can also be directly applied to individual warts. Regardless of the method for delivering profound hypothermia, it is important that the entire lesion be treated as well as the surrounding 3–4 mm of normal tissue. If this freeze/thaw cycle is unsatisfactory in achieving tissue necrosis, then a freeze/partial thaw/refreeze cycle should be employed that is more lethal to mammalian tissue. Cryosurgery for genital warts has been compared to cautery and chemical therapy.[13–16] In every instance, cryosurgery was equally or more effective. Moreover, the technique has been used in pregnant patients[17] with excellent results and minimal side effects.

Although, there has been little experience in eradicating premalignant vulvar disease, selected lesions can be treated by cryosurgery. First and foremost, invasive cancer must be excluded by colposcopy and tissue sampling. The lesion cannot be any larger than the 18-mm flat cryoprobe. Local anesthesia should be used. The iceball should extend 2–3 mm beyond the edge of the probe. Otherwise, evaluation, treatment, and posttreatment care is identical to that for benign HPV disease.

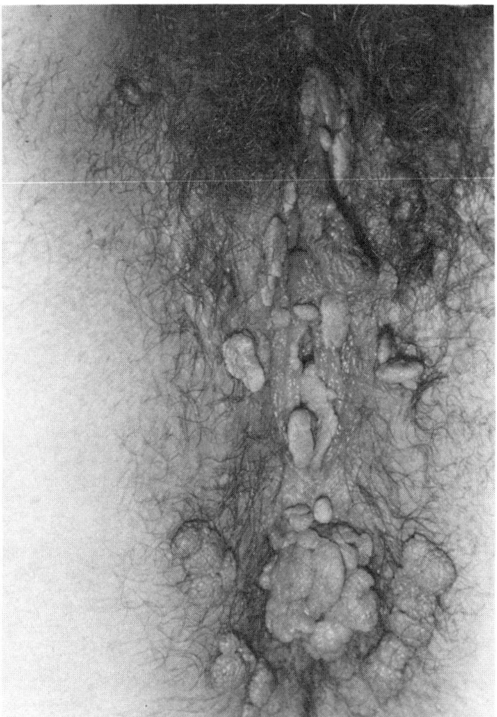

FIGURE 11–3 Extensive condyloma of vulva and anus.

VAGINA

Because of its relative inaccessibility and the lack of suitable probes, cryosurgery has not been extensively utilized for HPV infections of the vagina. However, individual sessile lesions that project into the vagina can be treated by profound hypothermia using a technique similar to that described for the vulva. This is virtually painless. The chance of freezing too deep and causing a fistula is remote because of the vascularity of the rectovaginal and vesicovaginal tissues. However, it is important not to freeze beyond 2 mm into the normal tissue, in order to minimize the risk of post treatment fistulas.

CERVIX

Cryosurgery is currently the most popular method of treating the benign and premalignant HPV lesions of the uterine cervix.[8,18–20] Any patient who has HPV infection of the cervix must be colposcoped and biopsied.[21] An endocervical curettage in nonpregnant patients is mandatory. There have been instances of so-called benign condylomas of the cervix being treated by freezing in patients in whom the lesion was a keratinizing invasive

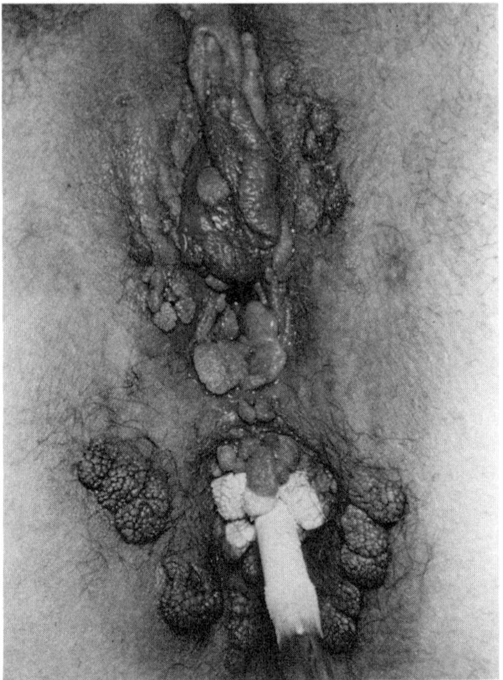

FIGURE 11–4 8-mm rod tip freezing anal condyloma.

cancer.[22] The technique of treating both the benign as well as premalignant lesions is similar.

Cryosurgery is best performed shortly after the cessation of menses. This will lessen the chance of freezing a patient just prior to menses and occluding the menstrual flow as well as reduce the chance of freezing the patient during pregnancy. Patients have been subjected inadvertently to cervical cryosurgery during the early phase of the pregnancy, and there have been no known deleterious effects. However, because of our highly litiginous society, it is best to avoid performing procedures during pregnancy when there is any chance of causing problems with the gestation. In performing cervical cryosurgery, a speculum as wide as the patient can tolerate is inserted and fully opened. The lesion must be confined to the visible portion of the ectocervix. A flat probe or a probe with a shallow convex surface is ideal. Freezing the endocervical canal may lead to cervical stenosis. A thin film of lubricating jelly is applied to the surface of the probe to provide a better probe surface to tissue surface contact. The lubricating jelly also improves the transfer of heat from the tissue to the boiler or probe tip. The probe is then seated onto the tissues, and it is made certain that

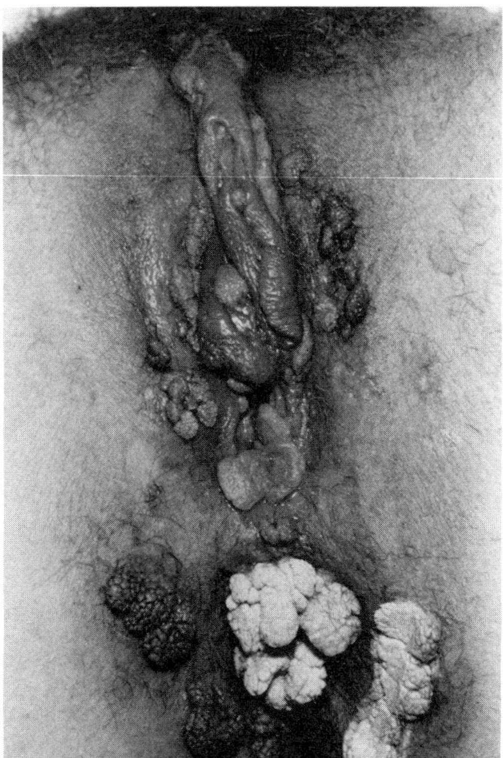

FIGURE 11–5 Immediately after freezing.

the probe completely covers the area to be treated. If the lesion is extensive and cannot be covered by the probe, the patient should be managed by other destructive means, ie, carbon dioxide laser.

After positioning the probe, refrigerant is circulated. Initially, ice crystallization will be noted on the back of the probe and then will begin to spread laterally from the edge of the probe. The freezing process is continued until the ice crystals are noted to extend at least 5–6 mm beyond the edge of the probe. The depth of tissue necrosis in these cases will be approximately 4–5 mm. It is important to freeze down to this depth because some HPV infections will extend well into the glands of the cervix. After the ice ball extends the necessary 5–6 mm, the probe is defrosted, and the patient is immediately reexamined to determine the success of the freezing session. Any areas that appear to be inadequately frozen should be immediately refrozen with the flat-tipped probe. The speculum is removed; the patients are provided with a sanitary napkin and given appropriate instructions, ie, no strenuous exercise and sexual activity for 3 weeks. This lessens the chance of spontaneous bleeding. Once the tissue thaws, a heavy dis-

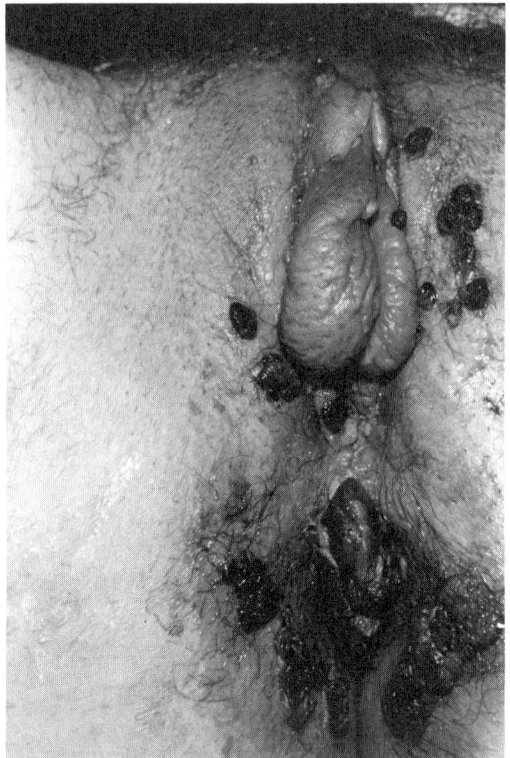

FIGURE 11–6 Five days after freezing—necrosis of lesion and edema of vulva.

charge ensues; most women require four to five pads a day for 3 weeks. The discharge at that time rapidly diminishes and will stop within a week. If patients are seen at 3–4 weeks after cryosurgery, a large necrotic bed will be noted, but most cervices are healed by 8 weeks. At 8 weeks, patients are carefully examined grossly, and, if any suspicious area is present, the patient is recolposcoped. Cytology is unnecessary at this time, and, in fact, if performed, false-positive reports are common. Patients return in another 3–4 months for a final checkup, and, if they had an intraepithelial neoplasia (CIN) lesion, cytology is carried out. If they were frozen for benign disease, they are placed on a regular gynecologic annual visit schedule. For CIN lesions, the patients are requested to return one additional time in 3–4 months for cytology; if that smear is normal, they are placed on the regular annual visit schedule.

The success of cryosurgery for HPV varies. In benign disease, recurrences will occur in those patients who have obvious infections of the vulva and vagina. As a consequence, these areas should be treated concomitantly or prior to the use of cryosurgery. Generally, chemical therapy is highly successful in controlling many areas of the female genital tract. Intravaginal

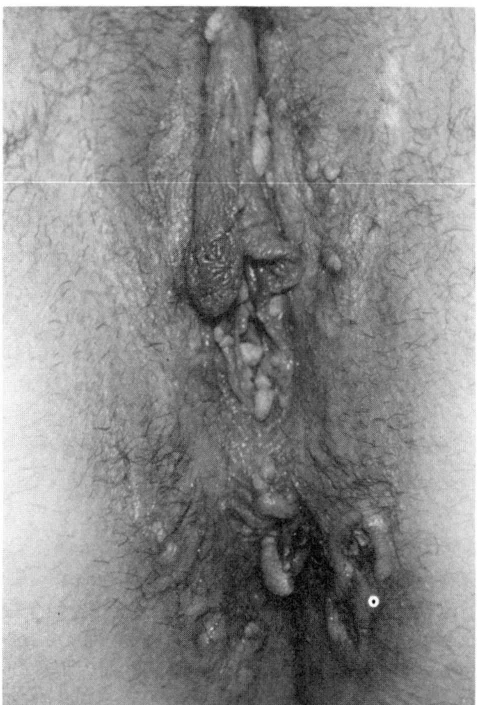

FIGURE 11–7 Three weeks after initial freezing—healing ulcers around anus. Remaining condylomas frozen in 2 weeks after photo.

5-FU for the vagina and trichloroacetic acid and podophyllin are preferred for external disease. Once the vaginal and vulvar lesions are brought under control, then the cervical disease can be managed. Concomitant therapy is usually unsatisfactory and awkward because of the excessive discharge that occurs following cervical cryosurgery. If more than 15% of patients develop recurrent HPV disease following cryosurgery, it is suggested that the patient intravaginally instill ¼ applicator full of 5% Efudex weekly beginning 3 weeks following the cryosurgical session. This is continued for 5–6 weeks. Persistent or recurrent disease may be retreated by freezing or alternative methods, ie, CO_2 laser.

When the HPV infection results in a lesion interpreted as CIN (dysplasia or carcinoma in situ), the success rates of cryosurgery are dependent on the size of the lesion rather than histologic diagnosis. A small ($<$¼ of the external surface area of the cervix) CIN III has a much higher success rate than a large ($>$½ of the external surface area of the cervix) CIN I.[23] The major factors that influence cryosurgical success are depicted in Table 11–1. Note that lesion size is the most important determinant with histologic diagnosis the least important.

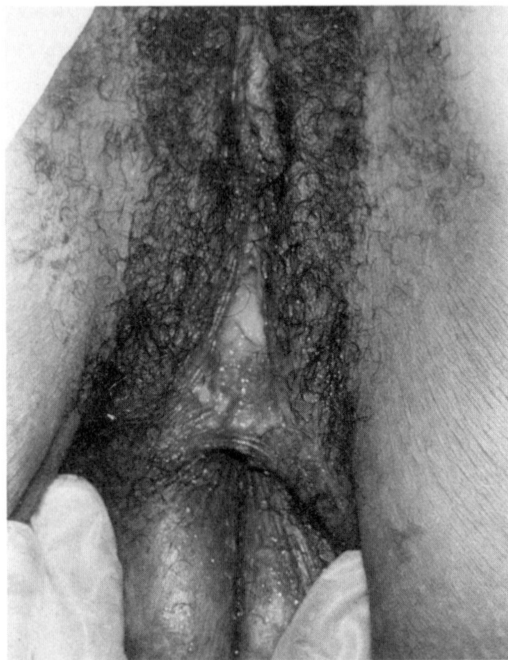

FIGURE 11–8 Vulva and anus after two cryosurgical sessions and 8 weeks after last freeze.

Cryosurgery as a therapeutic tool has been criticized as not lethal to the human papilloma virus. There have been no studies to date to substantiate this theoretical consideration, and the high cure rates associated with cryosurgery contradicted this opinion.

URETHRA

Intraurethral condyloma has been managed by cryosurgery. In an article by Sand et al,[24] the lesions were isolated with urethroscopy, and a very small cryoprobe was inserted into the urethra and the area was frozen with the ice ball extending 1 mm onto normal tissue. Success rates were high, and none of the patients suffered any stenosis.

TABLE 11–1. Factors that Affect Success of Cryosurgery for CIN Listed in Decreasing Importance

1. Lesion size
2. Tank pressure
3. Refrigerant
4. Probe tips
5. Histologic diagnosis

ANUS

Anal and perianal condyloma that are resistant to standard means of therapy can also be treated by cryosurgery. The technique of cryosurgery is similar to that for vulvar disease. The area that is to be treated should be thoroughly cleansed. Tissue sampling is conducted if there is even the slightest chance of a neoplastic process. As with the vulva, the lesions are moistened either with saline or lubricating jelly and the probe applied to the lesion. Freezing is commenced until the lesion as well as normal tissue has been frozen. Posttreatment of this area is similar to that of vulvar lesions with the addition of stool softeners until the tissues heal.

SUMMARY

The use of cold as a therapeutic tool has been utilized for decades. It is a highly successful method with minimal side effects. It is particularly cost effective and results in cure rates exceeding 90% for most areas of the female genital tract.

REFERENCES

1. Paloucek FP, Batayola W, Collins RH, et al: Historical aspects of cryotherapy in gynecology. J Cryosurg 1968;12:148.
2. Openchowski PH: Sur l'action localisee du froid, applique a la surface de la region corticale du cervau. Compt rend Soc de biol 1883;4:38.
3. Weitzner K: The treatment of endocervicitis with carbon dioxide snow (dry ice). Am J Surg 1940;48:620.
4. Hall FE: The use of quick freezing methods in gynecologic practice. A preliminary report. Am J Obstet Gynecol 1942;43:105.
5. Bobrow ML, Goldbaum A, Short V: Treatment of cervicitis by the carbon dioxide snow cauterization method. Obstet Gynecol 1961;18:726.
6. Cooper IS, Lee A St J: Cryothalamectomy—hypothermic congelation: A technical advance in basal ganglia surgery. Preliminary report. J Am Geriatr Soc 1961;9:714.
7. Collins RJ, Pappas HJ: Cryosurgery for benign cervicitis with follow up of six and one half years. Am J Obstet Gynecol 1972;113:744.7.
8. Collins RJ, Golab A: Cryosurgical treatment of uterine cervicitis. Preliminary report. Bull Mill Fill Hosp 1966;13:47.
9. Townsend DE, Ostergard DR: Cryocauterization for preinvasive cervical neoplasia. J Reprod Med 1971;6:171.
10. Crisp WE, Asadourian L, Romberger W: Application of cryosurgery to gynecologic malignancy. Obstet Gynecol 1967;30:668.
11. Ostergard E, Townsend DE, Hiroze FM: The treatment of chronic cervicitis by cryotherapy. Am J Obstet Gynecol 1968;102:426.
12. Townsend DE, Ostergard DR, Lickrish GM: Cryosurgery for benign disease of the uterine cervix. J Obstet Gynaecol Br Commonw 1971;18:667.
13. Ostergard DR, Townsend DE: The treatment of vulvar condyloma acuminta by cryosurgery. Cryobiol 1969;5:340.
14. Simmons PD, Langlet F, Thin RNT: Cryotherapy versus electrocautery in the treatment of genital warts. Br J Vener Dis 1981;57:273.

15. Ghosh AK: Cryosurgery of genital warts in cases in which podophyllin treatment failed or was contraindicated. Br J Vener Dis 1977;53:49.

16. Bashi SA, Ven D: Cryotherapy versus podophyllin in the treatment of genital warts. Int J Derm 1985;24:535.

17. Bergman A, Matsunaga J, Bhatia N: Cervical cryotherapy for condylomata acuminata during pregnancy. Obstet Gynecol 1987;69:47.

18. Creasman WT, Weed JC Jr, Curry SL, et al: Efficacy of cryosurgical treatment of severe cervical intraepithelial neoplasia. Obstet Gynecol 1973;41:501.

19. Kaufman RH, Strama T, Norton PK, et al: Cryosurgical treatment of cervical intraepithelial neoplasia. Obstet Gynecol 1973;42:881.

20. Tredway DR, Townsend DE, Hovland DN, et al: Colposcopy and cryosurgery in cervical intraepithelial neoplasia. Am J Obstet Gynecol 1972;114:1020.

21. Ostergard DR, Gondos B: Outpatient therapy of preinvasive cervical neoplasia. Selection of patients with the use of colposcopy. Am J Obstet Gynecol 1973;115:783.

22. Townsend DE, Richart RM, Marks EJ, et al: Invasive cancer following outpatient evaluation and therapy for cervical disease. Obstet Gynecol 1981;57:145.

23. Townsend DE: Cryosurgery for CIN. Obstet Gynecol Surv 1979;34:848.

24. Sand PK, Shen W, Bowen W, et al: Cryotherapy for the treatment of intraurethral condyloma acuminatum. J Urol 1987;137:874.

CHAPTER 12

Laser Therapy for Genital Warts

Michael S. Baggish, MD, FACOG, FACS

Women afflicted with genital warts wish to be rid of these unsightly growths. Although some cases of condyloma acuminata will spontaneously regress, only a minority of patients are willing to accept a wait-and-see attitude for an extended period of time. The most likely circumstance for the spontaneous remission of genital warts is following the termination of pregnancy.[1,2] Clearly, the 32–33-week gravida may be advised to forego therapy for 8–12 weeks with the expectation that her disease will improve or disappear after the delivery of her child. In the same vein, persons subjected to temporary immunodeficient states, eg, corticosteroid therapy, cancer chemotherapy may expect to witness wart regression after withdrawal of the drug(s). The opposite set of circumstances usually prevails with respect to the successful elimination of warts in individuals with acquired immune deficiency syndrome (AIDS), transplant drug-related immunosuppression, diabetes mellitus, and/or long-term cancer chemotherapy.[3,4] Interestingly, patients with severe states of malnutrition, who become anergic to a standard panel of skin tests, are prone to the deprivations of the human papilloma virus. Following hyperalimentation and reversal of skin anergy, the warts regress spontaneously. The CO_2 laser has proved to be an effective method of therapy for the removal of gross lesions produced by the human papilloma virus in genital and extra-genital locations. This surgical device has been used to treat genital warts for more than 10 years. In recent years, the popularity of laser methodology has increased, particularly for resistant and extensive wart disease.[4–11]

The most logical approach to laser therapy should include the setting of therapeutic goals, defining and staging the disorder(s) to be treated, specifying the methodology, and accurately identifying criteria for assessment of results.

Any treatment program that is prolonged, associated with substantial

Clinical Practice of Gynecology: **2,** 187–213, 1989
© 1989 Elsevier Science Publishing Co., Inc.
655 Avenue of the Americas, New York, NY 10010

ISSN 1043-3198/89/$3.50

and unpleasant side effects, and has the potential for unknown complications will never be popular. At the least, it should be embarked upon with a modicum of trepidation.

Treatment of normal tissues or a variation of normal anatomy may be expected to render excellent or inferior results, depending on the psyche of the patient undergoing such therapy. Sometimes the normal anatomic variant may be eliminated to the satisfaction of the therapist, only to be replaced by another even more vexing problem. Unfortunately, this is not hypothetical but is based on a not-insignificant number of actual cases. A prime example of this objectionable practice is the propensity for some gynecologists to treat the irregular projections of vestibular epithelium (known as papulosis) under the mistaken guise that these are warts. If the laser vaporization penetrates too deeply, the patient will have scarring, and subsequent dyspareunia. In other cases, where laser vaporization is properly performed, women are left with a chronic symptomatic vulvitis, sic "burning vulva syndrome." The latter is then attributed mistakenly and unfortunately to human papillomavirus (HPV). Finally, under the least unfortunate scenario, gross skin tags or projections are flattened and the patient gratified by the "cure." Likewise, the physician is satisfied by the rendering of a flat aspect to the vulvar anatomy.

THERAPEUTIC GOALS

The laser surgeon should aim to eliminate every visible wart as well as all nonpapillomatous warty tissue (flat warts) (Figure 12–1). This may be accomplished only with the aid of a combination of eyeglass mounted microscopes and/or the colposcope. Additionally, the operator should devise a plan for superficial destruction of epithelium neighboring warts and warty epithelium with a peripheral margin measuring 1–2 cm, depending on the anatomic location.[12,13] The treatment program should be designed carefully in order that scarring will not accrue after laser ablation.

DEFINITION OF LESIONS AMENABLE TO THERAPY

Obviously, one cannot treat what one cannot see. Only *gross disease* should be treated with the CO_2 laser. Treatment in the immediate vicinity of warts is scientifically sound, since recurrence and persistence have been identified most frequently in such locations.[12,13] Treatment of HPV DNA has never been shown to improve cure rates, and, indeed, such areas may not even contain infectious virus. In fact, women without any warty lesions have been demonstrated to have HPV DNA present in otherwise normal-appearing tissue. Similarly, no benefit has resulted after treating koilocytosis regardless of DNA typing positivity. Unfortunately, cytologists frequently tend to overread Papanicolaou smears, presuming that anything resembling koilocytosis is evi-

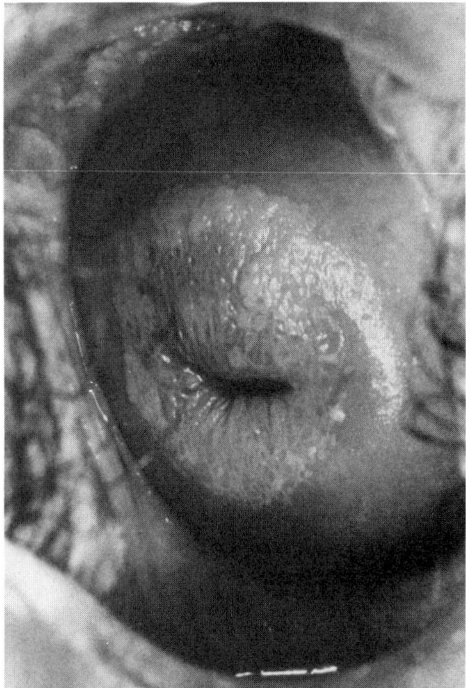

FIGURE 12–1 Flat wart disease is not uncommon on the cervix. It is diagnosed by careful colposcopic examination (before and after the application of 4% acetic acid) and directed biopsy.

dence of an active HPV infection. Therefore, treating a Pap smear suggestive of an HPV infection is to be decried. A better program would aim to follow these patients at regular intervals by cytology and colposcopy.

An area of great controversy converges on what to do with acetowhite epithelium, which on biopsy suggests an HPV infestation. Typically, such areas are diagnosed as showing condylomatous change or minimal condylomatous atypia or dysplasia. The latter is a disturbing phrase, since it implies intraepithelial neoplasia without fulfilling the necessary criteria to permit an accurate diagnosis. In such instances, viral typing utilizing, eg, the "Viratype" kit, may be helpful to determine the relative risk of subsequent neoplastic potential, prior to embarking on precipitate and often premature laser treatment.

METHODOLOGY

The most effective laser to treat lower-genital-tract neoplasia is the carbon dioxide (CO_2) laser. The CO_2 laser is a superb vaporizing device, which has a wide range of power and time settings. The system lends itself to delivery via handpiece or micromanipulator. Therefore, external surfaces

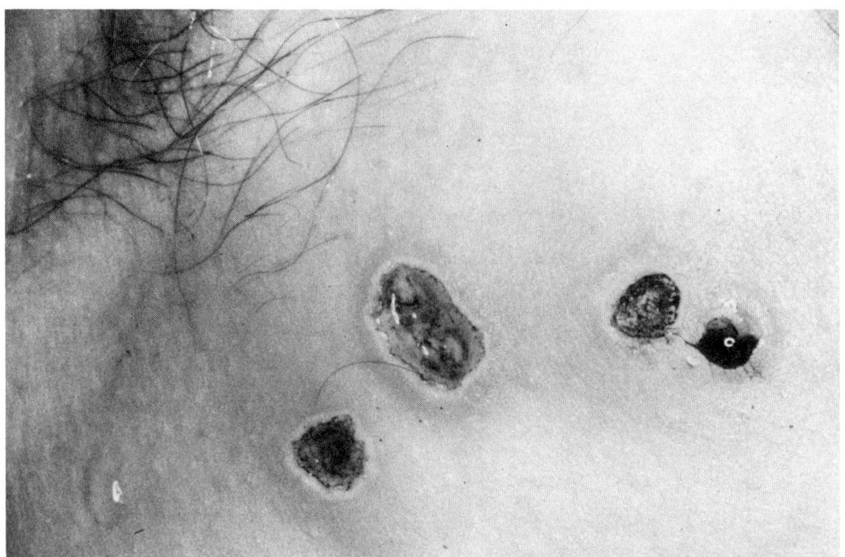

FIGURE 12-2 Warts should be vaporized to the level of the surrounding skin surface. The resulting wound extends into the superficial papillary dermis.

such as the vulva, perianal skin, or vestibule may be rapidly ablated with a high-power (>50 W), wide-diameter beam (≥ 3 mm). Use of the handpiece permits very rapid defocusing, ie, enlarged beam diameter and diminished power density. Additionally, the CO_2 laser permits the surgeon to select a variety of superpulse or continuous wave modes. This versatility translates into precision that is unavailable with other treatment regimes. For example, the laser can vaporize at continuous wave (CW) mode, cut at CW or superpulse (SP) mode. Superpulsing offers substantial advantages insofar as control and reduction of thermal action on tissue.[14] Continuous wave mode has the advantage of superior hemostasis in highly vascular areas. Tissue should be ablated only to the depth required to eliminate infecting virus. Deep treatment of infected epithelium adds to recovery time, pain, and complications such as scarring. It does not improve cure rates. The surgeon should be familiar with the depth of irreversible thermal effects at various tissue sites. For example, utilizing CW mode and varying the relative time of the laser beam on vulvar tissue, the operator can expect 300–500 μm or irreversible thermal injury beneath the zone of vaporization.

A most convenient plan stresses vaporization of warts to the surrounding surface normal skin level (Figure 12–2). This injury translates into tissue damage limited to the papillary dermis (in skin) and superficial injury within the vagina and cervix. When laser power densities are reduced to 100–200 W/cm^2, epithelium only is coagulated in tissues surrounding gross warts.[12,15] Stroma is completely spared, and even microscopic collagen deposition is ob-

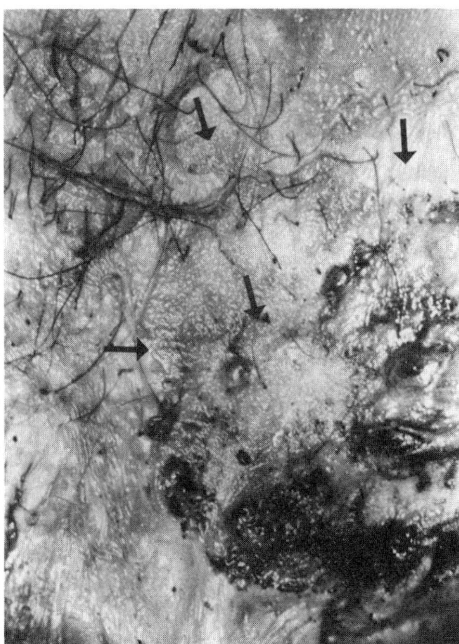

FIGURE 12–3 Skin surrounding gross warts is "brushed" at power densities of less than 300 W/cm². This superficial coagulation eliminates only the epidermis and spares the papillary dermis (arrows).

viated (Figures 12–3, 12–4). The zone of thermal injury may be diminished by utilization of the superpulse mode with low average powers. For example, with beam diameters of 0.5–1 mm and average powers ranging from 3–12 W, thermal injury below the zone of vaporization may be diminished to less than 200 μm. The only theoretical disadvantage to this technique relates to the shock wave action on cells created by the very-high peak powers associated with superpulsing. Under such circumstances, cells may be fractured with minimal thermal action, potentially allowing infected virus to survive and implant. The areas where superpulsing may be advantageous are clitoral, periurethral, and urethral skin. Additionally, superpulsing is advantageous for performing ultrathin excisions of vulvar skin, resulting in an available specimen for the pathologist as well as a lesion identical to one produced by superficial vaporization. Although other lasers may be utilized, eg, argon, KTP 532, and Nd-Yag (with sapphire tips), they offer no advantages to the patient or practitioner, and, in reality, they represent technology in search of an indication. Recently, some studies have suggested an advantage to utilizing the dye laser or gold vapor laser. The latter systems interact with the photoactive drug, hematoporphyrin derivative, to eliminate widespread clinical and subclinical HPV infections. Again, this complex technology remains investigational (personal communication).

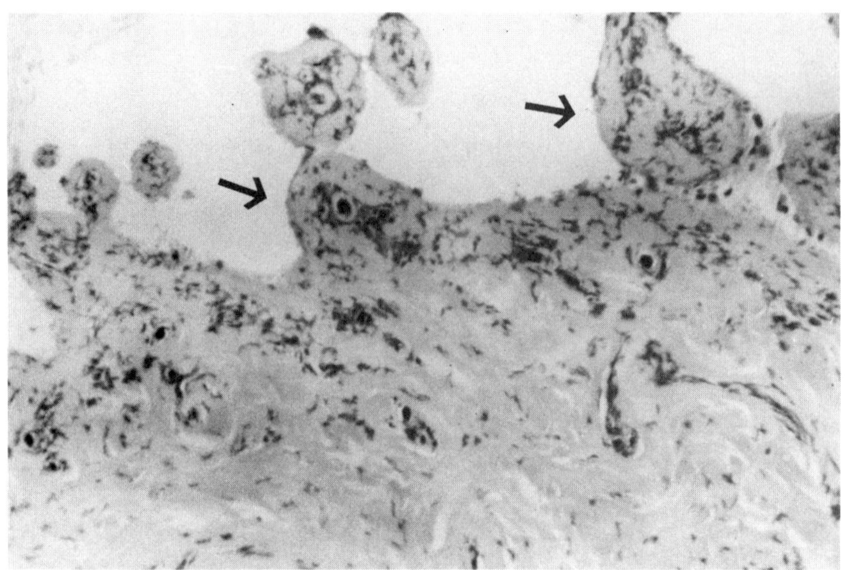

FIGURE 12–4 Histological section taken through "brushed" area reveals intact dermal papillae (arrows).

CRITERIA FOR ASSESSMENT OF TREATMENT RESULTS

What represents a cure of genital HPV infections? The clearest definition would be the elimination of gross condylomata and flat warty epithelium. This status could be said to have been accomplished only after the most careful scrutiny during follow-up examination with the colposcope. Follow-up periods should be measured in terms of at least 6 months and preferably 1 year. Disease appearing after 1 year is most likely the result of reinfection. A term preferable to cure is no evidence of disease (NED). I believe it is senseless and futile to attempt to render a patient so-called HPV DNA negative.

Obviously, one must be sure that warts are being treated in the first place. Unfortunately, in overdiagnosis, any bit of tissue protruding above an epithelial surface can be mistakenly called a wart. Another topic of concern are the vaginal rugae and other protrusions of epithelium that have been mistakenly diagnosed as condyloma. Patients who have had condyloma acuminata are similarly sensitized to view any protrusion as a wart and demand its removal. Aggressive retreatment or pronouncement of failure early in the follow-up period has mistakenly taken hypertrophied hair follicles to be incipient warts and has even progressed to improper vaporization of these appendages with resultant scar formation.

To date, no one has answered the question about how laser therapy eliminates warts. Obviously, the laser does not eliminate the infecting virus from tissue; this is too simplistic to be viable. Most certainly, the combination of destruction of proliferating lesions with an immunologic effort by the body defense system results in the elimination of disease.

PREPARATION

Every patient with genital warts must be evaluated thoroughly prior to laser treatment scheduling. Because many of these patients have already undergone treatment attempts with other techniques prior to referral for laser therapy, data regarding these other modalities and their effects on the patient should be documented. Interestingly, some patients no longer have any warts present. Since these women may have other serious underlying disorders, Venereal Disease Research Laboratory (VDRL), herpes simplex virus (HSV), and human immunodefiency virus (HIV) testing should be performed. At Syracuse Health Science Center, 3% of patients treated with laser for HPV genital infections have tested positive for HIV by both Western blot and ELISA. Additionally, all patients should be cultured for gonorrhea and chlamydia, and a Pap smear should be repeated.

Vulvar, vaginal, and cervical colposcopic examinations should be performed with the application of 4% acetic acid. Locations of warts and other types of lesions must be noted and mapped on the patient's record. Similarly, the urethra and anus should be examined for the presence of warts (Figure 12–5). Flat and pigmented warts should be sampled utilizing local anesthesia block. At least one wart should be sampled even in the face of all lesions appearing to be typical condyloma acuminata. Appropriate cervical and vaginal biopsies should be done when they are indicated to rule out neoplasia. Older women (50 yr) with flat vaginal warts arc at particular risk for an underlying squamous cell cancer. Such lesions should be multiply-sampled, since superficial biopsies may not show an underlying serious disorder. Extragenital sites, including the face, mouth, and extremities, should be carefully evaluated.

Every woman should be given a thorough, detailed description about the prospective laser treatment. The woman should be told specifically that the laser will create a wound that, when inflicted on an external surface such as the vulva or perianal skin, will result in postoperative pain. The intensity of the discomfort will vary depending on the surface area vaporized. Patients undergoing vaginal, cervical, and anal laser vaporization will not experience great discomfort.

The posttreatment regimen should be discussed with patients. Particularly, the mother of a child undergoing laser treatment should be instructed about the postoperative care of wounds. Immunodeficient patients should be given detailed information about effects, side effects, and reasons for adjuvant therapy, eg, 5-Fluoracil (5-FU) cream. Arrangements should also be made to have the patient's sexual partner(s) examined.

Those individuals who will require special anesthetics should be re-

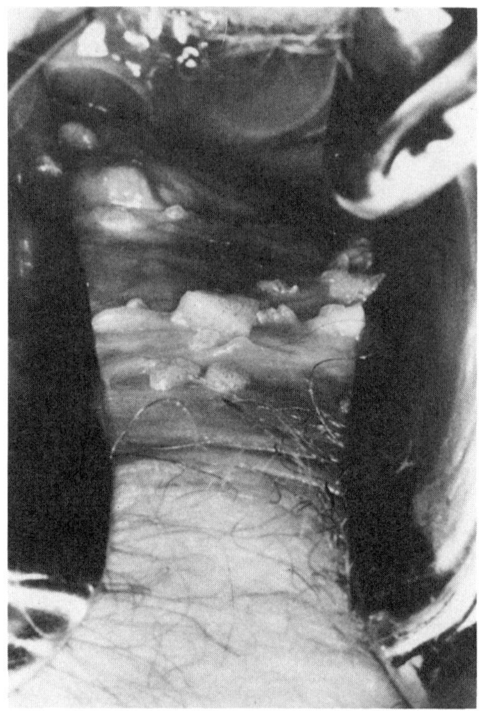

FIGURE 12–5 A laser speculum has been placed in the anus. Colposcopic view demonstrates numerous anal warts. Magnification is required if warts in the anus, vagina, and urethra are to be precisely located and mapped.

ferred for anesthesia consultation. Patients requiring antibiotic prophylaxis, eg, mitral valve prolapse, should be given appropriate prescriptions.

It is a principle at the SUNY Health Science Center and Crouse Irving Memorial Hospital that all patients undergoing laser treatment for condyloma acuminata have general anesthesia or regional block. Since our patients have moderate-to-extensive disease, the volume of local anesthesia required could produce significant toxicity as well as substantial discomfort.

All disease is staged according to the following classification:

Mild: − 10 warts
Moderate: 10–20 warts with or without confluence
Severe: ≥20 warts, confluence, extragenital site involvement (Figure 12–6).

LASER TECHNIQUE

The surgeon and assistants are gowned, gloved, and should don a special small-particle-filtering mask. The patient is placed in the dorsal lithotomy

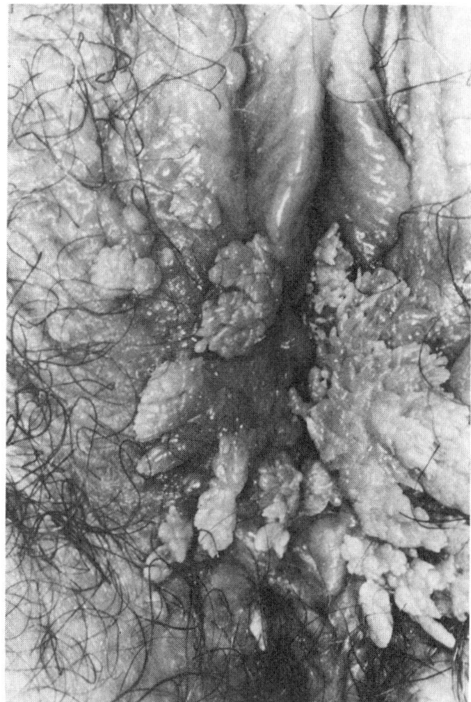

FIGURE 12–6 Severe warts are defined as 20 warts or more with confluence. Lesions should be biopsied prior to therapy to rule out neoplasia.

position after the induction of suitable general anesthesia. No preparatory solution is required. The perineum should be draped off with four moist linen towels. No paper drapes are used.

The smoke evacuator is readied by inserting a fresh cartridge filter. We always use equipment fitted with an ULPA filter in addition to the cartridge for vulvar vaporization. A plastic wand fitting is attached to the evacuation tubing. This must be held within 1–2 in. maximal distance from the laser treatment field. Special laser specula with smoke evacuation tubes are utilized for intravaginal and intraanal surgery. The laser equipment is test-fired prior to the induction of anesthesia to insure that the equipment is functioning properly. The usual routine fires a 1-mm focused beam into a wooden tongue depressor at 10 W, 0.1-second setting.

I utilize "Designs for Vision" ×3 magnification eyeglass-mounted microscopes for magnifications when using the laser freehand piece. Initially, laser power is set at 20–30 watts CW, and the handpiece is brought to an appropriate distance to deliver a 1.5-mm spot to the tissue target. The wart-bearing tissue is outlined by creating interrupted spots with a 2-cm margin around the warts. For confluent areas, the whole region, eg, the affected

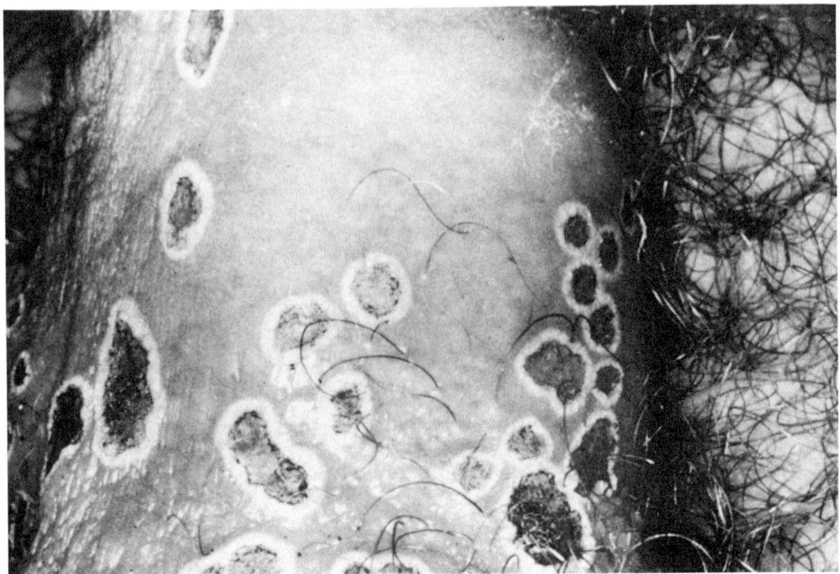

FIGURE 12–7 Vaporization of the penile shaft has been performed eliminating all visible warts. Note the superficial extent of vaporization.

labium majus or minus, is outlined. When an ultrathin excision is to be carried out, eg, in an area of flat warts, a special micromanipulator is attached to the operating microscope. This apparatus delivers a spot measuring 0.1685 mm in diameter.

Vaporization is performed at 40–60 W of power utilizing 2–4-mm spots in an effort to vaporize rapidly large tracts of wart-bearing tissue. The papillomatous extensions are vaporized in order to obliterate them to the level of the surrounding skin surface and no deeper. This specification translates to less than 1-mm depth of tissue vaporization. All visible warts are eliminated (Figure 12–7). Next, the handpiece is drawn back to defocus the beam so as to blanch white the skin surrounding the warts (in Caucasians), or black (in blacks). The key to this *brushing* technique is to coagulate the epidermis only, leaving the underlying papillary dermis untouched. I prefer to brush within a 2-cm radius around gross warts (Figures 12–3, 12–4). With high power and a 5–6-mm spot, the handpiece allows this operation to be completed in a few minutes. When excisions are desired, the laser is switched to super-pulse mode, 100 ppm, 0.4-ms width, average power 3 W. The special ultraspot micromanipulator delivers a power density of approximately 15,000 W/cm^2 and permits a deliberate and precise section of skin to be excised ≤ 1 mm in thickness (Figures 12–8, 12–9). This very thin section bleeds very little, and whatever bleeding that is present can be

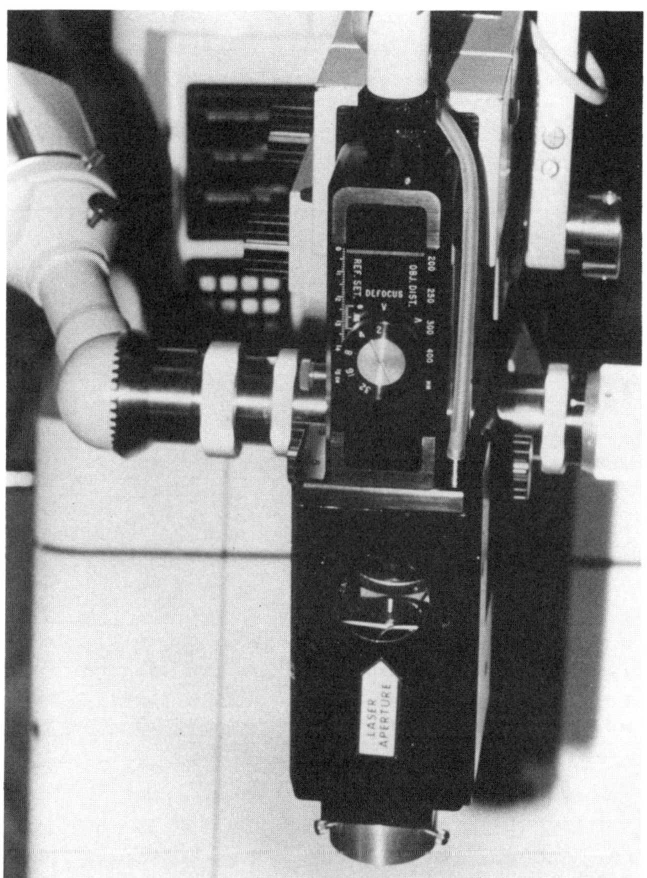

FIGURE 12–8 This specially designed micromanipulater delivers spots 0.2 mm in diameter.

managed easily by defocusing the beam and coagulating the vessel. The excised area heals without gross scar formation and is managed identically to a vaporized area. The technique described above creates no charring and less than one-half the thermal damage seen with CW vaporization (the thermally injured zone measures approximately 150 μm). When the vulva, perianal, and periclitoral skin have been treated, the laser is coupled to the microscope fitted with a standard micromanipulator. The vestibule is treated at 30–40 W with a 2-cm defocused spot. Brushing is accomplished by reducing power to 5W. A laser speculum is placed into the vagina. The cervix is swabbed with 4% acetic acid, and a colposcopic examination is repeated. If the cervix demonstrates a gross lesion, vaporization is carried out ablating the entire abnormal transformation zone to a measured depth of 3 mm, if coexisting

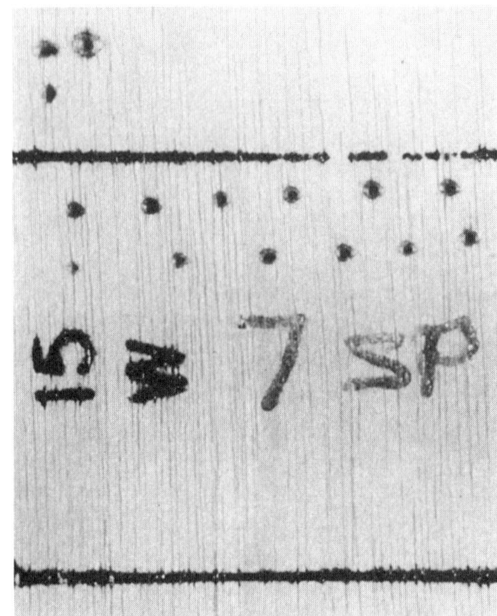

FIGURE 12–9 The 0.2-mm spots allow very-high-power densities to be obtained at relatively low powers. Split thickness excisions may be accomplished with little or no bleeding.

CIN is present, 5–7 mm, and brushing peripherally to 3–4 mm. This may be done with a setting of 30–40 W CW and a 1.5-mm spot. The vagina is carefully inspected for visible warts and is vaporized at 30 W, 1.5-mm spot. The surrounding tissue is brushed with a 2-cm radius at 100–200 W/cm^2 in a fashion analogous to that described for the vulva. Next, two laser hooks are placed at the external urethral meatus. Any warts visualized are vaporized at 15–20 W utilizing at 1.5–2-mm spot. A nasal speculum is then placed into the urethra and spread so as to allow inspection and treatment to the level of the urethral vesical junction.

A clean speculum is next inserted into the rectum. Inspection of the anus is carried out, and all visible warts are vaporized 20 W, 1.5-mm spot and brushed to a 1-cm radius at 100–200 W/cm^2. A wet 4 × 4 gauze sponge is placed into the rectum in order to isolate the laser field. Any affected extragenital sites are treated. All char material is cleared away with large swabs moistened in saline or 4% acetic acid. The perineum is dried. Silvadene cream is liberally applied to all externally lasered surfaces. If extensive vaporization has been performed, I prefer to place a pudendal nerve block, infiltrating 10 cc of 1% Carbocaine beneath each sacral spine. This short procedure results in the patient awakening from general anesthesia without any pain whatsoever.

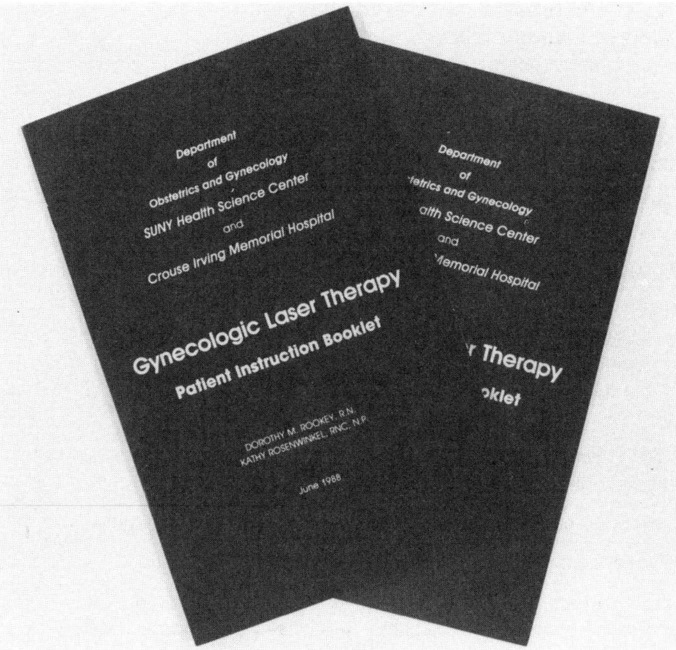

FIGURE 12–10 An instructional booklet provides easy to understand explanations of laser treatment at various sites as well as details about postoperative care.

Interestingly, these blocked patients complain of substantially less pain later in the postoperative period.

POSTOPERATIVE MANAGEMENT

All patients recover from anesthesia in the day-care recovery room. Children are admitted for postoperative management. When patients are ready to be discharged, they are given an instruction booklet. This booklet, prepared by our nurses, provides clear postoperative instructions for our patients (Figure 12–10). All women follow a regimen that has proved highly successful over the long test of time (Table 12–1). The application of ice packs to the vulva, which reduces edema, should be limited to the first 24 hours following laser surgery. Patients are sent home 3–4 hours following the completion of surgery and return to the office for the first examination 2 weeks later. Codeine (30 mg) and Motrin (400 mg) are prescribed every 4–6 hours for the first week. Antibiotics are *not* routinely prescribed.

Removal of a sample of tissue at the time of surgery is a highly worthwhile exercise. On two occasions, although the preoperative biopsy revealed benign condylomata acuminata, the intraoperative biopsy was

TABLE 12–1. Postoperative Management Routines Following Laser Vaporization of Condylomata Acuminata

Immediate
  Pudendal nerve block
  Ice pack to the vulva
  Silvadene cream or bio-occlusive dressing to vulva
  Sultrin or 5-FU cream into the vagina

Continuing
  Take sitz baths or soak in the tub in warm water for 15 min, 3 times or more per day.

  Add either:
  1. One cup Instant Ocean (available at our office or aquarium or pet stores)
  2. 1/4 cup epsom salts, or
  3. 1/4 cup table salt plus 1/4 cup baking soda, to approximately 3 in. of water in the tub

  After soaking, cleanse the area gently with 1/4 strength Betadine (available in drugstores); the proper mix is 1 part Betadine to 4 parts water

  Use a blow dryer on the "air" setting (no heat) to thoroughly dry the area

  Apply Silvadene cream or a bio-occlusive dressing if prescribed

  Do not wear sanitary pads; instead, wear all cotton underpants in a larger size than you normally wear to allow airflow; change 3–4 times per day or as needed

  If you have discomfort while urinating, try gently squirting warm water from a squeeze bottle down the perineum into the toilet, and drink lots of fluid to keep urine dilute; you may also void in the tub during your warm water soak

  Applications of a moistened tea bag for 10–30 min may help relieve burning or pain

  Your doctor may advise you to douche; specific instructions will be given if advised

diagnosed on one occasion as condylomata acuminata and on another as carcinoma in situ.

All patients are instructed to call immediately or come directly to the emergency room if a fever develops, or if they develop inordinate pain. Patients are instructed to call also if any bleeding occurs. Patients who have been taking oral contraceptives are advised to discontinue this medication and substitute contraceptive foam combined with condoms for a period of at least 6 months. No patient has accidentally gotten pregnant as a result of this regimen.

A colposcopic examination is performed at each office visit. These visits are routinely scheduled at 1–2 weeks, 4 weeks, 8 weeks, 12 weeks, 6 months, and 1 year. Obviously, in special circumstances visits are arranged as needed.

HEALING PATTERNS

One week following surgery, external surfaces are red and sore. Vaporization sites are covered with fibrin. Brushed areas are devoid of epidermis and sensitive. Maximal discomfort is experienced by the patient at this time. Pain is greatly ameliorated by preventing air drying of the exposed skin surfaces by frequent applications of Silvadene cream. If opposing surfaces of the labia minora have been treated by laser, these areas should be separated gently at each postoperative visit in order to prevent coaptation. Likewise, vaginal mucosa should be checked for coaptation. As with external surfaces, it is my policy to have intravaginal cream instilled following extensive laser vaporization. Patients should be instructed to separate the labia during soaking in the tub, since this is the best and least uncomfortable time to do this.

At the 2-week visit, the brushed areas are in an advanced state of healing, and the vaporized areas are epithelializing but still tender. Hair follicles are hypertrophied and appear as tiny cones that may be mistaken for incipient warts (Figure 12–11A,B). By 3 weeks, the brushed zones are healed; vaporized areas are covered with epithelium but remain red. At 4 weeks, tenderness has disappeared, and the vulva has a bright pink tinge.

Occasionally the vulva remains red and is associated with intense pruritus (Figure 12–12). This postlaser vulvitis is best treated with topical corticosteroid cream, eg, Mycolog or Kenolog, and a wetting agent such as Lachydrin. The skin responds favorably within 7 days after initiation of treatment. Under no circumstances should this irritated skin be retreated with the laser. Lachydrin should be applied routinely to the posterior fourchette area. Infections of the vulva, vagina, cervix, and anus are uncommon. If patients follow the above postoperative regimen, the vulva remains very clean and heals without scarring. In over 1000 cases, only one patient developed evident perianal scars following laser treatment.

RESULTS

Several series reported the successful elimination of warts in 87–91% of cases following laser vaporization.[4,7,8,10,12,16,17] Interestingly, poor outcomes attributed to laser ablation of condylomata acuminata are not commonly seen in the literature, whereas substantial documentation of mediocre results exists for other methods (Table 12–2). The author has participated in the treatment of and personally treated more than 1000 cases of genital warts. By and large, failures of the therapeutic method could be accounted in a select group of "high-risk" patients (Figure 12–13A,B). This group included diabetic, drug-suppressed, AIDS-afflicted women and men. The highest efficasy rates reported in published data are accrued when the epithelial surfaces neighboring gross warts are brushed, when patients are treated under general anesthesia, when extragenital wart sites are sought out and eliminated, when male consorts are treated, and when oral contraceptive drugs are withdrawn.[12]

Pregnancy presents a state of altered immunity. Laser ablation during the first trimester has been reported to have a 33% failure rate.[30] Clearly,

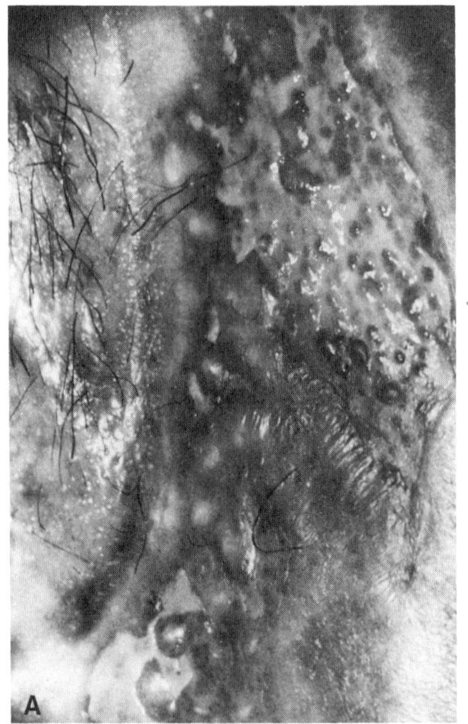

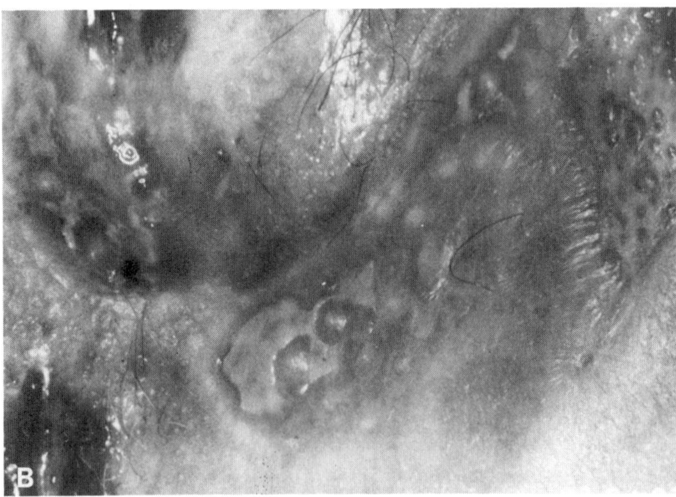

FIGURE 12–11 Vulva postlaser vaporization at 18 days reveals excellent healing. Hypertrophy of hair follicles is noted at the upper right of the picture.

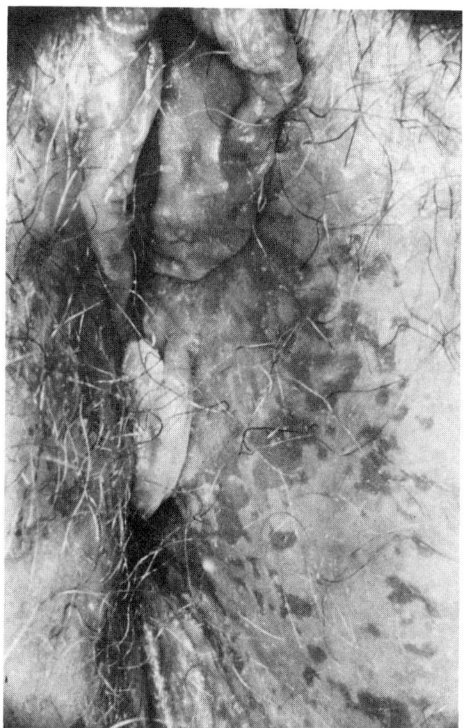

FIGURE 12–12 Vulvitis is characterized by erythema and pruritis. This picture was taken 4 weeks following laser vaporization of the vulva.

treatment in the third trimester is usually successful because the immune status of the patient will predictably change within a time limit of 3 months. Generally, second-trimester laser therapy can be expected to be successful in less than 80% of cases.

Male consorts of women afflicted with genital warts will be found to have lesions present on the penis and/or scrotum with a frequency ranging between 47–80%.[12,31] These males should be either referred to a urologist for diagnosis (magnification must be specified) and treatment, or the gynecologist should undertake to colposcope- and laser-ablate these males' lesions. The uncircumcised male presents a condition that is usually refractory to the elimination of warts; following circumcision, the disease can be satisfactorily treated.

Although a wide variety of other treatment methods has been widely published in the literature, scrutiny of the results reveal a rather dismal picture (Table 12–2). Recently, Krebs has published data advocating a combination of the CO_2 laser plus 5-FU cream for the treatment of extensive genital warts.[32,33] Ninety percent elimination of disease was reported in the

TABLE 12–2. Comparison of Nonlaser Methods for Treatment of Genital Warts

Method	Investigator(s)	Results (Cure %)
Trichloracetic acid (50%)	Gabriel and Thin[18]	28
Podophyllin (25%)	Simmons[19]	22
	Culp and Kaplan[20]	79.8
	Hage and Larsen[24]	21–64
Alpha interferon	FDA Bulletin (8/88)[22]	42
5-FU (topical cream)	Haye[23†]	10
	Ferenczy[24‡]	89.7
		50.0
Cryosurgery	Simmons, Langlet, and Thin[2/25§]	42
	Balsdon[26]	69
	Ghosh[27]	74
Electrocautery	Simmons, Lanlet, and Thin[25]	55
	Billingham and Lewis[28‖]	50
Autogenous vaccine	Powell, Pollard, and Jinkins[29]	83

*93% males
†External surfaces: penis, vulva, perianal.
‡Vaginal papillary warts versus flat vaginal warts.
§Males with anogenital warts.
‖Anal warts.

cohort of patients receiving this combination therapy.[32] Obviously, 5-FU must never be used in pregnant women.

Although infectious complications associated with the laser vaporization of genital warts have been rare, they do occasionally occur, and all women should be observed carefully for this complication. Toxic shock syndrome following laser treatment of the vulva and vagina was reported in 1986.[34]

Pain following extensive laser ablation should be expected. Strangely, the peak of discomfort occurs 4–7 days after treatment and may last for up to 2 weeks posttherapy. The discomfort may be ameliorated by a variety of remedies but consistently can be diminished by covering the raw exposed surface with biocclusive dressings or by the generous and frequent application of Silvadene cream (Figure 12–14). Scar formation results from overzealous treatment to depths unnecessary for the elimination of warts. Biopsies of vulvar skin taken during laser treatment have shown that depth may be estimated reasonably by visual perusal. This author has documented three levels that anyone can identify. *Level 1* is where vaporization may be induced by brushing, ie, blanching the skin white at 100–200 W/cm^2. At this level, the epidermis only is sacrificed, leaving behind intact dermal papillae. *Level 2* is hall-

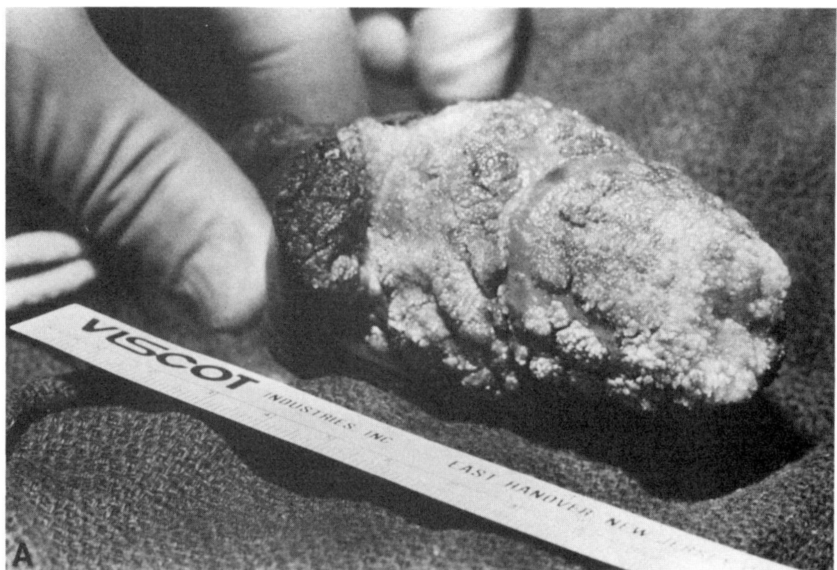

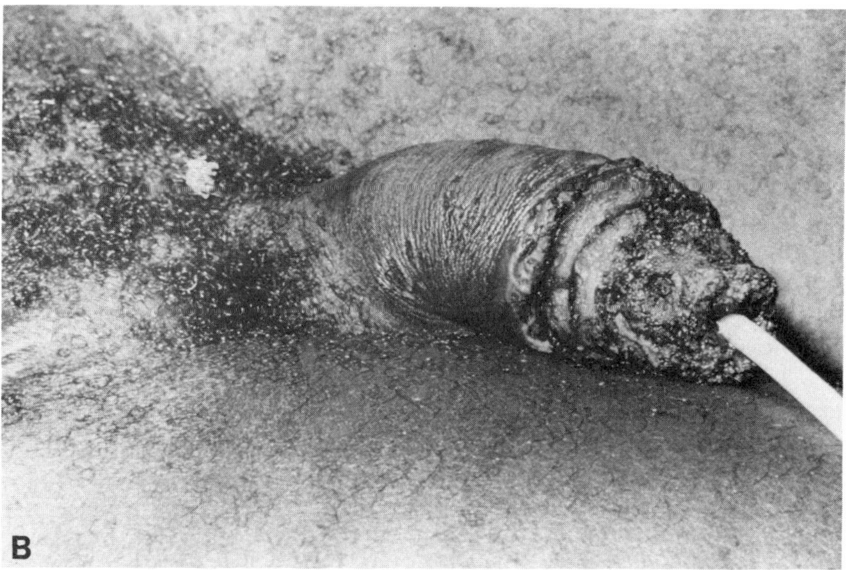

FIGURE 12–13 Extensive penile warts in this male with AIDS are unlikely to be eliminated with a single laser treatment. After three laser treatments, an HIV serological test was obtained and was positive by ELISA and Western blot.

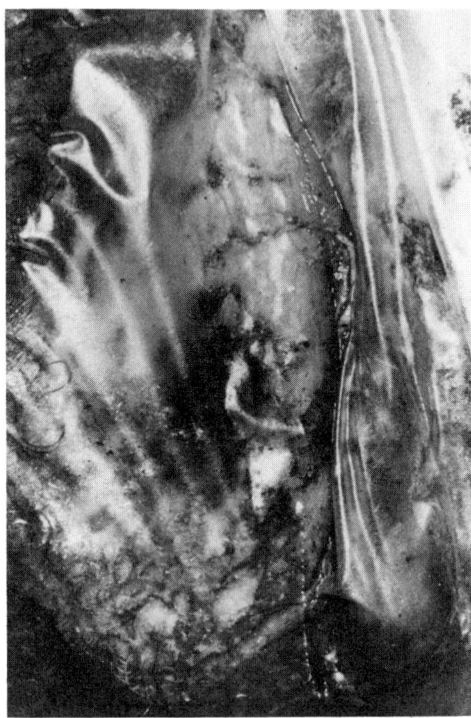

FIGURE 12–14 A biocclusive dressing has been applied to the laser-treated vulva. Pain may be greatly ameliorated by covering the raw, exposed surface.

marked by the appearance of yellow-tinged tissue (collagen), which is artifactually produced by the thermal interaction of the laser beam and dermis. It is impossible by eyeballing the wound to know whether one resides in the papillary or reticular dermal layer. Finally, *level 3* may be identified by the characteristic appearance of fatty tissue and denotes full thickness injury to the vulvar skin.

These layers can be demonstrated best after elimination of the residue char by wiping away the carbonized residue with saline or acetic acid-soaked swabs. A section taken through the dermis with the scalpel or the ultraspot micro-manipulator coupled with a superpulsed beam demonstrates pink-colored tissue, ie, the true color of dermis when not subjected to the heat artifact.

SPECIAL CONSIDERATIONS

Children

We have treated ten children ranging in age from 9 months to 4 years. Every patient had extensive genital warts, and one girl demonstrated nu-

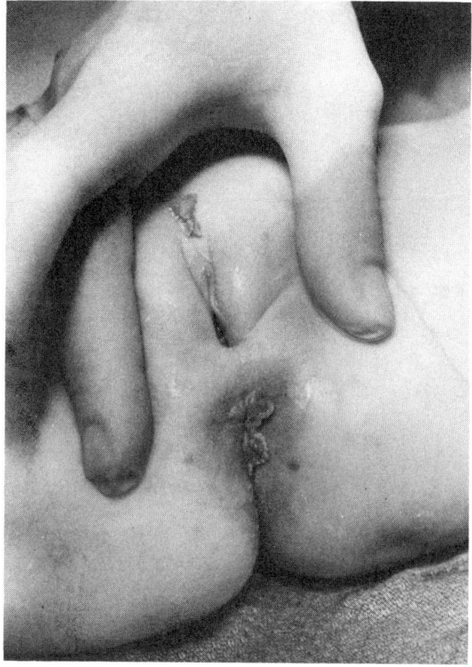

FIGURE 12–15 Perianal and vulvar warts are demonstrated in this 2-year-old child. Such cases should be investigated for sexual abuse.

merous soft warts on the extremities, trunk, and face (Figure 12–15). Every case was investigated by social services for sexual abuse. In two instances, the youngster had been abused by a live-in male consort of the child's mother. No evidence of sexual tampering was found in the remaining eight cases. The lesions were characteristic of condyloma acuminata. All children were admitted to the pediatric service prior to laser therapy. The techniques and specifications for treatment were identical to those described under Methodology. Following laser vaporization and brushing, the children were returned to the pediatric floor for a mean length of stay of 48 hours. During the hospitalization, mothers were instructed about postoperative care of the laser wounds. Healing progressed very rapidly and without complications in these youngsters. The vulva skin was completely epithelialized at 2 weeks and totally healed in 4 weeks. Interestingly, in the case described above with extensive extragenital warts, treatment of the child's genitalia and the mother's fingers led to spontaneous regression of the child's extremity, facial, and trunk lesions (Figure 12–16). Eight of the ten mothers were found to have typical verrucae on their fingers, hands, or feet.

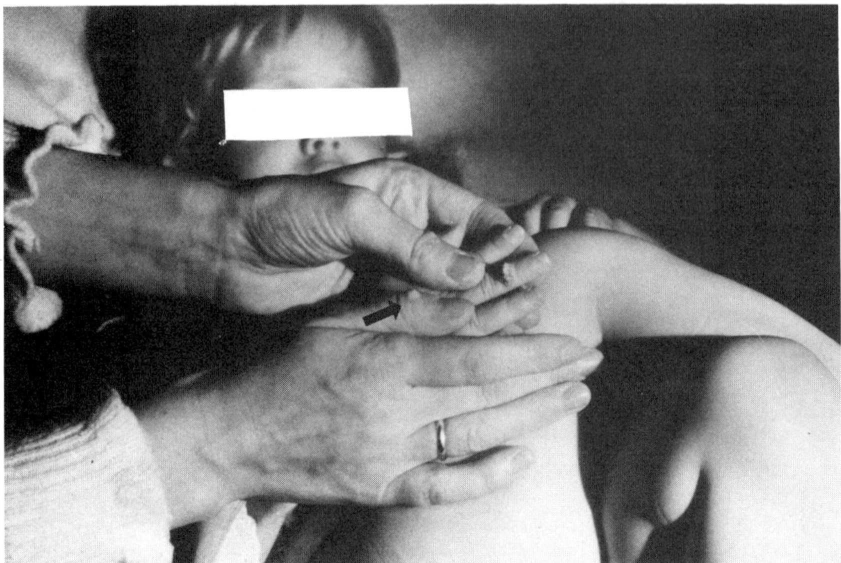

FIGURE 12–16 Children with condylomata acuminata are frequently infected by their mothers. Note the wart on this mother's thumb (arrow).

Pregnancy

Seventy-two out of 1025 cases of condyloma acuminata were associated with pregnancy states. We, as well as others, have observed rapid and stubbornly persistent growth of these lesions during pregnancy (Figure 12–17).[35] The chance of eliminating warts during early pregnancy is approximately 50%. The best time to utilize the laser for treatment is between 20–32 weeks gestation. Prior to 20 weeks, the failure rate is unacceptably high, and after 32 weeks bleeding as well as other complications are common. Laser vaporization of the cervix is risky anytime during pregnancy. Labor may be stimulated perhaps by the secondary liberation of endogenous prostaglandins. Although it is an uncommon complication, careless laser surgery could penetrate the amniotic sac. Particular care should be focused on the vagina after laser surgery because of the risks of infection and delayed bleeding. A lower range of power densities and large spots are recommended for vaginal wart vaporization.

One peculiar risk associated with pregnancy focuses on the infant who delivers through grossly warty tissue. The hazard is related to the subsequent development of juvenile papillomas growing on the vocal cords.[36,37] The latter is a serious condition that can lead to subsequent asphyxia if untreated and multiple recurrences posttreatment. Shah et al[38] in a multicenter study demonstrated that juvenile papillomas are rare with an estimated risk of transmission between 1:80–1:1500. Interestingly, out of 109 collected cases,

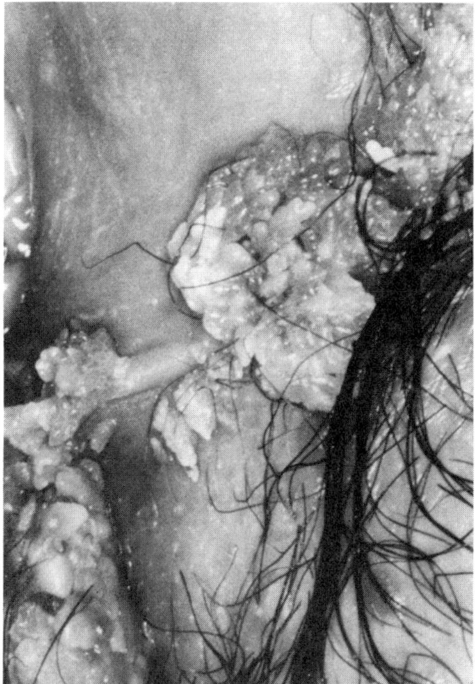

FIGURE 12–17 The growth of warts accelerates during pregnancy and in turn usually regress after the termination of the gestation.

only one occurred in a child who was delivered by cesarean section. The rate for cesarean section during the study period would predictably have approached $\times 5$–20 that number.

The CO_2 laser is the safest and most reasonable alternative for the therapy of genital warts during pregnancy. Podophyllin, trichloracetic acid, and 5-FU cream should be avoided during pregnancy.[39]

Immunosuppressed and Diabetics

This subset of patients has the highest treatment failure rate for any group except those persons afflicted with the human immune deficiency virus. In our series, this group had greater than 50% failure rate and almost universally needed repetitious treatment for persisting warts. Because of the high risk of treatment failure, this group of patients will benefit from combination therapy. Combining laser vaporization with twice-monthly instillation of 1.5 gm of 5-FU cream into the vagina for 4–6 months has improved our results in elimination of disease in these patients.

LASER SMOKE

Recent reports in the literature have fully documented the hazards of breathing laser vapor. Baggish and Elbakry[40] demonstrated that the fine particulate matter dispersed in laser smoke produced interstitual pneumonia, bronchial epithelial hyperplasia, lymphocytic infiltration, and emphysema in the lungs of rats. A second series of experiments by Baggish et al[41] found that this particulate matter was not trapped by production model smoke evacuators equipped with cartridge filters, ie, the fine particles in the smoke were smaller than 0.5 μm. Nezhat et al,[42] utilizing a marble cascade impactor, determined that the median aerodynamic diameter of 32 plume samples was 0.31 μm (range 0.1–0.8 μm). Baggish et al[41] utilized a special smoke evacuator employing an ULPA filter capable of trapping particles less than 0.1 μm in size. Every rat breathing filtered smoke was protected from the ravages of the smoke; the sacrificed animals' lungs were identical to normal controls.

Garden et al[43] collected smoke generated from vaporizing four bovine fibropapillomas. Hybridization with bovine papilloma DNA probes revealed intact BPV DNA in the laser vapor in every case. Seven patients undergoing CO_2 laser vaporization for plantar warts were also studied. Two of the seven patients showed intact HPV DNA in the vapor.

Although papilloma virus DNA was found to be present in laser plume, the question of whether intact and infectious virus can be transmitted in laser smoke remains unanswered. Some viral particles are less than 0.1 μm in diameter; however, these viruses are attached to intact or fragmented cells, which may well be trapped in suitable filters.

SUMMATION

Although the CO_2 laser is an excellent surgical tool for the elimination of condyloma acuminata, failure to take advantage of its best features relegates the instrument to base value. Those unique properties peculiar to laser technology include nontouch surgery, selective beam diameter, and precise-tissue-depth adjustment. Variations of power density as well as magnification should be employed to attain the desired action, eg, brushing or vaporization. Knowledge of mode characteristics, ie, continuous wave and various superpulse modes, is necessary to maximize thermal relief when ultrathin tissue excisions are taken. The latter is recommended highly when one wishes to combine treatment and at the same time supply the pathologist with a specimen. The end result is identical to a vaporization procedure, ie, little or no blood loss, no suture closure, and no subsequent scarring.

A detailed search must be made to uncover all potential sites of wart infestation. When warts are seen, they and surrounding tissues must be removed. Blasting away at warts with a fixed continuous wave mode and a limited range of power will not suffice. This type of gross surgery will never produce the optimal results capable with sophisticated laser technology. Poor results are invariably the end product of poor technique, hurried appraisal, and careless attention to therapeutic and diagnostic details.

Follow-up is of equal import to treatment. Recognizing persistent warts and eliminating them in a timely fashion is not only good medical practice, but it is also important for the patient's morale. Restraint should be exercised to avoid incorrect and overzealous sacrifice of normal healing tissue, skin folds and tags, and other normal epithelial variants.

Finally, knowledge of the anatomy of the disorder and action of the laser beam on tissues at various genital and extragenital locations, as well as the effects of altered immune states on treatment results, is critical to success.[44,45] Recent data have shown that oncogenic transformation of HPV groups may depend on the interaction of the virus and certain immunosuppressive steroids, eg, dexamethasone and oral contraceptives.[46] Underlying human immune deficiency viral infection should be considered possible in every case of genital warts presented for laser therapy.

REFERENCES

1. Oriel D: Genital warts in sexualy transmitted diseases. In Caterall RD, Nicol CS, eds. London; Academic, 1976;186.
2. Almedia JD: Virus disease II. Genital warts in sexually transmitted disease. In: Caterall RD, Nichol CS, eds. London; Academic, 1976;135
3. Seski JC, Reinhalter ER, Silva J: Abnormalities of lymphocyte transformations in women with condylomata acuminata. Obstet Gynecol 1978;51:188.
4. Baggish MS: Condylomata acuminata genital infections treated by the CO_2 laser. In: Baggish MS, ed. Basic and advanced laser surgery in gynecology. Norwalk, CT: Appleton-Century-Crofts, 1985;261.
5. Baggish MS: Carbon dioxide laser treatment for condylomata acuminata venereal infections. Obstet Gynecol 1980;55:711.
6. Baggish MS: Treating viral venereal infections with the CO_2 laser. J Reprod Med 1982;27:737.
7. Hahn GA: Carbon dioxide laser surgery in treatment of condyloma. Am J Obstet Gynecol 1981;141:1000.
8. Calkins JW, Masterson BJ, Magrina JF, et al: Management of condylomata acuminata with the carbon dioxide laser. Obstet Gynecol 1982;59:105.
9. Stanhope CR, Garth DP, Stuart GC, et al: Carbon dioxide laser surgery. Obstet Gynecol 1983;61:624.
10. Ferenczy A: Using the laser to treat vulvar condylomata acuminata and intraepithelial neoplasia. Can Med Assoc J 1983;128:135.
11. Bellina JH: The use of the carbon dioxide laser in the management of condyloma acuminatum with eight-year follow-up. Am J Obstet Gynecol 1983;147:375.
12. Baggish MS: Improved laser techniques for the elimination of genital and extragenital warts. Am J Obstet Gynecol 1985;153:545.
13. Ferenczy A, Mitao M, Silverstein SP, et al: Latent papillomavirus and its relationship to recurrence of genital warts following laser surgery. N Engl J Med 1985;313:784.

14. Baggish MS, Elbakry MM: Comparison of electronically superpulsed and continuous-wave CO_2 laser on the rat uterine horn. Fertil Steril 1986;45:120.
15. Reid R, Elfont EAH, Zirkin RM, et al: Superficial laser vulvectomy. Am J Obstet Gynecol 1985;152:261.
16. Kryger-Baggensen N, Larsen JF, Pedersen PH: CO_2 laser treatment of condylomata acuminata. Acta Obstet Gynecol Scan 1984;63:341.
17. Krebs HB, Wheelock JB: The CO_2 laser for recurrent and therapy-resistant condylomata acuminata. J Reprod Med 1985;30:489.
18. Gabriel G, Thin RNT: Treatment of anogenital warts. Br J Vener Dis 1983;59:124.
19. Simmons PD: Podophyllin 10% and 25% in the treatment of ano-genital warts. Br J Vener Dis 1981;57:208.
20. Culp OS, Kaplan IW: Condylomata acuminata. Ann Surg 198;120:251.
21. Hage E, Larsen PO: Condylomata acuminata. Ugeskr Laeger 1975;137:679.
22. FDA Drug Bulletin: Alpha interferon for venereal warts. 1988;18:19.
23. Haye KR: Treatment of condylomata acuminata with 5% 5-fluorouracil (5-FU) cream. Br J Vener Dis 1974;50:466.
24. Ferenczy A: Comparison of 5-fluorouracil and CO_2 laser for treatment of vaginal condylomata. Obstet Gynecol 1984;64:773.
25. Simmons PD, Langlet F, Thin RNT: Cryotherapy versus electrocautery in the treatment of genital warts. Br J Vener Dis 1981;57:273.
26. Balsdon MJ: Cryosurgery of genital warts. Br J Vener Dis 1978;54:352.
27. Ghosh AK: Cryosurgery of genital warts in cases in which podophyllin treatment failed or was contraindicated. Br J Vener Dis 1977;53:49.
28. Billingham RP, Lewis FG: Laser versus electrical cautery in the treatment of condylomata acuminata of the anus. Surg Gynecol Obstet 1982;155:865.
29. Powell IC, Pollard M, Jinkins JL: Treatment of condyloma acuminata by autogenous vaccine. South Med J 1970;63:202.
30. Ferenczy A: Treating genital condyloma during pregnancy with the carbon dioxide laser. Am J Obstet Gynecol 1984;148:9.
31. Ferenczy A: Evaluation and management of male partners of condyloma patients. Colpo Gynecol Laser Surg 1986;2:15.
32. Krebs HB: Combination of laser plus 5-fluorouracil for the treatment of extensive genital condylomata acuminata. Lasers Surg Med 1988;8:135.
33. Krebs HB: Prophylactic topical 5-fluorouracil following treatment of human papillomavirus-associated lesions of the vulva and vagina. Obstet Gynecol 1986;68:837.
34. Bowen LW, Sand PK, Ostergard DR: Toxic shock syndrome following carbon dioxide laser treatment of genital tract condyloma acuminatum. Am J Obstet Gynecol 1986;154:145.
35. Wilson J: Extensive vulvar condylomata acuminata necessitating caesarean section. Aust NZ J Obstet Gynaecol 1973;13:121.
36. Fearon B, Macrae D: Laryngeal papillomatosis in children. J Otolaryngol 1976;5:493.
37. Quick CA, Krzyzek RA, Watts SL, et al: Relationship between condylomata and laryngeal papillomata. Ann Otol 1980;89:467.
38. Shah K, Kashima H, Polk BF, et al: Rarity of casarean delivery in cases of juvenile-onset respiratory papillomatosis. Obstet Gynecol 1986;68:795.
39. Slater GE, Rumack RH, Peterson RG: Podophyllin poisoning. Obstet Gynecol 1978;52:94.
40. Baggish MS, Elbakry M: The effects of laser smoke on the lungs of rats. Am J Obstet Gynecol 1987;156:1260.
41. Baggish MS, Baltoyannis P, Sze E: Protection of the rat lung from the harmful effects of laser smoke. Lasers Surg Med 1988;8:248.
42. Nezhat C, Winer WK, Nezhat F, et al: Smoke from laser surgery: Is there a health hazard? Lasers Surg Med 1987;7:376.
43. Garden JM, O'Banion K, Shelnitz LS, et al: Papillomavirus in the vapor of carbon dioxide laser-treated verrucae. JAMA 1988;259:1199.

44. Reid R, Laverty CR, Coppleson M, et al: Non-condylomatous cervical wart virus infection. Obstet Gynecol 1980;55:476.

45. Reid R, Greenberg M, Jenson B, et al: Sexually transmitted papillomaviral infections. Am J Obstet Gynecol 1987;156:212.

46. Pater MM, Hughes GA, Hyslop DE, et al: Glucocorticoid dependent oncogenic transformation by type 16 but not type 11 Human papilloma virus DNA. Nature 1988;335:832.

CHAPTER 13

Management of the Male Partner

Alex Ferenczy, MD and Christine Bergeron, MD, PhD

Recent epidemiologic-colposcopic-histologic correlations together with molecular hybridization confirmed the sexually transmitted nature of human papillomavirus (HPV) infections.[1–4] Sexual contact rates range between 65% and 85% in most reported series.[1–5] In today's practice, genital HPV infection is rampant, particularly between the ages of 20–25 years, and it is the most common form of sexually transmitted disease in North and South America and Europe.[6] In addition to the sexually transmitted nature of HPV, some infections, ie, types 16 and 18 and related viruses, have been strongly associated with lower anogenital squamous cell carcinogenesis.[7,8] Approximately 10% of clinically asymptomatic males carry HPV-DNA in penile skin and urethra,[4,9–11] and one-third of male partners of HPV-infected women were found to have HPV type 16 and 33 positive penile lesions.[4,10,11] While penile cancers in Western countries are rare,[12] squamous cell carcinoma of the cervix is frequent. Annually, close to 500,000 women develop this disease worldwide.[13] Thus, it appears that a significant number of males carry high-carcinoma-risk, virus-containing lesions of the penis and are a source for potential cancer development in their female consorts.[4,5,9,13–16] Equally important are recent observations that maintain 60–70% of all genital HPV infections in the male are in a subclinical form and are detected only by high magnification (androscopy/colposcopy) following the application of 5% acetic acid.[4,5,17–26] Finally, in male receptive homosexuals, anal condylomata are strongly associated with squamous cell carcinoma with a relative risk of 33, compared to anal cancer in women engaged in ano-receptive intercourse.[27]

Up to today, it is not possible to prevent genital HPV infections. Physicians involved in this challenging field of medicine should use means that are meaningful to control viral transmission and infections as much as possible; by doing so, it is hoped that morbidity and mortality associated with

ISSN 1043-3198/89/$3.50

Clinical Practice of Gynecology: **2,** 214–232, 1989

squamous cell carcinoma of the cervix and other lower-genital cancer will be reduced. The role of the male partner in genital HPV infections has only recently been recognized; careful, and preferably systematic examination of the anogenital skin of the male sexual partners with an androscope (colposcope) is recommended.[3,4,10,11,15,16,18,19,22,24–26] Once detected, and when appropriate, histologically, and/or virologically (hybridization)[10] verified, genital HPV infections are managed according to their size, location, HPV content, and sexual habits of the patient.

In this chapter, the authors' clinical experience with over 400 male patients with anogenital HPV infections is reviewed with emphasis on diagnostic and therapeutic means that are available in today's practice for their management.

DIAGNOSING HPV INFECTIONS IN THE MALE

There are three types of HPV infections in the male anogenital skin: One is the raised, papillary, cauliflower-type condyloma acuminatum (Figure 13–1); the second is the slightly raised papular condyloma with often granular surface or punctations (Figure 13–2); and the third, more frequent, variant is the flat condyloma (planum) seen only with the androscope after the application of 5% acetic acid. They appear as white focal lesions with or without punctation (Figure 13–3). Most HPV infections, regardless of clinical presentation, are located on the penile shaft, 2–3 cm from the corona of the glands (Table 13–1). However, condylomata are also relatively frequent on the perianal skin and may also be found in the fossa navicularis[16,28] (Figure 13–4), the scrotum, mons pubis, and even the groin. Since most HPV-related lesions are not seen by the naked eye and without the application of acetic acid solution, an appropriate androscopic examination includes in addition to naked eye inspection, androscopy at $\times 4$–30 magnifications and the application of an acetic acid-soaked dressing gauze on the penis (Figure 13–5), the scrotum as well as the perianal skin. Unless the patient has severely irritated anogenital skin, 5% acetic acid will not cause discomfort. The meatus of the urethra (fossa navicularis) is also examined with the androscope by gently dilating it with an endocervical speculum. A 5% solution of acetic acid is then applied with a cotton-tipped swab. The vast majority (99%) of either flat or acuminate condylomata are located within the view of an androscope (1 cm or less from the external ostium)[22,28] and routine urethroscopy or cystoscopy is, therefore, not recommended. Those patients with extensive urethral warts, limits of which are not visualized with the androscope, should be examined by a urologist using urethrocytoscopy. Approximately one-fourth of heterosexual males and 90% of homosexual males with perianal condylomata acuminata have intraanal lesions (Figure 13–6). As a result, the anal canal should be examined in all cases of perianal warts. This can be achieved on an outpatient

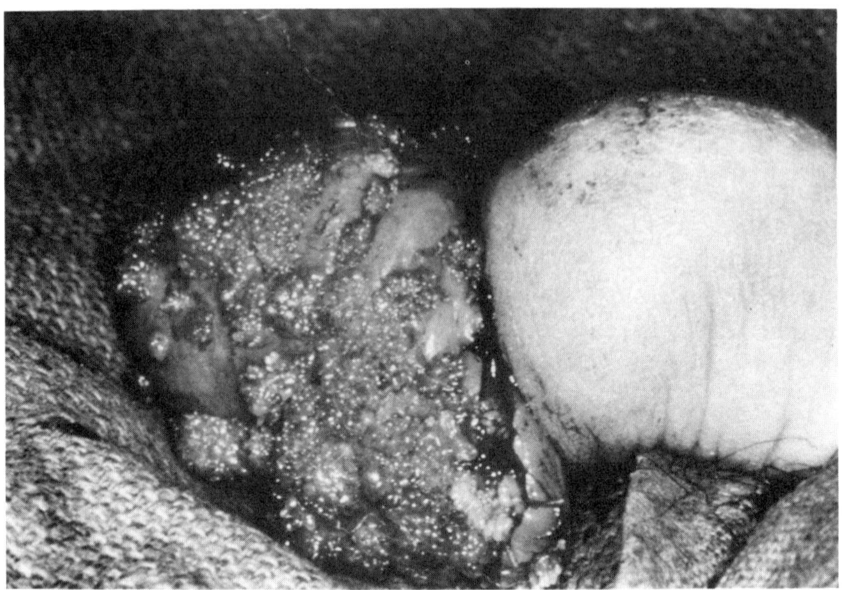

FIGURE 13-1 Extensive, coalescent, papillary condylomata acuminata with granular surface involving the glans and prepuce of the penis.

FIGURE 13-2 Acetowhite, papular condylomata located on the preputial skin.

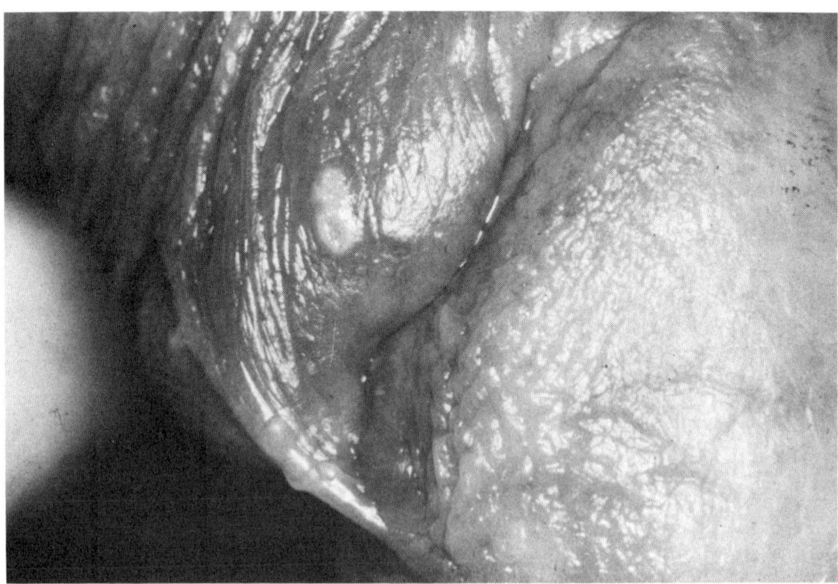

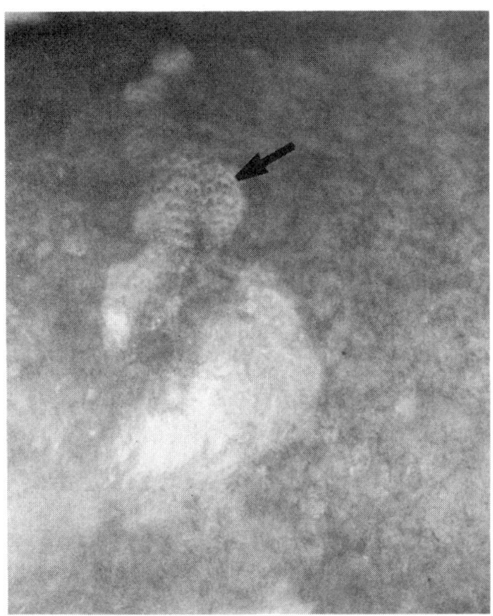

FIGURE 13–3 Androscopic view of flat, macular condylomata with minute surface asperities (arrow) after the application of 5% acetic acid (vinegar).

FIGURE 13–4 Androscopic view of acetowhite acuminate condyloma in the fossa navicularis of the urethra.

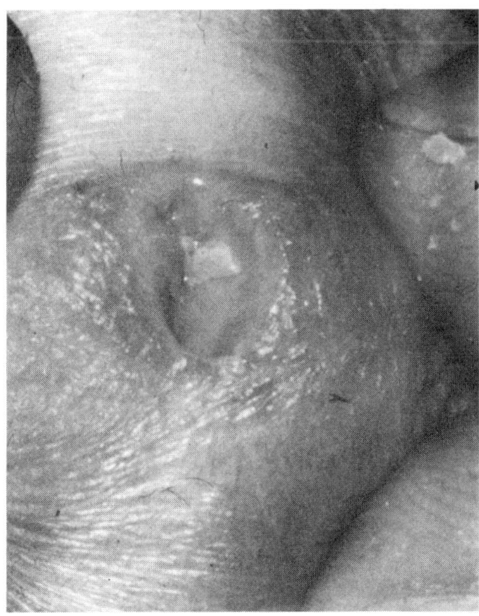

TABLE 13–1. Relative Distribution of Anogenital Condylomata in Heterosexual Males*

Site	No. Cases	%
Prepuce including frenulum	309	70
Proximal shaft and mons pubis	44	10
Anus alone	40	9
Urethra alone	25	6
Glands, scrotum, groin	23	5
Total	438	100

*Including acuminate, papular, and macular condylomata.

basis by applying 20% benzocaine ointment (Astra Pharmaceuticals) over the anal sphincter area circumferentially, 5 minutes prior to gently dilating the sphincter with a nasal speculum in heterosexuals and an anal speculum (Figure 13–6) in homosexuals. With the use of androscopy, the anal canal is then visualized up to 5 cm; in nearly all cases, condylomata are located within 3 cm from the external orifice and are concentrated on each side of the external anal sphincter.

Not all lesional tissues on the male anogenital skin are necessarily

FIGURE 13–5 A vinegar-soaked dressing gauze is applied to the entire penile shaft, glands, and dorsal scrotum for 1–3 minutes.

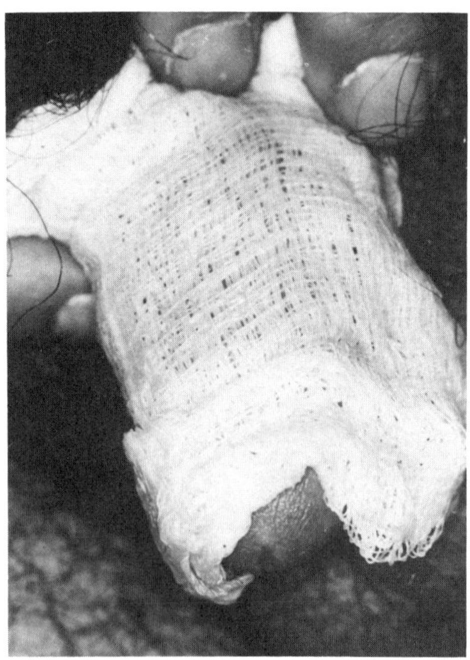

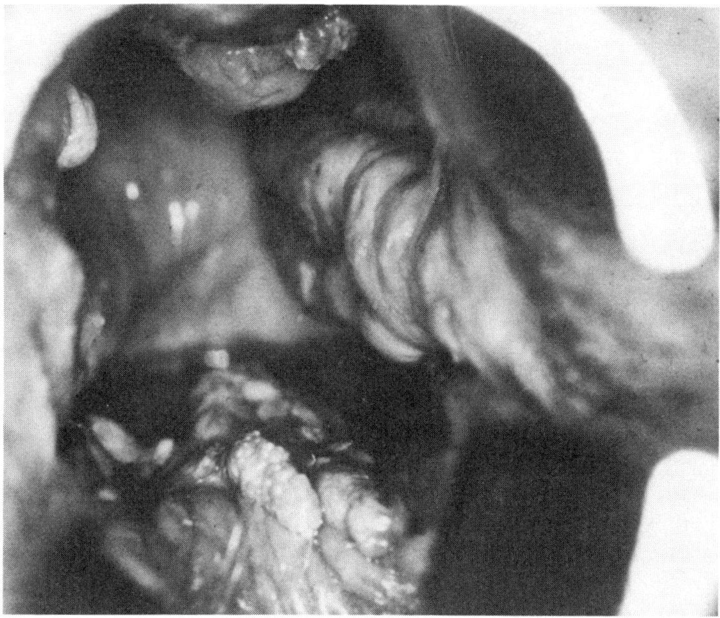

FIGURE 13–6 Androscopic view of anal canal dilated with an anal speculum. Several acuminate condylomata are seen at the external sphincter region, circumferentially.

TABLE 13–2. Conditions Resembling Genital Condylomata*

Penile intraepithelial neoplasia (Bowenoid papulosis)
Invasive squamous cell carcinoma including verrucous carcinoma (Buschke–Lowenstein)
Molluscum contagiosum
Micropapillomatosis glandis (pearly penile papules)
Nevi
Seborrheic keratosis (over 35 years old)
Epidermal inclusion cyst (mainly scrotum)
Condylomata lata
Candidiasis
Contact dermatitis
Psoriasis
Folliculitis
Recent intercourse
Herpes
Nonspecific urethritis

*Including acuminate, papular, and flat.

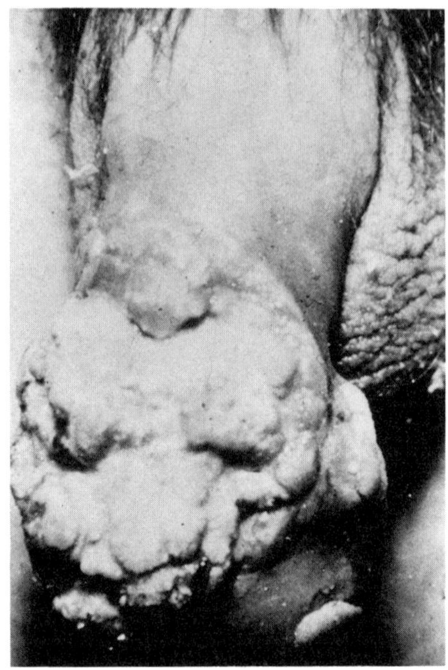

FIGURE 13–7 Invasive, exophytic, squamous cell carcinoma of preputial skin with necrotic surface.

condylomata (Table 13–2). All grossly atypical lesions are to be biopsied to rule out possible mimics, including the rare invasive carcinoma (Figure 13–7). Multiple, brown-red, or acetowhite papules with punctation resistant to topical treatment may be penile intraepithelial neoplasia (PIN), also referred to as Bowenoid papulosis[29–31] (Figure 13–8). Molloscum contagiosum (Figure 13–9) are often confused with condylomata acuminata as are the so-called micropapillomatosis glandis (pearly penile papules).[32] The latter are subepithelial angiofibromata[33] typically located on the corona of the glans and each side of the glands-frenulum junction. They are seen in about 10% of male patients.[22] They may occasionally be infected by HPV[34]; they appear prominent and acetowhite (Figure 13–10). Among the frequent flat, acetowhite condylomata mimics are candidiasis (Figure 13–11), folliculitis, contact dermatitis secondary to heat and sweat particularly in the obese patient, recent intercourse (within 3 hours from examination), balanitis xerotica (lichen sclerosus), and *Chlamydia trachomatis.*

Lesions of the penile and perianal skin may be conveniently biopsied with a Kevorkian punch biopsy forceps or similar instruments. Local anesthesia is obtained in a supine position by slowly infiltrating 1% Xylocaine

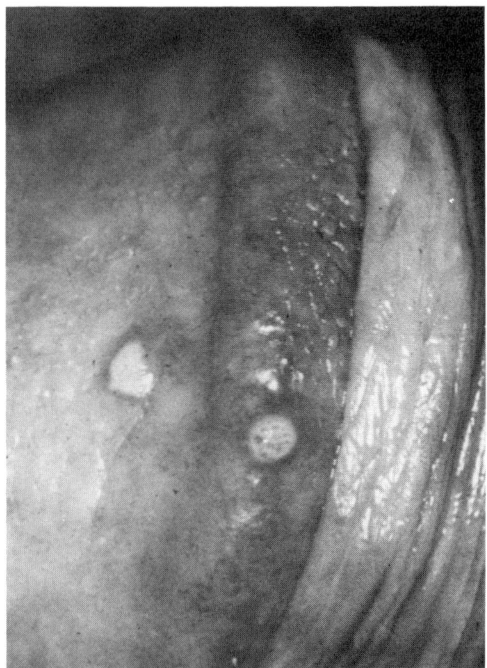

FIGURE 13–8 Androscopy of two acetowhite papules on glands of penis with irregular, coarse punctation. Biopsy contained penile intraepithelial neoplasia.

solution underneath the lesional tissue using a 30-gauge dental needle in a dental syringe (Figure 13–12). Biopsies of the penis should be shallow, preferentially carried out under androscopic guidance. Indeed, the penile epidermis is supported only by a thin (.25 mm) collagen table, and penetration deeper than 1 mm may injure the underlying fascia, producing delayed, painful healing and scarring. Biopsy of the glands should be avoided whenever possible because of significant discomfort produced by local anesthesia and hemorrhage may develop after biopsy.

TREATMENT OF HPV INFECTIONS OF THE ANOGENITAL SKIN

Condylomata

Many therapeutic modalities are available for the treatment of genital warts.[22,35–47] Unfortunately, their success rates are difficult to analyze because their use in terms of dose, duration, and frequency is highly variable from one report to another, as are the number, location, and duration of anogenital condylomatous lesions.

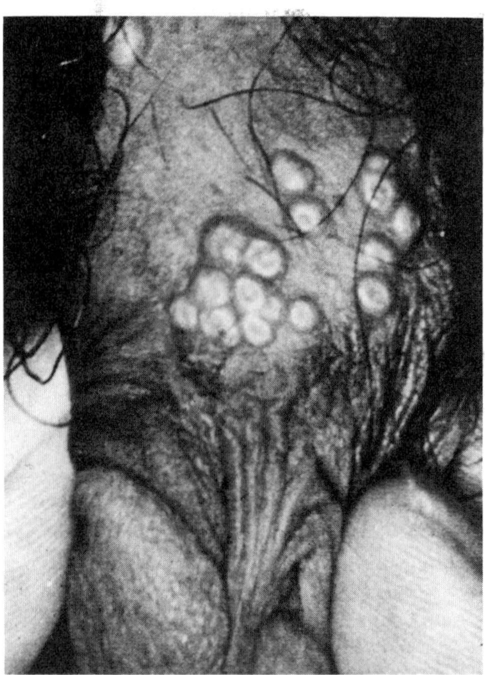

FIGURE 13–9 Clusters of smooth-surfaced papules with central umbilication typical of pox-virus positive molluscum contagiosum.

The choice of therapy for condylomata is based on the number, morphology, and distribution of anogenital condylomata. Acuminate and papular lesions involving no more than a total of 5 cm^2 area of the penile shaft, preputial skin, perianal skin, and scrotal skin are treated with 50% trichloroacetic acid (TCA) in 70% ethanol solution applied topically twice a day for 3 days. If, at the end of the 4-week therapy, partial or no response is obtained, the patient is given 80% TCA in 70% ethanol solution applied topically, twice a day for 3 consecutive days per week for a total of 3 weeks. Persistent condylomata are removed by cytodestructive means with either excisional biopsy, electro- or cryocautery, or laser vaporization. The advantages of TCA over other conservative topical treatment modalities, including 25% podophyllum resin[44] in compound tincture of benzoin or liquid nitrogen freezing, or both, are less discomfort during application and that TCA can safely be applied by the patient himself, reducing cost of treatment. The patient with acuminate or papular condylomata is instructed to apply the solution as follows:

1. Wash area thoroughly with soap and water.
2. Rub surface of warts gently with an abrasive such as an emery board or a pumice stone.

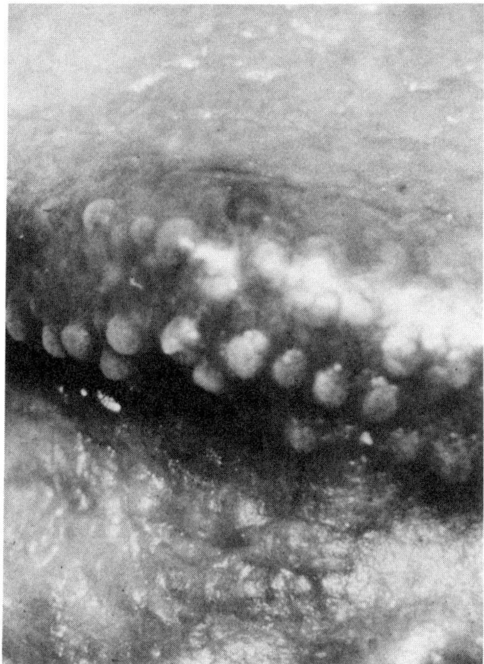

FIGURE 13–10 Micropapillomatosis glandis (pearly penile papules) arranged in an Indian-file pattern along the corona glandis. According to the patient whose female partner had vulvar condylomata, the acetowhite papules recently became enlarged, and histology contained hyperkeratosis and dot blot hybridization HPV type 6.

3. Apply solution on top of each lesion with a cotton tip applicator.
4. Allow to dry (a white layer is produced in 30 seconds accompanied by mild to moderate discomfort lasting 2–5 minutes).
5. Apply another layer of solution on top of the already treated area.
6. Protect adjacent skin with vaseline or 5% lidocaine ointment.
7. Do not wash off TCA.
8. Keep bottle tightly closed in the refrigerator (can last without crystallization of salt for 6 months.
9. Repeat TCA application as instructed (prescription contains 10 cc, 50% TCA in 70% ethanol, topical application b.i.d. × 3 days/week × 3 weeks or 5 cc, 80% TCA in 70% ethanol, topical application, b.i.d. × 3 days/week × 3 weeks.

The lesional tissue usually falls off layer by layer. TCA oxidizes rapidly when exposed to air and is not absorbed into deep tissue layers or the vascular system. In responders, a shallow ulcer will be formed at the treated site that heals within 3 weeks without leaving scar. However, about one-

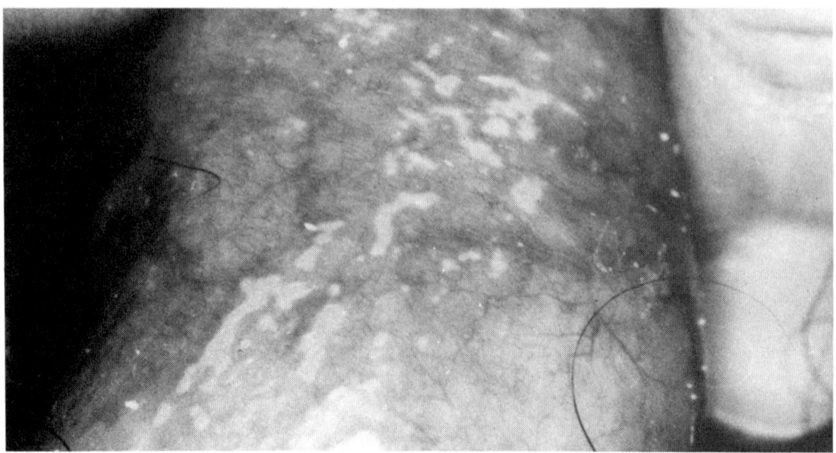

FIGURE 13–11 Androscopic view of acetowhite macular ("flaky") lesions of the preputial skin. The patient's sexual partner had candidiasis, HPV-DNA hybridization was negative, and anticandidiasis treatment of 2 weeks duration cleared the lesions.

FIGURE 13–12 A dental syringe with a 30-gauge needle and 1% xylocaine (Astra Pharmaceuticals) in cartouche and a Kevorkian biopsy punch (EuroMed, California) are used for local anesthesia and histologic sampling of the penis, respectively.

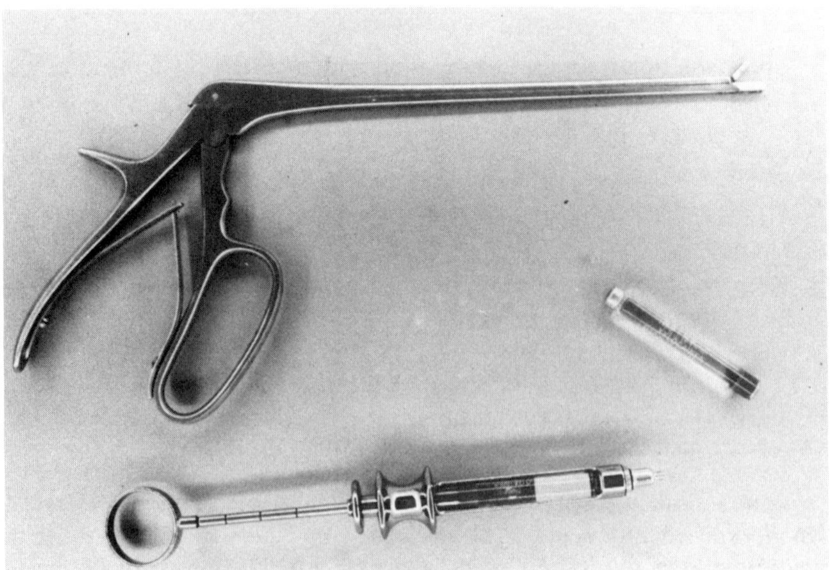

TABLE 13–3. Cytotoxic Treatment–Results of Anogenital Condylomata* in Male Patients (N = 300)**

Treatment	Failures (%)	Recurrences (%)
50% TCA	30	5
80% TCA***	15	0
25% podophylin	40	15
Liquid nitogen	21	9
5% 5-FU cream (Efudex)	50	4

   * Excluding urethral and intraanal condylomata.

  ** Follow-up 6 months to 8 years, mean 28 months.

***Only partial or non-responders to 50% TCA.

third of patients fail to reacquire melanin pigmentation and developed vitiligo in the areas treated. To achieve high patient compliance, it is useful to have a treatment demonstration in the office and have 10 cc 50% and 5 cc 80% TCA on hand, stored in a refrigerator. In the rare patients in whom TCA produces severe discomfort (of Mediterranean Sea origin), other treatment should be tried, since they will not be compliant with the treatment prescribed. Although treatment results with TCA are not significantly better than with podophyllum or liquid nitrogen given in drops (Table 13–3), the fact that it is self-administered at home makes it a comparatively cheaper treatment approach. The use of other keratolytic agents, such as 5–20% salicylic acid and 5–20% lactic acid in flexible colloidon (Duofilm), 40% salicylic acid plaster, cantharidin (Cantharone), a mitochondrial poison, is not recommended for the treatment of genital warts. These agents are used for common skin warts with relative success, but no scientific data are available as to their therapeutic effectiveness for anogenital warts. Recent experimental studies found 0.5% pure podophyllotoxin (Condyline) self-treatment highly successful in eradicating penile warts.[46] If confirmed, Condyline may be an attractive alternative treatment modality for anogenital warts. The compound is currently being tested in the United States under the name of Podofilox.

Five percent 5-fluouracil (5-FU) in the form of cream (Efudex) is preferred for treating flat (macular) condylomata as well as all forms of condylomata on the glans of the penis and the meatus of the urethra (Table 13–4). Efudex treatment is also acceptable for clustered papular lesions that failed 50–80% TCA therapy.[35,47] In the authors' experience, Efudex therapy is ineffective for extensive acuminate condylomata. Akin to TCA, Efudex may also be applied by the patient himself. For flat condylomata of the penis involving the glands, a thin film of Efudex cream is applied (in patients with fair skin, blue eyes, and blond or red hair) one to three times a week for 6 weeks; the cream is retained on epithelial surfaces by using a condom (snug fit) for 3 hours and a "micropore" tape (for anal warts), after which the cream is washed off. For perianal and urethral disease, Efudex is

TABLE 13–4. 5% 5-Fluorouracil (Efudex) Treatment–Results of Flat (Macular) and Papular Anogenital Condylomatosis in the Male Patient (N = 138)*

Site of Condyloma	Failures (%)	Recurrences (%)
Penis (N = 64)	18	16
Perianal skin (N = 42)	23	7
Urethra (N = 32)	8	2

*Follow-up 6–30 months, mean: 18 months.

applied tri-weekly with a cotton swab and clean fingers, respectively. Patients with intrameatal warts are hydrated so the cream is washed off by urinating 3–4 hours after each application. Lesional tissues that fails to respond by 6 weeks of Efudex therapy is unlikely to respond to longer treatment sessions and are removed by cytodestructive type of treatment such as electrocautery or, preferably, laser vaporization. Efudex, if used over-aggressively, may produce chemical dermatitis with painful erosion and hyperpigmentation. However, if it is applied once to three times a week, discomfort is none to moderate in the vast majority of the cases. When one is applying Efudex on the penis, the scrotal skin has to be protected by zinc oxide or other occlusive ointment to prevent contact dermatitis. 5-fluoracil is a pyrimidine antagonist and an antimetabolite. It forms abnormal nucleotides, inhibits thymidilate synthetase, and produces abnormal growth and division of cells. In general, Efudex produces irreversible cell injury, and the dead cells are sloughed off. However, 5-FU, by virtue of its pharmacologic characteristics, may be a DNA-splitter and, theoretically at least, may be associated with an increased carcinoma risk. Long-term follow-up of patients treated for skin carcinoma (basal cell carcinoma) or carcinoma precursors (CIS, actinic keratosis) as well as CIS of penis failed to demonstrate an increased incidence of carcinoma in these patients including the immunosuppressed.[35,48]

Extensive penile and anal condylomatosis are best treated with cytodestructive means.[25,37–40,45] The various treatment modalities and their respective success rates are presented in Table 13–5. The comparatively better results with the CO_2 laser are largely due to the fact that vaporization is performed under high-magnification androscopy,[40] and the vaporization margins are extended 10–15 mm from lesional tissues rather than to the laser itself. Indeed, androscopy helps the operator to include all minute satellite lesions into the treatment field. Laser vaporization of these subclinical lesions prevents their later growth masquerading as "recurrences" or treatment-failed disease. Extended laser vaporization of 10 and occasionally 15 mm beyond lesional tissue margins of normal skin destroys persistent but clinically unexpressed (latent) human papillomaviruses (HPVs). Latent HPV has been shown by Southern blot hybridization in 45%

TABLE 13–5. Cytodestructive Treatment–Results of Anogenital Condylomata in the Male Patient*

Treatment	Failures (%)	Recurrences (%)
Excisional biopsy	2.0	35.0
Electrocautery including electrodessication	2.0	27.0
Cryocautery with nitrous oxide	8.0	20.0
Laser vaporization	1.5	7.5

*Data based on personal experience (400 patients) and literature review. Failures are persistent disease; recurrences are new disease.

of female and male patients with anogenital HPV infections[49], in over 70% of patients with cervical cancer[50], and the mucus membrane of the larynx of patients treated many years previously for juvenile laryngeal papillomata.[51] The fact that 67% of 20 patients with latent HPV-DNA recurred compared to 1 (11%) of 20 patients with HPV-negative laser margins supports the latent HPV concept. Also, the comparatively better treatment results (7.5%) obtained with extended laser vaporization of adjacent normal skin (laser epidermectomy) compared to that of no or narrow (less than 5 mm) skin margins (22%)[45] emphasizes the role of latent HPV in producing "recurrent disease" or "treatment-failures."

As has been suggested earlier, laser vaporization is done under androscopic guidance. Lesions located on the penile shaft exclusively (glands not involved) may be lasered under local anesthesia with 1% xylocaine solution (penile block at the level of the base of the shaft), whereas cases in which the glands as well as the anus are involved, are treated under general anesthesia. Large exophytic lesions are excised with the laser beam at their base. The laser's power density ranges between 350 to 750 cm^2, using 2–5-mm spot sizes and depth of penetration does not exceed 1.0 and 0.5 mm at the site of lesional tissue and the adjacent normal epithelium, respectively.[22,40] Most recurrences occur during the first 6 weeks after vaporization, are few in number, and are retreated either with the laser or 50% TCA solution. Superficial laser ablation of the penile skin heals rapidly without significant discomfort. In patients with extensive perianal and anal warts, topical anesthetic ointment and analgesics control severe pain during the first 2 weeks after therapy. In general, cosmetic results are excellent (Figure 13–13). Hypo- or hyperpigmentation may occur, however, and the patients should be told about this possible side effect prior to therapy. Complications are rare and include phymosis (1/113 patients with penile warts) and perianal abscess (1/98 patients with anal warts).[22,40]

Treatment of male patients with chronically recurrent anogenital warts, particularly in homosexuals and immunosuppressed patients, is frustrating and, more often than not, provides unsatisfactory treatment results. The most successful therapeutic approach to this particular patient population in the authors' experience is laser vaporization followed immediately by

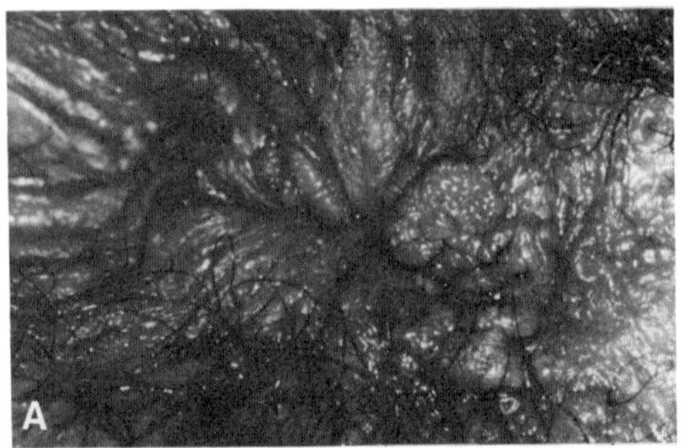

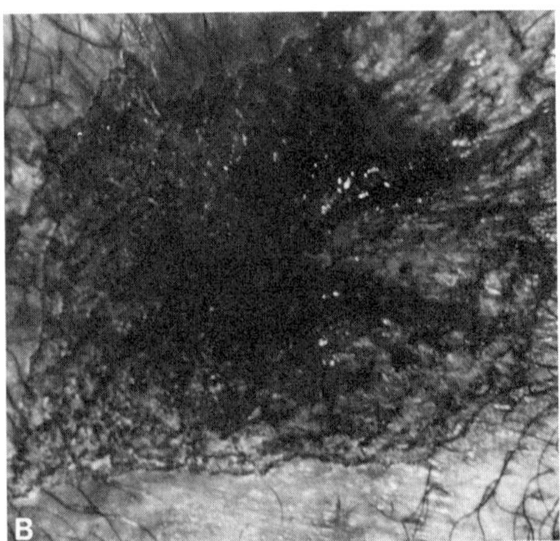

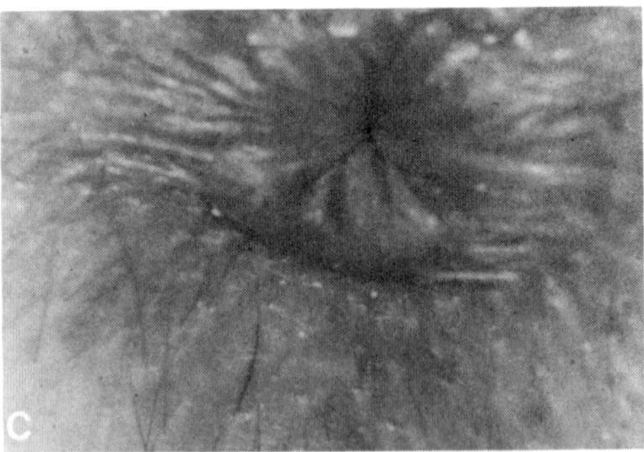

FIGURE 13–13 Extended laser epidermectomy: (A) Perianal condylomata acuminata before laser vaporization. (B) Perianal skin after laser vaporization with 1-mm deep extension into the underlying connective tissue at the lesional tissue level and 0.3-mm deep laterally of the surrounding 1-cm normal epithelium. (C) The same perianal skin 8 weeks after laser therapy for condylomata.

topical application of 5% Efudex cream in the treated areas and once a week thereafter for 6–10 weeks. Although controls are not available, in the first 20 patients with intractable penile and anal condylomata, complete response for a mean follow-up of 8 months has been obtained in 10 patients and partial response in 2 (unpublished observations). Other desperate therapies include the use of immunomodulating agents such as the topical application of 2,4 dinitrochlorobenzene (DNCB) directly to the warts in patients previously sensitized to the agent. Delayed cellular hypersensitivity reaction in all respects similar to contact dermatitis is responsible for the disappearance of the disease. Today, no randomized, double-blind study appeared to indicate the real value of this form of therapy. Immunization with autologous vaccines in the treatment of genital warts[36] has been abandoned because of the use of only partially inactivated, possibly oncogenic viruses, and because of lack of obtaining better therapeutic results than in the placebo group. Polyclonal and recombinant interferons, alpha, beta, and gamma, have been used for the past few years in the form of both intra- and perilesional injections and subcutaneous/intramuscular injections.[41–43] In most of the studies, complete response rates have been lower than 50%, and long-term follow-up is not available. In one study, significantly better treatment results were obtained with HPV-6- than HPV-16/18-containing lesions.[43] The treatment is carried out over a 4–8-week period and the higher-dose regimens are associated with cumbersome side effects, including flulike symptoms, headache, myalgia, etc. Lower doses of interferons given systemically by subcutaneous injections have negligible side effects; but failure rates are similar to those obtained with placebo (personal observations).

Intraepithelial Neoplasia

Clinically, this form of HPV infection is relatively rare,[29–31] although a significant proportion of macular and some papular (Figure 13–8) lesions[4,5] contain the potentially oncogenic type 16 and 33 HPVs.[4] Penile (PIN) and perianal (PAIN) intraepithelial neoplasias are best treated with CO_2 laser vaporization, although superficial electrodessication also provides acceptable treatment results. Laser treatment is carried out for PIN and PAIN as for flat (macular) condylomata[22], and, provided that the 1.0 cm adjacent normal skin is selectively removed as well, treatment results are excellent (Table 13–6).

In all patients treated for anogenital warts, we recommend the use of condoms made of latex at least until healing is completed and, if appropriate, until their female sexual partners being treated as well for genital HPV infections have cytologic and colposcopic evidence of cure. Although data on the true effectiveness of condom use in the prevention of HPV transmission are not available, theoretically at least, the latex meshwork of today's

TABLE 13–6. Laser Treatment–Results of Penile and Perianal Intraepithelial Neoplasia*

	Failures (%)	Recurrences (%)
PIN (N = 9)**	0	0
PAIN (N = 4)	0	1

*Follow-up 1–8 years, mean 2 years.
*Four of nine and two of four patients, respectively, received two treatments.

condoms is so dense and complex with blind loops as to prevent transfer of viruses.[52,53] The same may not apply for condoms made of natural lambskin.[52] Patients should be discouraged from using petrolatum or vegetable-based lubricants on condoms because of the great risk of break.[54]

ACKNOWLEDGEMENTS

This research was supported by SD-Path-4 Research Fund of the Sir Mortimer B. Davis Jewish General Hospital.

REFERENCES

1. Oriel JD: Genital warts. Sex Transm Dis 1981;8:326–329.
2. Meisels A, Morin C, Casas-Cordero M: Human papillomavirus infection of the uterine cervix. Int J Gynecol Pathol 1982;1:75–94.
3. Campion MJ, Singer A, Clarkson PR, et al: Increased risk of cervical neoplasia in the consort of men with penile condylomata acuminata. Lancet 1985;i:943–945.
4. Barrasso R, De Brux J, Croissant O, et al: High prevalence of papillomavirus-associated penile intraepithelial neoplasia in sexual partners of women with cervical intraepithelial neoplasia. N Engl J Med 1987;317:916–923.
5. Zanardi C, Guerra B, Martinelli G, et al: Papillomavirus-related genital lesions in male partners of women with genital condyloma or cervical intraepithelial neoplasia: Diagnostic approach. Cervix 1988;6:127–134.
6. Munoz N, Bosch X, Kaldor JM: Does human papillomavirus cause cervical cancer? The state of the epidemiological evidence. Br J Cancer 1988;57:1–5.
7. Howley PH: On human papillomaviruses, editorial. N Engl J Med 1986;315:1089–1090.
8. Zur Hausen H: Papillomaviruses in human cancer. Cancer 1987;59:1692–1696.
9. Grussendorf-Conen EI, de Villiers EM, Gissmann L: Human papillomavirus genomes in penile smears of healthy men, letter to the editor. Lancet 1986;ii:1092.
10. von Krogh G, Syrjanen SM, Syrjanen KJ: Advantage of human papillomavirus typing in the clinical evaluation of genitoanal warts. J Am Acad Dermatol 1988;18:495–503.
11. Campion MJ, McCance DJ, Mitchell HS, et al: Subclinical penile human papillomavirus infections and dysplasia in consorts of women with cervical neoplasia. Br J Gen Urin Med, in press.
12. Narayana AS, Olney LE, Loening SA, et al: Carcinoma of the penis. Analysis of 219 cases. Cancer 1982;49:2185–2191.
13. WHO Meeting: Control of cancer of the cervix uteri. Bull WHO 1986;64:607–18.
14. Zunzunegui MV, King MC, Conia CF, et al: Male influence on cervical cancer risk. Am J Epidemiol 1986;123:302–304.
15. Krebs HB, Schneider V: Human papillomavirus-associated lesions of the penis: Colposcopy, cytology and histology. Obstet Gynecol 1987;70:299–304.

16. Boon ME, Schneider A, Hogewoning CJA, et al: Penile studies and heterosexual partners. Peniscopy, cytology, histology and immunocytochemistry. Cancer 1988;61: 1652–1659.

17. Levine R, Crum C, Herman E, et al: Cervical papillomavirus infection and intraepithelial neoplasia: A study of male sexual partners. Obstet Gynecol 1984;64:16–20.

18. Sand P, Bowen L, Blischke S, et al: Evaluation of male consorts of women with genital human papillomavirus infection. Obstet Gynecol 1986;68:679–681.

19. Sedlacek T, Cunnane M, Carpiniello V: Colposcopy in the diagnosis of penile condyloma. Am J Obstet Gynecol 1986;154:494–496.

20. Schneider A, Sawada E, Gissmann L, et al: Human papillomaviruses in women with a history of abnormal Papanicolaou smears and in their male partners. Obstet Gynecol 1987;69:554–562.

21. Campion MJ, McCance DJ, Jenkins J, et al: Subclinical penile human papillomavirus infection: The clue to the high risk male. Colp Gyn Laser Surg 1987;3:11–22.

22. Ferenczy A: Evaluation and management of male partners of condyloma patients. Colp Gyn Laser Surg 1986;2:15–24.

23. Bistoletti P, Lidbrink P: Sexually transmitted diseases including genital papillomavirus infection in male sexual partners of women treated for cervical intraepithelial neoplasia III by conization. Br J Obstet Gynecol 1988;95:611–613.

24. Rosenberg SK, Reid R: Sexually transmitted papillomaviral infections in the male: I. Anatomic distribution and clinical features. Urol 1987;29:488–492.

25. Rosenberg SK, Greenberg MD, Reid P: Sexually transmitted papillomaviral infection in men. Obstet Gynecol Clin North Am 1987;14:495–512.

26. Comité SL, Castadot MJ: Colposcopic evaluation of men with genital warts. J Am Acad Dermatol 1988;18:1274–1278.

27. Daling JR, Weiss NS, Hislop TG, et al: Sexual practices, sexually transmitted diseases and the incidence of anal cancer. N Engl J Med 1987;317:973–977.

28. Murphy WM, Fu YS, Lancaster WD, et al: Papillomavirus structural antigens in condyloma acuminatum of the male urethra. J Urol 1983;130:84–85.

29. Wade TR, Kopf AW, Ackerman AB: Bowenoid papulosis of the genitalia. Arch Dermatol 1979;115:306–308.

30. Gross G, Ikenberg H, DeVilliers EM, et al: Bowenoid papulosis: A venerally transmissible disease as reservoir for HPV 16, In Peto R, zur Hausen H (eds): Viral Etiology of Cervical Cancer. Banbury Report 27. Cold Spring Habor, NY, Cold Spring Harbor Laboratory, 1986:149–165.

31. Obalek S, Jablonska S, Beaudenow S, et al: Bowenoid papulosis of the male and female genitalia: Risk of cervical neoplasia. J Am Acad Dermatol 1986;14:433–444.

32. Somogyi L, Malpica CC: Carbon dioxide laser treatment of male external genitalia with human papillomavirus (HPV) infection. Colp Gyn Laser Surg 1986;2:209–216.

33. Ackerman AB, Kornberg R: Pearly penile papules. Acral angiofibromas. Arch Dermatol 1973;108:673–675.

34. Schneider A, Kirchmayr R, De Villiers E-M, et al. Subclinical human papillomavirus infections in male sexual partners of female carriers. J Urol (in press).

35. von Krough G: 5-fluorouracil cream in the successful treatment of therapeutically refractory condylomata acuminata of the urinary meatus. Acta Derm-Venereol (Stockh) 1976;56:297–301.

36. Abcarian H, Smith D, Sharon N: The immunotherapy of anal condyloma acuminatum. Dis Col Rect 1976;19:237–244.

37. Gosh AK: Cryosurgery of genital warts in cases in which podophyllin treatment failed or was contraindicated. Br J Vener Dis 1977;53:49–53.

38. Thompson JPS, Grace RH: The treatment of perianal and anal condylomata acuminata. J R Soc Med 1978;71:180–185.

39. Fuselier HA Jr, McBurney EI, Brannan W, et al: Treatment of condylomata acuminata with carbon dioxide laser. Urol 1980;15:265–266.

40. Ferenczy A: Laser therapy of genital condylomata acuminata. Obstet Gynecol 1984;63:703–707.

41. Eron LJ, Judson F, Tucker S, et al: Interferon therapy for condylomata acuminata. N Engl J Med 1986;315:1059–1064.

42. Gross G, Roussaki A, Brzoska J: Low doses of systemically administered recombinant interferon-gamma effective in the treatment of genital warts, abstracted. J Invest Dermatol 1988;90:242.

43. Schneider A, Papendick U, Gissmann L, et al: Interferon treatment of human genital papillomavirus infection: Importance of viral type. Int J Cancer 1987;40:610–614.

44. Beutner KR: Podophyllotoxin in the treatment of genital human papillomavirus infection: A review. Sem Dermatol 1987;6:10–18.

45. Ferenczy A: Laser treatment of patients with condylomata and squamous carcinoma precursors of the lower female genital tract. Ca 1987;37:334–347.

46. von Krogh G: Podophyllotoxin for condylomata acuminata eradication. Acta Dermat Venerol 1981;98 (suppl):1.

47. Debenedictis TJ, Marmar JL, Praiss DE: Intraurethral condylomas acuminata: management and review of the literature. J Urol 1977;118:767–769.

48. Ott F, Eichenberger-DeBeer H, Storck H: The local treatment of precancerous skin conditions with 5-fluorouracil ointment. Dermatol 1970;140:109.

49. Ferenczy A, Mitao M, Nagai N, et al: Latent papillomavirus and recurring genital warts. N Engl J Med 1985;313:784–788.

50. Macnab JCM, Walkinshaw SA, Cordiner JW, et al: Human papillomavirus in clinically and histologically normal tissue of patients with genital cancer. N Engl J Med 1986;315:1052–1058.

51. Steinberg BM, Topp WC, Schneider PS, et al: Laryngeal papillomavirus infection during clinical remission. N Engl J Med 1983;308:1261–1264.

52. Van de Perre P, Jacobs D, Sprecher-Goldberger S: The latex condom, an efficient barrier against sexual transmission of AIDS-related viruses. AIDS 1987;1:49–52.

53. Steben M. Condoms: what you should know. Contemp Obstet Gynecol 1988;57–68.

54. White N, Taylor K, Lyszkowski A, et al: Dangers of lubricants used with condoms, correspondence. Nature 1988;335:19.

CHAPTER 14

Interferon Therapy of Genital Human Papillomavirus Infection

Stephen K. Tyring, MD, PhD

Condyloma acuminatum (CA), also known as venereal or genital warts, is not only a very widespread, sexually transmitted disease but also a benign tumor of known viral etiology with a potential for malignant transformation. Over 60 types of human papillomaviruses (HPV) have been described; at least 23 of these types are associated with anogenital lesions. The incidence of CA is increasing rapidly and is at least the third-most-common sexually transmitted disease in the United States (after nongonococcal urethritis and gonorrhea). Some authorities, however, believe that CA is actually the most prevalent sexually transmitted disease but is underreported greatly. The relatively recent awareness of the association between CA and cervical carcinoma, as well as a number of other anogenital malignancies,[1] has stimulated much interest in the treatment of HPV infections.

In the past, treatment of CA was limited to surgical excision of the infected tissue or to cytodestructive and/or antimitotic preparations, such as podophyllin, cryotherapy, bichloracetic acid, trichloracetic acid, or 5-fluorouracil (5-FU). Recently, however, several reports in the literature have documented the efficacy of various interferon preparations for the treatment of CA. Interferons, as opposed to other treatment modalities, can not only rid the patient of CA lesions but also have the unique potential to eradicate the responsible virus.[2] This property of interferons is a result of their antiviral, antiproliferative, and immunomodulatory activities.[3]

CLINICAL TRIALS WITH INTERFERONS

Most investigations of interferon for the treatment of CA have concerned interferon alpha (IFNα). The first reports of any interferon being employed in the therapy of CA was in 1975 with topical preparations of relatively impure natural IFNα known as leukocyte interferon.[4–6] Encouraging results

Clinical Practice of Gynecology: **2,** 233–244, 1989
© 1989 Elsevier Science Publishing Co., Inc.
655 Avenue of the Americas, New York, NY 10010

ISSN 1043-3198/89/$3.50

were obtained with vulvar and vaginal warts treated five times per day with an ointment containing 4000 U IFNα/g.

Topical treatment was also employed by Vesterinen et al[7] in 1984 for flat vaginal condylomas with mild to moderate dysplasia. A cream containing 2×10^6 IU/g of partly purified human leukocyte IFN (IFNα) was applied intravaginally for four 2-week-treatment courses 1 week apart. Of eight patients treated with IFN, five had colposcopic remissions; two of these responding patients relapsed 2 months after completion of the study. Cytologic evidence of HPV infection remained in all the patients. No remissions were observed in five additional patients treated with a placebo cream. No overt side effects were reported in any patient.

Intralesional treatment of CA with fibroblast interferon (IFNβ) was first reported by Scott and Csonka.[8] Minimal clinical results were obtained with single injections of penile warts with only 300 U IFNβ. Intramuscular therapy of CA with IFNβ was demonstrated to be effective by Schonfeld et al.[9] Nine of 11 patients with previously untreated CA had disappearance of lesions within 6 weeks after completion of therapy with IFNβ at 2×10^6 U for 10 consecutive days. This result was in contrast to only two placebo-treated patients who experienced a complete remission of their lesions. After 3 months, eight of the nonrespondents were treated with the same regime of IFNβ, and all achieved a complete response.

The intramuscular route of administration of natural IFNα was also used by Einhorn et al[10] to produce complete regression of CA in one reported patient. A highly purified preparation of natural IFNα, human lymphoblastoid interferon (Wellferon) was evaluated by Gall et al[11] against CA. Patients with resistant and persistent CA were treated daily from 14 to 28 days with intramuscular injections of IFNα, followed by 2–4 weeks of injections with the same dose three times per week. Nonresponders were then given intralesional injections twice weekly for 4 weeks. Although all patients initially treated with 5×10^6 U/m^2 had to have the dosage reduced because of side effects, 69% of these persons had a complete response to therapy. Five of 37 patients treated with 3×10^6 U/m^2 also required a reduction in dosage, but 57% experienced a complete response. The complete response rate was 43% in patients who received 1×10^6 U/m^2; none of these persons required a dosage reduction. Additional therapy with excision or cryotherapy of persons who experienced $\geq 50\%$ decrease in lesion areas (but no complete response) with IFNα increased the complete cure rate to greater than 90%. The influence of HPV type on the response to IFNα was not clear, since pretreatment biopsy specimens were only examined with probes to HPV 6.[12] Subtypes of HPV 6 were identified in specimens from 13 of 17 patients examined.

Most recently, the results of a randomized double-blind, placebo-controlled, multicenter trial demonstrated the efficacy of intralesional treatment of CA with highly purified natural IFNα (Alferon).[13] Eighty-six patients were treated with IFNα, and 72 patients received a placebo. Eighty-six percent and 89%, respectively, of these patients had received previous therapy for CA. All lesions present at the initiation of therapy were injected twice weekly for 8 weeks or until all treated warts disappeared. The median initial IFNα dose was 1.2×10^6 IU, while the median total dose was 14.3 $\times 10^6$ IU. At the end of the 8 weeks, 29% of the IFNα-treated patients had experienced a complete response; 3 months following completion of therapy, however, a total of 62% of the IFNα-treated patients were free of lesions. In contrast, in the placebo treatment group, a complete response was seen in only 9% at the conclusion of therapy and in 21% 3 months later. Complete responders in both groups were followed for relapses for up to 1.5 years. Twenty-seven of 36 IFNα-treated patients evaluated, and 10 of 13 placebo-treated subjects, were still free of lesions. The mean time until relapse was 4 months for IFNα-treated persons and 2 months for the placebo group. Determination of HPV types was not reported in this study.

Results of intralesional therapy with recombinant alpha-2 IFN (Intron A) in the treatment of CA was reported by Vance et al[14] from a multicenter double-blind study in which a single wart on each patient was injected with 10^6 IU of IFNα, 10^5 IU of IFNα, or placebo three times weekly for 3 weeks. During those 3 weeks of treatment, no significant differences between these three groups were observed. Two weeks following completion of therapy, a significant difference was first seen between the high-dose IFNα group and the placebo group. At the ninth week following conclusion of therapy, patients having received 10^6 IU of IFNα had significantly more complete responses than did members of either other group. In this high-dose group, complete regression of the treated lesion was observed in 16 (53%) of 30 patients in contrast to only six (19%) of 32 patients who received 10^5 IU of IFNα per injection ($P < .01$) and in contrast to four (14%) of 29 persons treated with placebo ($P < .01$). No significant differences in the response of uninjected warts, however, were seen between the three groups. Determination of HPV types was not done.

A larger, placebo-controlled, multicenter, randomized, double-blind trial of interferon alpha-2b (Intron A) for the treatment of CA was reported subsequently by Eron et al.[15] Up to three warts per patient were each injected with placebo or 10^6 IU of IFNα three times weekly for 3 weeks. A significant difference was first observed between the two groups at the completion of the 3 weeks of therapy. Maximal differences in clinical response were seen 1 week later. Patients who received IFNα experienced a 62.4% mean decrease in wart area in contrast to a 1.2% increase in wart area in subjects treated with placebo ($P < .001$). Lesions continued to clear throughout the 16-week study period in both groups. At the end of this time, all treated warts had completely regressed in 36% of the IFNα-treated patients and in 17% of the placebo-treated subjects ($P < .001$). The rates of clearing of untreated warts were the same in the IFNα-treated patients

(17%) as in the placebo group (18%). Although perianal CA tended to respond less well than did penile or vulvar lesions, the differences were not significant. The response to IFNα appeared to be independent of the sex of the patients, the number of warts treated, or history of previous therapy. None of nine patients who were antibody positive for the human immunodeficiency virus (HIV) experienced a complete response to IFNα therapy.[15,16] The response to IFNα was inversely related to the pretreatment size of the warts and to the age of the wart. The former point was in contrast to the finding of Geffen et al.[17] Since there was very little effect of placebo treatment of warts present for more than 24 months, it was concluded that IFNα therapy may be particularly indicated for these lesions.

To determine if differences exist in the efficacy and toxicity of intralesionally administered IFNs, Reichman et al[18] evaluated three IFN preparations in 76 patients with biopsy-proven CA. All patients had persistent or recurrent lesions despite previous conventional therapy. One wart per patient was injected three times per week for 4 weeks with either 10^6 IU of recombinant alpha-2b interferon (Intron A), natural lymphoblastoid IFNα (Wellferon), IFNβ, or with placebo. Complete regression of CA was observed at 16 weeks after initiation of therapy in 47% of IFN-treated patients in contrast to 22% of placebo recipients ($P = .009$). No differences in the rates of response or in the development of side effects were noted among the three IFN treatments. Although the rate of complete response of uninjected warts was greater in IFN recipients than in placebo-treated patients, the difference was not significant. Complete resolution of all monitored warts was noted in 42% of patients whose injected wart completely resolved. Factors that were independent of the clinical response included the following: the location of the CA, the sex or sexual preference of the patients, the size and age of the lesions, and the history of persistence or recurrence. Neither HPV typing nor the HIV antibody status of the patients was reported. After initial resolution of the injected wart, 9/27 (33%) of IFN-treated lesions recurred in contrast to 0/4 (0%) of placebo-treated warts. The mean time to recurrence was 46 days following initial resolution. Only one patient among 16 persons who experienced complete resolution of all lesions had a recurrence.

Evidence for the efficacy of recombinant gamma interferon (IFN-γ) in the treatment of refractory, biopsy-proven CA has been obtained in three phase II studies at the University of Washington, Seattle.[19] In the first study, 11 patients were treated with up to two 10-day cycles of daily intramuscular IFN-γ at doses of 2×10^5, 1×10^6, and 2×10^6 U/m²/day. An 8-week observation period followed the first 10-day cycle. Five patients experienced partial responses following the first 10-day cycle, with an additional three following the second cycle, for an overall response rate of 8/11. In the second study, 17 patients were treated either three times weekly for 6 weeks (at 2×10^5 or 1×10^6 U/m²/day) or once per week for 10 weeks (at 1×10^6 U/m^2/day). Ten of the 17 patients experienced at least partial responses. In the third study, six patients were treated with IFN-γ (1×10^6 U/m^2) administered subcutaneously on a three times per week schedule for 6 weeks. Two patients experienced responses, including one complete and one partial response. Thus, the overall response rate for these studies was 20/34 (59%).

ADVERSE SIDE EFFECTS OF INTERFERON THERAPY FOR GENITAL HPV INFECTION

Almost all patients treated intralesionally or systemically with doses of IFNs high enough to be effective report some adverse side effects. In patients treated intralesionally, a common complaint is the pain of injection, although this is rarely significant and is well tolerated by most patients, especially when a 27–30-gauge needle is used and a small volume (ie, 0.1 cc) is injected. Adverse reactions are reported by the majority of patients who receive IFN at $\pm 10^6$ per injection. The most common of these side effects are fever and a flulike syndrome. The fever is usually mild and lasts only a few hours. Tolerance to the fever often develops after the second or third injection of a three-times-per-week schedule of injections. Somewhat less common adverse reactions include myalgias, chills, headache, malaise, gastrointestinal discomfort (uncommonly including nausea and vomiting), somnolence, and emotional lability (rarely). These adverse reactions are observed in patients given placebo, but at a much lower incidence. It is rare for any of these IFN-related adverse effects to be so severe for a patient to withdraw from a study. This is true especially for patients who have previously failed traditional modes of therapy. Laboratory changes that are associated occasionally with IFN treatment include leukopenia and thrombocytopenia. These changes are rarely of clinical significance and are reversible after completion of therapy.

SERUM NEUTRALIZING FACTORS IN IFN-TREATED PATIENTS

In the few studies in which the presence of neutralizing antibodies to IFN have been reported, their incidence has been very low and of questionable clinical significance. Friedman-Kien et al[13] reported that no such antibodies could be detected in the serum of 48 patients tested after being treated with natural IFNα. Only two of 147 recombinant alfa-2b IFN (Intron A) patients reported by Eron et al[15] developed interferon-neutralizing factors in the serum. One of these patients responded to treatment, while the other person did not. Spiegel et al[20] reported the incidence of serum-neutralizing factors in patients having received recombinant alfa-2b (Intron A) for either CA, cancer, or a number of other conditions to be very low. Only 2.4% of

537 patients who received systemic IFNα therapy, and <1% of 1326 subjects who received intranasal IFNα or of 154 persons who received intralesional IFNα administration, developed these antibodies. Clinical responses were observed in two of ten patients with cancer in whom neutralizing factors were detected. None of the patients with serum-neutralizing factors experienced any side effects attributable to immune-complex phenomenon.

FACTORS AFFECTING THE EFFICACY OF INTERFERONS

The studies presented in this chapter indicate that IFNα or IFNβ can be expected to produce a complete eradication of CA lesions in approximately 50–60% of patients especially when they are used intralesionally, in dosages $\geq 10^6$ IU/injection and when treatment is given at least three times per week for 3–4 weeks (Table 14–1). Furthermore, the side effects of systemic or intralesional IFN administration, most commonly fever and a flulike syndrome (Table 14–2), are well tolerated by almost all patients. In addition, tolerance to these adverse reactions develop in most persons by the end of the first week of treatment. It must be noted that in most reported investigations, the odds may have been stacked against IFN by the fact that most patients had previously failed traditional modes of therapy for CA. Treatment of these resistant lesions, however, is precisely where IFN therapy has the most potential value. Recurrences of CA after traditional modes of therapy have eradicated the original lesions have been linked closely to the existence of latent HPV in "clinically normal" skin adjacent to the lesion.[21] Evaluation of the efficacy of IFN treatment, however, is complicated by at least two factors: the difficulty in differentiating recurrences from reinfections and the finding that approximately 20% of CA lesions will completely regress with injections of placebo. This later finding is probably a combination of the known spontaneous regression of these lesions plus inflammation resulting from the trauma of injection.

Many questions remain concerning IFN treatment of CA. Key among these issues is the question of how patients whose lesions respond completely to IFN differ from patients whose warts respond incompletely or not at all. One factor that has previously been mentioned is the presence of antibodies to HIV, which is associated with a poor response to recombinant alfa-2b interferon.[16] Very few clinical investigations of IFN treatment of CA have reported the HPV type present in the lesions. The findings of Schneider et al,[22] however, indicate that this may be an important parameter in determining the efficacy of IFN. They found that women with HPV 16 or HPV 18 had a poorer response rate to IFN than did those who were infected with HPV 6 or HPV 11. Interestingly, it is the former HPV types that are much more closely associated with dysplasia and neoplasia.[1]

Although the precise immune deficit in otherwise healthy persons who

TABLE 14–1. Summary of Large, Controlled Clinical Studies of Intralesional and Systemic Interferon in the Treatment of Condyloma Acuminatum

Study	Interferon Preparation	Dose	Route/Schedule	Complete Patient Responses (%) with IFN	Complete Patient Responses With Placebo (%)
Schonfeld et al (1984)	IFNβ	2×10^6 U	i.m. daily $\times$ 10 days	9/11 (82)	2/11 (18)
Gall et al (1985)	IFNα nl*	5×10^6 U	i.m. daily $\times$ 4–28 days followed	11/16 (69)	ND**
Gall et al (1985)	IFNα nl*	3×10^6 U	by 3$\times$ weekly 2–4 wk	17/30 (57)	
Gall et al (1985)	IFNα nl*	1×10^6 U		6/14 (43)	
Friedman-Kien et al (1988)	IFNα nl	1.2×10^6 U	Intralesional, 2$\times$ weekly $\times$ 8 wk	41/66 (62)	14/66 (21)
Vance et al (1986)	IFNα r***	1×10^6 U	Intralesional, 3$\times$ weekly $\times$ 3 wk	16/30 (53)	4/29 (14)
		1×10^5 U		6/32 (19)	
Eron et al (1986)	IFNα r	1×10^6 U	Intralesional, 3$\times$ weekly $\times$ 3 wk	42/116 (36)	20/116 (17)
Reichman et al (1988)	IFNα nl	1×10^6 U	Intralesional, 3$\times$ weekly $\times$ 4 wk	7/15 (45)	4/18 (22)
	IFNα r	1×10^6 U		11/23 (48)	
	IFNβ	1×10^6 U		10/20 (50)	

*nl, natural.
**ND, not done.
***r, recombinant.

TABLE 14–2. Adverse Reactions to Alpha Interferon Therapy

Clinical	Study (% of Patients Reporting any Degree of These Reactions)	
	Summation: Vance et al (1986); Eron et al (1986) IFNα r*	Friedman-Kien et al (1988) IFNα nl**
Fever or chills	56	46
Fatigue	18	3
Headache	47	35
Myalgias	44	5
Local reactions	28	8
Impaired concentration	1	NR***
Gastrointestinal discomfort (ie, nausea, etc)	17	9
Significant pain at injection site	1	5
Laboratory		
Leukopenia ($<3000/mm^3$)	2	0
Thrombocytopenia ($<74,000$ but $>50,000/mm^3$)	1	NR***

*Recombinant interferon alfa-2b (Intron A).
**Natural leukocyte interferon alfa (Alferon N).
***NR, not reported.

have recurrent and/or treatment-resistant CA is not known, patients who have general immunosuppression from systemic disease or from medication often are plagued by highly aggressive CA and other HPV-associated lesions. Such patients have generally been excluded from large studies of IFN treatment of CA. Therefore, the potential usefulness of IFNs in these patients remains unknown. Conflicting reports of the immune status of otherwise healthy CA patients have appeared in the literature. Gall et al[23] reported that T cell helper/suppressor ratios and mitogenic stimulation of lymphocytes from CA patients were normal. In contrast, Carson et al[24] reported that patients with the genital neoplasia-papilloma syndrome had reduced T cell helper/suppressor ratios and diminished blastogenic responses to mitogens. They defined this syndrome as the occurrence of HPV-associated lesions in multiple organ sites, in which at least one lesion is an intraepithelial or invasive neoplasm of squamous epithelium. Cauda et al[25] observed that lymphocytes from otherwise healthy CA patients exhibited decreased interleukin-2 and IFNγ production, depressed natural killer cell activity, and a reduced T cell helper/suppressor ratio (associated with a marked increase in suppressor T cells). These apparent differences in immune status may be secondary to such factors as differences in HPV types responsible for the lesions, different immunologic techniques employed, possible concomitant subclinical infections, or to associated drug use (including ethanol and tobacco). Whatever the factor(s) responsible, it remains an enigma that some patients can have massive numbers of recurrent and/or treatment-resistent CA lesions and still be otherwise clinically healthy.

THE FUTURE OF INTERFERONS IN THE TREATMENT OF CONDYLOMA ACUMINATUM

Although several IFN preparations, dosages, routes of administration, and schedules have been evaluated for the treatment of CA, much remains to be determined concerning the role of IFNs in the therapy of HPV infections. At this time, IFNs would appear to be indicated for the treatment of CA resistant to more traditional modes of therapy. The time, expense and discomfort of multiple injections of each CA lesion would probably preclude use of injectable IFN as first-line therapy. A topical preparation of IFN that could be self-administered would be far preferable, but the initial enthusiasm for the efficacy of IFN cream[5] has so far not been supported by subsequent studies. Since the complete response rate to injectable IFN appears to be 50–60%, and since the complete response is not usually seen until after the third or fourth week of IFN therapy, it might be useful to predict future responders in order to select appropriate therapy. One parameter that appears useful is activation of natural killer (NK) cell activity.[26] Although no pretreatment differences in NK activity existed, persons who eventually responded to intralesional IFNα-2b (Intron A) for CA were found to have a significantly greater boosting of NK activity than did nonresponders. This difference in NK activity between responders and nonresponders was maintained following completion of therapy.

Further studies are needed to determine more thoroughly optimal parameters for the use of IFNs in the therapy of HPV-associated lesions in order that an efficacious therapy of minimal cost and discomfort to the patient may be found. While recombinant IFNα, natural IFNα, or natural IFNβ given by the same route, schedule, and dosage appear equivalent[18] for the treatment of CA, comparisons with the efficacy of IFNγ have not yet been reported. Although IFNγ is known to act synergistically with IFNα or with IFNβ in antiviral activities, cytostasis and cytolysis, and in immunomodulatory actions,[3] no reports of IFNγ combined with IFNα or IFNβ for the therapy of CA have yet been published.

In June 1988, the Schering Corporation received approval from the Food and Drug Administration (FDA) for the use of Intron A (IFNα) in the treatment of CA. They recommend that Intron A be injected into each lesion three times per week on alternate days, for 3 weeks. This drug has approval for use in as many as five lesions per treatment. Therefore, the highest recommended dosage is 5×10^6 U per patient per treatment, although higher dosages have been employed safely in the treatment of various malignancies. If a complete response is not observed by 2–3 months following completion of initial therapy, the same schedule and dosage of Intron A may be repeated. No well-controlled studies of the safety and effectiveness of Intron A for the treatment of patients under 18 years of age, of pregnant women, or of nursing mothers have been reported. Therefore, this drug should be used in these patients only if the potential benefits clearly outweigh the potential risks.

Because of the probability of such adverse experiences as fever and other "flulike" symptoms, particular caution should be employed if Intron A is to be used in patients with such debilitating medical conditions as severe cardiovascular or pulmonary diseases, ketoacidosis-prone diabetes mellitus, coagulation disorders, or severe myelosuppression. While the monitoring of such laboratory parameters as a complete blood count and serum liver enzymes (especially SGOT) may be considered in otherwise healthy patients with HPV infections treated with Intron A, such monitoring is indicated clearly in patients with major medical problems.

While IFNα has received Food and Drug Administration (FDA) approval for intralesional therapy of as many as five HPV-associated lesions per treatment, questions still remain as to the role of IFN(s) in the treatment of patients with numerous lesions, of patients with very large lesions, and of patients who fail to completely clear even after a second course of IFN therapy. In such cases, more IFN is not necessarily better. More adverse side effects will be experienced by the patient receiving greater than 5×10^6 U of IFN, but greater clinical benefit may not be observed. This is true especially for patients with individual CA lesions greater than 1 cm^3 in size. We have observed in such patients, however, that IFNα has as much potential as adjunct therapy. When patients having multiple (ie, >5) HPV-associated lesions, such as CA or intraepithelial neoplasia, are treated with such cytodestructive and/or antimitotic agents as bichloracetic acid, trichloracetic acid, 5-FU, podophyllin, or cryotherapy, concomitant IFN therapy produces rates of complete regression of these lesions that are semiadditive to additive.[27] Specifically, one of these topical agents can be applied to all lesions weekly for at least 3 weeks while IFN is administered three times per week intralesionally or even subcutaneously in the center of a cluster of lesions. In such patients, doses of IFN should be at least 5×10^6 U per treatment, but higher dosages may be considered if constitutional symptoms and laboratory parameters are not prohibitive.

An especially difficult problem is seen in patients with large (ie, ≥ 1 cm^3) CA lesions. Surgical (including laser) excision of such lesions results in an unacceptably high recurrence rate. We have found that injection of IFNα at 5×10^6 U intralesionally into a single large lesion, three times per week for 3 weeks, results in a low rate of complete remission.[27] If residual CA lesions are excised subsequent to this regimen of IFN therapy, the recurrence rate is lower than that observed following excision without IFNα but is still unacceptably high. We have found that optimal therapeutic results with such multiple, large HPV-associated lesions can be achieved by first reducing the viral and tumor load by excision of all visible lesions. IFNα therapy can then successfully eliminate latent HPV responsible for recurrences observed following surgery alone. Immediately following excision of these lesions, a 3–6-week course of IFNα therapy can be initiated three times per week with 5×10^6 U given subcutaneously in the region of the former lesions. In the case of widespread lesions, the injection site should be alternated between involved quadrants of the genitalia. This treatment regimen of surgical excision followed by local subcutaneous IFN therapy can result in a synergistic reduction in recurrence rates.[27]

Clearly, interferons are important agents in the treatment of HPV-associated lesions,[28,29] but further clinical trials are indicated. These studies should examine further the efficacy and toxicities of combinations of IFNα and IFNγ, of IFN(s) combined with traditional cytodestructive and/or antimitotic therapies, of IFN(s) combined with retinoids, and possibly of IFN(s) combined with other biologic response modifiers. Such investigations should explore various dosages, routes, and schedules, and they should include determinations of HPV type as well as evaluations of the immune status of the patient.

REFERENCES

1. Gissman L, Boshart M, Durst M, et al: Presence of human papillomavirus in genital tumors. J Invest Dermatol 1984;83:26s–28s.
2. Turek LP, Byrne JC, Lowy DR, et al: Interferon induces morphologic reversion with elimination of extrachromosomal viral genomes in bovine papillomavirus-transformed mouse cells. Proc Natl Acad Sci USA 1982;79:7914–7918.
3. Tyring SK: Antitumor actions of interferons: Direct, indirect, and synergy with other treatment modalities. Int J Dermatol 1987;26:549–556.
4. Ikic D, Bosnic N, Smerdels, et al: Double blind clinical study with human leukocyte interferon in the therapy of condylomata acuminata. Proc Symposium Clin Use Interferon. Zagreb: Yugoslav Acad Sci Arts, 1975.
5. Ikic D, Brnobic A, Jurkovic-Vukelic V, et al.: Therapeutical effect of human leukocyte interferon incorporated into ointment and cream on condylomata acuminata. Proc Symposium Clin Use Interferon. Zagreb: Yugoslav Acad Sci Arts, 1975.
6. Ikic D, Orescanin M, Krusic J, et al: Preliminary study of the effect of human leukocyte interferon on condyloma acuminata in women. Proc Symposium Clin Use Interferon. Zagreb: Yugoslav Acad Sci Arts, 1975.
7. Vesterinen JE, Meyer B, Purola E, et al: Treatment of vaginal flat condyloma with interferon cream. Lancet 1984; i:157.
8. Scott GM, Csonka GW: Effect of injections of small doses of human fibroblast interferon into genital warts. A pilot study. Br J Vener Dis 1979;55:442–445.
9. Schonfeld A, Schattner A, Crespi M, et al: Intramuscular human interferon-β injections in the treatment of condyloma acuminata. Lancet 1984; i:1038–1042.
10. Einhorn N, King P, Strander H: Systemic interferon alpha treatment of human condylomata acuminata. Acta Obstet Gynecol Scand 1983;62:285–287.
11. Gall SA, Hughes CE, Trofatter K: Interferon for the therapy of condyloma acuminatum. Am J Obstet Gynecol 1985;153:157–163.
12. Gall SA, Hughes CE, Mounts P, et al: Efficacy of human lymphoblastoid interferon in the therapy of resistant condyloma acuminata. Obstet Gynecol 1986;67:643–651.

13. Friedman-Kien AE, Eron LJ, Conant M, et al: Natural interferon alfa for treatment of condyloma acuminata. JAMA 1988;259:533–538.
14. Vance JC, Bart BJ, Hansen RC, et al: Intralesional recombinant alpha-2 interferon for the treatment of patients with condyloma acuminatum or verruca plantaris. Arch Dermatol 1986;122:272–277.
15. Eron LJ, Judson F, Tucker S, et al: Interferon therapy for condylomata acuminata. N Engl J Med 1986;315:1059–1064.
16. Douglas JM, Rogers M, Judson FN: The effect of asymptomatic infection with HTLV-III on the response of anogenital warts to intralesional treatment with recombinant α_2 interferon. J Infect Dis 1986;154:331–334.
17. Geffen JR, Klein RJ, Friedman-Kien AE: Intralesional administration of large doses of human leukocyte interferon for the treatment of condylomata acuminata. J Infect Dis 1984;150:612–615.
18. Reichman RC, Oakes D, Bonnez W, et al: Treatment of condyloma acuminatum with three different interferons administered intralesionally: A double-blind, placebo-controlled trial. Ann Intern Med 1988;108:675–679.
19. Kirby P, Wells D, Kiviat N, et al: A phase 1 trial of intramuscular recombinant human gamma interferon for refractory genital warts. J Invest Dermatol 1986;86:485a.
20. Spiegel RJ, Spicehandler JR, Jacobs SL, et al: Low incidence of serum neutralizing factors in patients receiving recombinant alfa-2b interferon (Intron A). Am J Med 1986;80:223–228.
21. Ferenczy A, Mitao M, Nagai N, et al: Latent papillomavirus and recurring genital warts. N Engl J Med 1985;313:784–788.
22. Schneider A, Papendick U, Gissmann L, et al: Interferon treatment of human genital papillomavirus infection: Importance of viral type. Int J Cancer 1987;40:610–614.
23. Gall SA, Hughes CE, Trofatter K, et al: Lymphoblastoid interferon for the therapy of condylomata acuminata: An inter-study comparison of two dose regimens. In: Howley PM, Broker TR, eds. Papillomaviruses: Molecular and Clinical Aspects. New York: Alan R Liss, Inc, 1985;201–215.
24. Carson LF, Twiggs, LB, Fukushima M, et al: Human genital papilloma infections: An evaluation of immunologic competence in the genital neoplasia-papilloma syndrome. Am J Obstet Gynecol 1986;155:784–789.
25. Cauda R, Tyring SK, Grossi CE, et al: Patients with condyloma acuminatum exhibit decreased interleukin-2 and interferon gamma production and depressed natural killer activity. J Clin Immunol 1987;7:304–311.
26. Tyring SK, Canda R, Ghanta V, et al: Activation of natural killer cell function during interferon-α treatment of patients with condyloma acuminatum is predictive of clinical response. J Biol Regul Homeost Agents 1988;2:29–32.
27. Tyring SK, Whitley R, Hatch K, et al: Treatment of large condyloma acuminatum with alpha-2 interferon. Presented at the 17th World Congress of Dermatology, Berlin, West Germany, May 1987.
28. Tyring SK, Cauda R, Baron S, et al: Condyloma acuminatum: Epidemiological, clinical and therapeutic aspects. Eur J Epidemiol 1987;3:209–215.
29. Weck PK, Brandsma JL, Whisnant JK: Interferons in the treatment of human papillomavirus diseases. Cancer Metastasis Rev 1986;5:139–165.

CHAPTER 15

Chemotherapeutic Management of Human Papillomavirus Infections

Linda Van Le, MD and Jeffrey L. Stern, MD

Human papillomavirus (HPV) infection of the lower genital tract has reached epidemic proportions in the United States. A sixfold increase in the incidence of HPV has been observed, and the Centers for Disease Control (CDC) estimate that over a million new cases occur each year.[1] To answer demands for treatment, health care providers must have access to a variety of treatment regimens that will allow them to tailor their therapy to histologic type and lower genital tract infection site. Several therapeutic modalities are presently available for the treatment of lower genital tract infections, such as topical chemotherapy, local excisional or destructive procedures, and immunotherapy. These are associated with variable success rates, costs, and morbidity. Topical chemotherapy is an attractive choice because of its low cost and ease of use. Podophyllin, halogenated acetic acids, 5% 5-fluorouracil (5-FU), and retinoids are topical agents presently available for treatment. Various regimens for treatment of lower genital tract HPV infections in women and men are discussed.

CHEMOTHERAPEUTIC AGENTS

Podophyllin

Podophyllin is a cytotoxic keratolytic resin that has been widely used in the treatment of condylomata acuminata for the past 40 years.[2] Its active component is podophyllotoxin; however, it is the resin that is usually available in a 25% concentration in tincture of benzoin. Its action is thought to be twofold: inhibition of cellular mitotic activity and destruction of keratinized epithelial cells. Application of podophyllin has not been without side effects, and there are numerous cases documenting its toxicity.[3–5] Toxic side effects may result from applying a large quantity of podophyllin to

Clinical Practice of Gynecology: **2,** 245–251, 1989
© 1989 Elsevier Science Publishing Co., Inc.
655 Avenue of the Americas, New York, NY 10010

ISSN 1043-3198/89/$3.50

open, friable condylomata or epithelial mucosal surfaces. Mild toxic symptoms include nausea and vomiting, while severe toxicity is characterized by the onset of neurologic symptoms. Because of these potential complications, patients are required to wash areas treated with podophyllin 6 to 8 hours after application. Since podophyllin can be absorbed and in experimental situations has been shown to result in birth defects, it should not be used in pregnancy.[3,6]

Trichloroacetic Acid

Trichloroacetic acid (TCA) and bichloroacetic acid, both halogenated acetic acids, are keratolytic agents widely used for the treatment of genital HPV infections. The former may be ordered in concentrations of 50, 80, or 85% through local pharmacies. Trichloroacetic acid (85%) is also sold under the name of Nevitol (Nevitol Co, Monrovia, CA). When applied to epithelium, these keratolytics react quickly and destroy the epithelium by denaturing cellular proteins. Systemic toxicity does not occur, as it is not absorbed, and treated areas do not need to be washed after application. Despite its widespread use, there is a paucity of studies documenting its clinical efficacy, and conclusions are mostly based on unpublished clinical experience. Its popularity is due to its ease of use and lack of systemic toxicity.

5-Fluorouracil

Five-percent 5-fluorouracil is an antimetabolite commonly used for a variety of epithelial malignancies. It has been used since the early 1960s for a variety of dermatologic conditions, including actinic keratosis, basal and squamous cell carcinomas, and other potentially malignant epithelial neoplasms. A pyrimidine analog, it competes with thymidilate synthetase and substitutes for uracil, thereby impairing DNA and RNA synthesis. Its success in the treatment of lower genital tract HPV-related lesions is due to its ability to penetrate epithelial surfaces without causing systemic toxic side effects.[7] Concentrations of 1% and 2% are available, but most regimens utilize the 5% concentration. It is commercially available as Efudex Cream (Roche Labs, Div. of Hoffman-La Roche, Inc., Nutley, NJ) in one size, a 25-g tube. Because of the unknown teratogenic effect of vaginal absorption of 5% 5-FU in pregnancy, careful contraceptive counseling should be offered for women using 5% 5-FU for vaginal lesions.

Retinoids

Retinoids, organic compounds derived from vitamin A, have been useful for a number of dermatologic disorders because of antiproliferative and keratolytic activity upon epithelial tissues. In animal experiments, retinoids have been reported to delay tumor formation and suppress neoplastic changes stimulated by carcinogens.[8] HPV infections of nongenital tissues, such as epidermodysplasia verruciformis and nongenital warts, have been treated effectively with retinoid derivatives.[9] As a result, retinoids have been considered by some to be a treatment option for lower-genital-tract HPV infections. To date, information regarding their usefulness and efficacy has been limited to treatment of cervical lesions.[10]

TREATMENT FOR SPECIFIC AREAS OF THE LOWER GENITAL TRACT
Vulvar and Perineal HPV Infection

HPV infection of the external genitalia may vary in gross and microscopic findings as well as in location and extent. Treatment of these lesions should be tailored according to their clinical appearance. For instance, keratinized lesions, such as condylomata acuminata, are generally treated with topical keratolytic agents. A solution of 25% podophyllin (25% podophyllin resin in tincture of benzoin) may be applied weekly with a cotton-tipped applicator. Application two or three times a week may dissolve lesions more rapidly. Cure rates of acuminate lesions range from 2–98% when treated with podophyllin.[2,11,12] These widely disparate response rates may reflect several clinical variables. Relatively new, soft, papillary condylomata with thinner keratinized surfaces respond more readily than thick, well-keratinized older acuminata. Additionally, therapy of warts in previous studies may have neglected to treat the surrounding margin of infected epithelium. HPV-DNA has been found in normal appearing epithelium 10 mL distant from grossly obvious lesions, and a 5–10-mL area of surrounding epithelium should also be treated.[13] The area of application should be washed 6 to 8 hours after application. If external genital lesions have not resolved after three or four treatments, another form of treatment should be instituted.

Trichloroacetic acid is probably the therapeutic agent of choice for small keratinized lesions. A very effective regimen is 85% TCA applied focally with a cotton-tipped applicator on a weekly basis. One to four applications of TCA are usually required to eradicate visible lesions. Protective vaseline jelly can be applied to the surrounding area to prevent unintended contact. A local burning sensation usually occurs and lasts for several minutes. Application of local anesthetic jelly, such as 2% Xylocaine (Astra Pharmaceutical Products, Inc., Westborough, MA) Americaine jelly (Penwalt Corporation, Rochester, NY), or use of topical anesthetic sprays such as Dermoplast (Ayerst Corporation, New York, NY) or Americaine spray (Penwalt) improves temporary pain. Mild soreness may persist a few days; however, this does not interfere with normal activity. Intercourse may be resumed when the treated areas heal, usually in 10–14 days. Permanent

TABLE 15–1. Vulvar and Perianal Topical Chemotherapy

1. Apply 50, 80, or 85% TCA focally to each condylomata. A margin of at least 5 m of normal skin should also be treated. Repeat once or twice a week as needed. Depending on the extent of the area treated, protective jelly may be used on the surrounding skin; 50% TCA can be applied to areas of flat condyloma occurring at the introitus with a cotton-tipped applicator. Large areas in this region can be treated in one sitting.

   Dermoplast (Penwalt), Americaine (Penwalt) topical anesthetic spray, and/or Xylocaine (Ayerst) jelly may be applied before or after application of TCA to decrease immediate pain.

2. 25% podophyllin may be applied to highly keratinized condylomata acuminata. Weekly applications are the minimum, and twice-a-week application improves resolution rates. Podophyllin should not be applied to large areas, friable open acuminata, or mucosal surfaces.

3. If 5% 5-FU is chosen to treat less keratinized vulvar lesions, apply a light layer of cream to the area nightly for 5–7 nights. Patients need to wash their hands carefully after applying the cream using their fingertips. If burning occurs before reaching a full course, patients should discontinue application for the rest of that cycle. Patients should refrain from intercourse on these nights and for 7 days thereafter. Contraception should be used during treatment.

4. For prophylactic use, light weekly or biweekly application of 5% 5-FU to vulvar areas may reduce occurrences. The precautions and guidelines described above should be followed.

ulceration has not been associated with its use, and most areas heal without scarring. Another treatment plan should be initiated if lesions persist despite numerous applications. Unlike podophyllin, TCA has no associated systemic effect and may be used in pregnancy if necessary. The less keratinized lesions such as the flat condyloma or micropapillary spicular lesions involving the introitus can also be treated with 50% or 85% solution of TCA. It should be noted, however, that in a study of 29 patients with these lesions, no HPV DNA was isolated using Southern blot technique (L Van Le and JL Stern, unpublished data). Topical therapy for vulvar, perineal, and perianal HPV infection is summarized in Table 15–1.

The use of 5% 5-FU on highly keratinized vulvar lesions is controversial. It has been observed to eradicate effectively thick epithelial lesions of various dermatoses; however, its ability to adequately penetrate the thick, keratinized exterior of condylomata acuminata has been suspect.[7,14] Topical application of 5% 5-FU to individual condyloma for 5–7 consecutive days has resulted in resolution in some cases. Woodruff has reported up to a 75% cure rate in selected cases with topical 5% 5-FU.[15] Response rates appear to be higher in newer, less keratinized lesions.

It has also been used to treat less keratinized acuminata of the vulvar introitus and posterior fourchette. Application of topical 5% 5-FU for 5–7 days has resulted in resolution in a few cases. Patients using 5% 5-FU in this fashion have not noted significant local irritation. As might be anticipated, if topical 5% 5-FU has been used to the extent that ulceration results, cure rates have been higher. If resolution of lesions does not occur, another cycle can be repeated in 3–4 weeks. Alternatively, 5% 5-FU applied weekly or biweekly for 3–6 months may be effective in a few cases. Fair-skinned patients are thought to be more sensitive to 5% 5-FU irritation; decreasing the number of treatment days in these patients is suggested.

It has been suggested that application of 5% 5-FU may have prophylactic use in the treatment of vulvar HPV infections. In a study of immunocompetent and immunocompromised patients, those receiving 5% 5-FU had significantly less recurrences than control patients.[16] For prophylactic use, 5% 5-FU is applied to the affected area, either once or three times a week every 1–2 weeks for 3–6 months.

Cervix

Human papillomavirus DNA has been detected in several abnormalities of cervical epithelium implicating the virus in the pathogenesis of cervical condyloma and neoplasia. Eradication of all epithelial changes thought to be HPV-related, including condylomata without atypia and intraepithelial neoplasia of mild, moderate, or severe degree, is recommended to reduce the risk of later developing invasive lower-genital-tract neoplasms. The usual therapeutic choices include destructive modalities such as cryosurgery, laser ablation, or conization. Although not a conventional therapeutic option, the use of topical chemotherapeutic agents for cervical HPV infections has been explored. Several investigators have studied cervical application of 5% 5-FU as a therapeutic option relying on its ability to denude the cervical epithelium to effect cure. After an application of 2.5–5 g of 5% 5-FU per vagina on a daily basis for 7–10 days, neoplastic epithelium may be lifted off, either spontaneously or with instrumentation.[7,17] Colposcopic evaluation concluded that the cervical lesion had resolved in 70–100% of treated patients; however, persistent disease was detected in the subsequent cone specimens from these patients.[17,18] Another drawback to cervical 5% 5-FU use was the observation that several treatment sessions were required as compared to the single visit required for destructive therapeutic modalities. Experience with topical cervical application of retinoic acid has been restricted to trials evaluating its efficacy in treating cervical intraepithelial neoplasia. Transretinoic acid applied via a cervical cap resulted in a response rate of only 47%.[10]

Cervical application of TCA to remove cervical intraepithelial neoplasia has also been reported. Application of 85% TCA to the squamocolumnar junction and affected ectocervical epithelium resulted in an overall resolution rate of 86%; however, two or more applications were required in 60% of the patients.[19]

When one compares the success rates and number of visits required for topical treatment of cervical lesions to those of destructive methods, there does not appear to be any major benefit to topical chemotherapy of cervical lesions at present. Minimal risks appear to be associated with the topical application of these agents, however, in situations where destructive procedures are not available (Third World countries, rural communities), topical therapy may be a practical option.

Vagina

Vaginal condyloma acuminata, flat condylomas, and vaginal intraepithelial neoplasia can also be effectively treated with chemotherapeutic agents. The nonkeratinized, thin, squamous epithelium of the vagina is particularly responsive to topical 5% 5-FU. Studies regarding the use of 5% 5-FU in vaginal intraepithelial neoplasias have demonstrated that in doses of 2.5–5 g either weekly for 12 weeks or sequentially for 1–10 days can produce cure rates of 70–80%.[20–24] The efficacy of 5% 5-FU in treating benign vaginal HPV infections is extrapolated from this experience. An 80% resolution rate has been observed when 1.5 g of 5% 5-FU was applied to the vagina weekly for 10 weeks in cases of vaginal warts.[25] In another study comparing the success of laser ablation to 5% 5-FU vaginal application, 90% of vaginal condyloma were eradicated with one 5% 5-FU application, while 69% of lesions were eliminated with laser. For flat condyloma treated with 5% 5-FU, only 50% of these lesions were observed to resolve, suggesting that these lesions may be more resistant to 5% 5-FU therapy.[26]

A regimen for the use of 5% 5-FU in the treatment of vaginal HPV-related lesions is outlined in Table 15–2. Five percent 5-FU is inserted into the vaginal canal with a plastic applicator such as that used for antifungal treatment of vaginitis. Insertion of one-third to one-half of an applicator into the vagina nightly for 5 nights is tolerated and is effective. This regimen may be repeated every 3–4 weeks as needed, and one to two cycles of treatment is usually sufficient. It is important to prevent the development of an erosive vulvar dermatitis, which may result from leakage of 5% 5-FU from the vagina. A tampon should be inserted just past the introitus after insertion of 5% 5-FU at bedtime. Zinc oxide or petroleum jelly should be applied to the vulva at bedtime, again in the morning, and as necessary throughout the day. The patient is instructed to remove the tampon in the morning and allow drainage of residual 5% 5-FU to occur in the shower. Douching in the morning is also effective in preventing the occurrence of

TABLE 15–2. Vaginal Chemotherapy

1. Apply 85% TCA with a cotton-tipped applicator to focal regions followed with 2% Xylocaine jelly or anesthetic spray as necessary. Reapplication can be performed weekly if necessary. Podophyllin is not recommended for vaginal lesions.

2. Insert one-third to one-half applicator of 5% 5-FU into the vagina for 5 consecutive nights. Insert a tampon just past the introitus to prevent leakage. Zinc oxide or petroleum jelly should be applied to the introitus, vulva, and perineum to protect the skin from chemical ulceration. In the morning, remove the tampon and allow the excess cream to drain in the shower. Thoroughly wash the external genitalia. Douching should be encouraged. A panty liner should be worn and changed frequently if discharge continues throughout the day. The discharge may continue for up to 14 days after the last application of cream. If external irritation occurs, Silvadine cream with 2% Xylocaine jelly, mixed in a 1:1 concentration may be prescribed t.i.d. and q.i.d. Soaking in a warm bathtub provides relief as well. Refrain from intercourse for 2 days after prophylactic use and for 2 weeks after therapeutic use of 5% 5-FU.

3. For prophylactic use of 5% 5-FU in vaginal disease, insert one-third to one-half applicator every 1–2 weeks for 3–6 months.

vulvar erosive dermatitis from the leaking cream. Throughout the day, a panty liner should be worn to catch the excess drainage as well. The patient should be advised to change the liner frequently to prevent prolonged vulvar exposure. Drainage of the cream may persist up to 10 days after its last application, and patients should continue using topical protective agents for up to a week after the last application. Patients should refrain from intercourse for 2 weeks after finishing a 5-day treatment course. Again, fair-skinned patients are postulated to be more sensitive to 5% 5-FU, and adjustment in duration of treatment is recommended. Some patients may have a marked reaction to topical vaginal 5% 5-FU, resulting in areas of granulation tissue. The appearance of vaginal endometriosis and adenosis after vaginal 5% 5-FU use has also been observed (JL Stern, unpublished data). The occurrence of vaginal adhesions after 5% 5-FU use has recently necessitated vaginal adhesiolysis.

Continuing treatment with 5% 5-FU in a prophylactic fashion may prevent vaginal recurrences. One-third to one-half of an applicator of 5% 5-FU cream inserted into the vagina once every 1–2 weeks for 3–6 months is suggested as a prophylactic regimen. Prophylactic use of 5% 5-FU has been shown to significantly decrease the recurrence rate of vaginal condylomata without causing significant morbidity or inconvenience.[16,27]

Other keratolytic agents such as TCA and podophyllin have not been extensively studied for lesions involving the vagina. TCA may be applied to solitary small vaginal lesions with impunity, and some lesions may resolve. Podophyllin, however, has been associated with toxic neurologic effects when applied to mucosal surfaces and should probably not be used on the vaginal mucosa.[4]

Penile HPV Infection

Penile condylomata and intraepithelial neoplasia are HPV-related, sexually transmitted diseases.[28,29] Podophyllin has been previously regarded as the mainstay of treatment for penile warts. Initial excitement regarding podophyllin stemmed from an early study showing a high resolution rate with topical application.[2] Since then, numerous studies have observed a cure rate of only 22–50% with weekly topical application.[30,31] Treatment of warts with a combination of 50% TCA and 25% podophyllin does not appear to be more efficacious than 25% podophyllin alone.[11]

Eighty-five percent TCA alone works extremely well for small lesions. Condylomata acuminata, as well as flat condyloma and macular lesions, respond well to its keratolytic effect. It may be applied to any region of the penis except the urethra, and moderately large areas can be treated at each visit. Several repetitive applications are usually required for multiple or moderate-size lesions. Application generally results in a few minutes of local burning, which resolves rapidly, and analgesia is not required afterwards. Topical application of 2% Xylocaine jelly applied immediately after TCA may relieve burning. Patients should refrain from intercourse until treated areas have healed, usually in 10–14 days. Treated areas may become hypopigmented after healing, and patients should be informed of this before initiating TCA treatment. Tub soaks are encouraged afterwards to keep treated areas clean and help relieve the minor soreness that may result after treatment.

Topical 5% 5-FU has been one of the mainstays of treatment for smaller acuminate and nonacuminate penile HPV lesions. In contrast to the poorer response observed when 5% 5-FU is used to treat vulvar keratinized warts, studies show that 40–60% of penile acuminata resolve after daily 5% 5-FU therapy.[30,31] Topical use in our experience, however, has resulted in only variable success that does not correlate with extent or morphology of lesions. If 5% 5-FU is chosen for treatment, it can be applied in several ways. For papillary lesions, topical 5% 5-FU can be applied to individual lesions with a cotton-tipped applicator for 5–7 consecutive nights. For treatment of flat condyloma, 5% 5-FU may be applied with the fingertips in a thin layer once or twice a week. Treatment should continue for 3 months before declaring a treatment failure. Patients are instructed to wash their hands after each application and to refrain from intercourse while undergoing treatment. It must be emphasized that the cream should be applied in a thin layer to prevent the occurence of an erosive dermatitis. Patients are asked to place a tissue or gauze in the area between the penis and the scrotum and wear tight-fitting underwear to keep this in place, so the scro-

TABLE 15–3. Chemotherapy of Penile HPV Lesions

1. Apply 85% TCA with a cotton-tipped applicator to focal areas followed with 2% Xylocaine jelly or anesthetic spray as necessary. Reapplication can be performed weekly or monthly depending on lesion morphology. Podophyllin can also be applied this way; however, more frequent application is recommended.

2. 5% 5-FU cream applied nightly for 5 nights may be applied to focal condylomata acuminata with a cotton-tipped applicator. If larger areas of flat warts are present, 5% 5-FU may be applied in a light layer with the fingertips once or twice weekly for 3–6 months.

   If burning occurs before achieving 5 nights of application, applications should be discontinued. If excessive cream is used and ulceration results, soaking in warm water, use of Silvadine cream, supportive care is recommended. Ulcers will heal with time without scarring.

3. Place gauze or tissue between the penis and scrotum to avoid skin irritation. Silvadine cream with 2% Xylocaine jelly mixed in a 1:1 concentration may be applied or soaking in a bathtub may provide relief if needed. Refrain from intercourse for 7 days after use.

tum can be protected from excessive 5% 5-FU exposure. Silvadine (Flint Labs, Deerfield, IL) cream mixed with 2% Xylocaine jelly in a 1:1 concentration provides relief and should be applied as needed. Sitz baths also provide relief and assist healing. If mild ulceration occurs, areas usually heal spontaneously over several weeks without significant scarring, and only supportive care is needed. Patients are reevaluated in 4 weeks if lesions are acuminate or 3 months if HPV lesions are flat. Treatment regimens are shown in Table 15–3.

Other Lesions of the Genital Tract

Distal urethral lesions in women or men can be successfully treated with 5% 5-FU (see Table 15–4). Meatal application of the cream nightly for 7–14 days resulted in disappearance of almost all condylomata treated.[32-36] Medication can be applied with either a cotton-tipped applicator or the fingertips. Insertion of 1% 5-FU through the tip of a 1-cc syringe is an alternative method. Dysuria may be experienced, but it is usually temporary. Denuded meatal tissue may heal, resulting in partial distal urethral agglutination. This presents as a diversion of urinary stream and can be easily treated with urethral sounding. Long-term strictures have not been a significant complication, and systemic side effects have not been reported.

Anal condylomata may be successfully treated with topical trichloroacetic acid or 5% 5-FU. Eighty-five percent TCA may be used successfully on smaller lesions, while 5% 5-FU applied intraanally using a fingercot for 5 consecutive days is recommended for anal lesions. Because of the risk of systemic toxicity, we again recommend against the extensive use of topical podophyllin on mucosal surfaces. Perirectal condylomata can be success-

TABLE 15–4. Topical Chemotherapy for Urethral and Rectal Lesions

1. Apply 5% 5-FU cream to meatal lesions with cotton applicator for 3–5 days depending on tolerance. Void in 3–4 hours after applying cream. If unable to void, drinking fluids will help. Application in the morning is practical to avoid late night voiding.

2. Refrain from intercourse for 7 days after each use.

3. 5% 5-FU may be applied topically to intraanal lesions with a fingercot or with a cotton applicator. A protective perineal lining should be worn to prevent distributing cream to other areas unintentionally. It should be applied for 3–5 nights.

fully treated with either topical podophyllin, TCA, or 5% 5-FU. Treatment regimens are similar to those used to treat vulvar disease.

SUMMARY

Topical treatment of lower-genital-tract infections is usually inexpensive and associated with minimal morbidity. Regimens specific for certain histologic types and lower-genital-tract locations, as discussed above, are fairly effective for minimal to moderate amount of disease and should be offered initially. When topical therapy fails, patients may then be offered destructive or ablative treatment. In unique cases or in the face of extensive disease, topical therapy may be skipped and ablative and destructive treatment offered primarily. However, because of low costs, ease of use, and acceptable success rates, topical treatment is a popular and desirable treatment choice for lower-genital-tract lesions.

REFERENCES

1. Centers for Disease Control. MMWR 1983;32:306.
2. Culp MOS, Kaplan CIW: Condylomata acuminata: two hundred cases treated with podophyllin. Ann Sur 1944;120:251.
3. Chamberlain MJ, Reynolds AL, Yeoman WB: Toxic effect of podophyllum application in pregnancy. Br Med J 1972;3:391.
4. Montaldi DH, Giambrone JP, Courey NG, et al: Podophyllin poisoning associated with the treatment of condylomata acuminatum: A case report. Am J Obstet Gynecol 1974; 119:1130–1131.
5. Slater GE, Rumack BH, Peterson RG: Podophyllin poisoning systemic toxicity following cutaneous application. Obstet Gynecol 1978;52:94.
6. Karol MD, Conner CS, Watanabe AS, et al: Podophyllum: Suspected teratogenicity from topical application. Clin Toxicol 1980;16:283.
7. Sillman FH, Sedlis A, Boyce JG: A review of lower genital intraepithelial neoplasia and the use of topical 5-fluorouracil. Obstet Gynecol Survey 1985;40:190.
8. Gassenmaier A, Lammel M, Kleiner E, et al: Treatment of bovine-papillomavirus-type-1 (BPV)-transformed mouse cells with aromatic retinoid and retinoic acid. Arch Dermatol Res 1985;81:79.
9. Lutzner MA, Blanchet-Bardon C, Orth G: Clinical observations, virologic studies, and treat-

ment trials in patients with epidermodysplasia verruciformis, a disease induced by specific human papillomaviruses. J Invest Dermatol 1984;83:s18.

10. Weiner SA, Meyskens FL, Surwit EA, et al: Response of human papilloma-associated diseases to retinoids (vitamin A derivatives). Retinoids in cervical dysplasia. In: Papillomaviruses: Molecular and clinical aspects. New York. Alan R. Liss, Inc, 1985;249.

11. Gabriel G, Thin RNT: Treatment of anogenital warts. Br Vener Dis 1983;59:124.

12. Simmons PD: Podophyllin 10% and 25% in the treatment of ano-genital warts: A comparative double-blind study. Br J Vener Dis 1981;57:208.

13. Ferenczy A, Mitao M, Nagai N, et al: Latent papillomavirus and recurring genital warts. N Engl J Med 1985;313:784.

14. Friedrich EG Jr: Vulvar Disease. In: Major problems in Obstetrics and Gynecology Philadelphia: W.B. Saunders Company, 1983;9:194.

15. Woodruff JF: Identifying and treating the acuminate wart. Contemp Obstet Gynecol 1976;7:125.

16. Krebs HB: Prophylactic topical 5-fluorouracil following treatment of human papillomavirus-associated lesions of the vulva and vagina. Obstet Gynecol 1986;68:837.

17. Pride GL, Chuprevich TW: Topical 5-fluorouracil treatment of transformation zone intraepithelial neoplasia of the cervix and vagina. Obstet Gynecol 1982;60:467.

18. Townsend DE, Marks EJ: Cryosurgery and the CO_2 laser. Cancer 1981;48:632.

19. Malviya VK, Deppe G, Pluszczynski R, et al: Trichloroacetic acid in the treatment of human papillomavirus infection of the cervix without associated dysplasia. Obstet Gynecol 1987;70:72.

20. Ballon SC, Roberts JA, La Gasse LD: Topical 5-fluorouracil in the treatment of intraepithelial neoplasia of the vagina. Obstet Gynecol 1979;54:163.

21. Cagler H, Hertzog RW, Hreshchyshyn MM: Topical 5-fluorouracil treatment of vaginal intraepithelial neoplasia. Obstet Gynecol 1981;58:580.

22. Petrilli ES, Townsend DE, Morrow CP, et al: Vaginal intraepithelial neoplasia: biologic aspects and treatment with topical 5-fluorouracil and the carbon dioxide laser. Am J Obstet Gynecol 1980;138:321.

23. Piver MS, Barlow JJ, Tsukada Y, et al: Postirradiation squamous cell carcinoma in situ of the vagina: treatment by topical 20 percent 5-fluorouracil cream. Am J Obstet Gynecol 1979;135:377.

24. Stokes IM, Hawthorne JHR: A new regimen for the treatment of vaginal carcinoma in situ using 5-fluorouracil. Br J Obstet Gynecol 1980;87:920.

25. Krebs HB: Treatment of vaginal condylomata by weekly topical application of 5-fluorouracil. Obstet Gynecol 1987;70:58.

26. Ferenczy A: Comparison of 5-fluorouracil and CO_2 laser for treatment of vaginal condylomata. Obstet Gynecol 1984;64:773.

27. Krebs HB, Schneider V, Hurt WG, et al: Genital condylomas in immunosuppressed women: A therapeutic challenge. South Med J 1986;79:183.

28. Levine RU, Crum CP, Herman E, et al: Cervical papillomavirus infection and intraepithelial neoplasia: a study of male sexual partners. Obstet Gynecol 1984;64:16.

29. Barrasso R, De Brux J, Croissant O, et al: High prevalence of papillomavirus-associated penile intraepithelial neoplasia in sexual partners of women with cervical intraepithelial neoplasia. N Eng J Med 1987;15:916.

30. Haye KR: Treatment of condylomata acuminata with 5 percent 5-fluorouracil (5-FU) cream. Br J Vener Dis 1974;50:466.

31. von Krogh G: Podophyllotoxin for condylomata acuminata eradication: clinical and experimental comparative studies on podophyllum lignans, colchicine, and 5-fluorouracil. Acta Derm Venereol [Suppl] (Stockh) 1981;98:1.

32. Debenedictis TJ, Marmar JL, Praiss DE: Intraurethral condylomas acuminata: management and review of the literature. J Urology 1977;118:767.

33. Dretler SP, Klein LA: The eradication of intraurethral condyloma acuminata with 5 percent 5-fluorouracil cream. J Urology 1975;113:195.
34. Wallin J: 5-fluorouracil in the treatment of penile and urethral condylomata acuminata. Br J Vener Dis 1977;53:240.
35. Wein AJ, Benson GS: Treatment of urethral condyloma acuminatum with 5-fluorouracil cream. Urology 1977;9:413.
36. Weimer GW, Milleman LA, Reiland TL, et al: 5-fluorouracil urethral suppositories for the eradication of condyloma acuminata. Urology 1978;120:174.

Index

Sure to become a classic!

Series Editor: **Michael S. Baggish, MD,** Professor and Chairman, Department of Obstetrics and Gynecology, SUNY Health Science Center, Syracuse, New York

The CLINICAL PRACTICE OF GYNECOLOGY Series

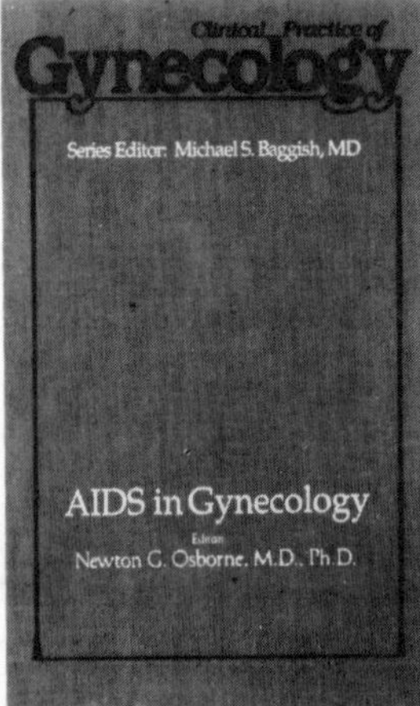

Volume One, 1989:

Issue 1: **AIDS in Gynecology**
Editor: **Newton G. Osborne, MD, PhD,** State University of New York

Issue 2: **Human Papillomavirus Infections**
Editors: **Barbara Winkler, MD,** and **Ralph M. Richart, MD,** Columbia University College of Physicians and Surgeons

Issue 3: **Pediatric and Adolescent Gynecology**
Editor: **Donald P. Goldstein, MD,** Harvard Medical School

Focusing exclusively on gynecology

- Each issue devoted to a single, timely topic in gynecology
- Edited by noted experts in the field
- Written by top authorities
- Complete with photos, drawings and diagrams
- Presented in a concise, accessible format, three times a year
- Filled with information **most relevant to you in your practice** — from diagnosis and treatment options to special problems and ethical questions

Why wait? Become a subscriber by ordering the series on the business reply card below and save 10%!

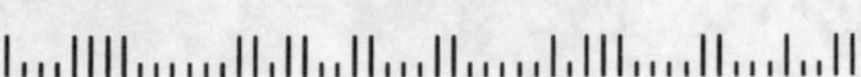